PEDIATRIC DIAGNOSTIC MEDICINE

A Collection of Cases

T0176507

PEDIATRIC DIAGNOSTIC MEDICINE

A Collection of Cases

Andrew J. White, MD

James P. Keating, MD Professor of Pediatrics
Washington University in St. Louis School of Medicine
St. Louis Children's Hospital
St. Louis, Missouri

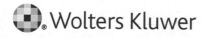. Wolters Kluwer

Philadelphia • Baltimore • New York • London
Buenos Aires • Hong Kong • Sydney • Tokyo

Acquisitions Editor: Colleen Dietzler
Development Editor: Thomas Celona
Editorial Coordinator: Christopher George Rodgers
Editorial Assistant: Victoria Giansante
Marketing Manager: Kirsten Watrud
Production Project Manager: Justin Wright
Design Coordinator: Stephen Druding
Manufacturing Coordinator: Beth Welsh
Prepress Vendor: TNQ Technologies

Printed in China

Library of Congress Cataloging-in-Publication Data

ISBN-13: 978-1-975159-47-4

Cataloging in Publication data available on request from publisher.

---

shop.lww.com

CCS0521

This collection is dedicated to the memory of James P. Keating, MD.

Contributors

Miriam Ben Abdallah, MD
Pediatric Resident
Department of Pediatrics
Children's Hospital Colorado
Aurora, Colorado

Shannon C. Agner, MD, PhD
Assistant Professor
Department of Neurology
Washington University School of Medicine
St. Louis, Missouri

Anne Marie Anderson, MD
Resident Physician
Department of Pediatrics
Washington University in St. Louis
St. Louis, Missouri

Kevin T. Barton, MD
Assistant Professor of Pediatrics
Division of Pediatric Nephrology
Department of Pediatrics
Washington University in St Louis
St. Louis, Missouri

Kevin Baszis, MD
Associate Professor
Department of Pediatrics
Washington University School of Medicine
St. Louis, Missouri

Marie L. Batty, MD
Pediatric Chief Resident
St. Louis Children's Hospital
St. Louis, Missouri

Susan J. Bayliss, MD
Professor of Dermatology and Pediatrics
Washington University School of Medicine
St. Louis, Missouri

Nicole Benzoni, MD, MPHS
Critical Care Fellow
Department of Medicine
Washington University in St Louis
St. Louis, Missouri

Tarin M. Bigley, MD, PhD
Rheumatology Fellow
Department of Pediatrics
Washington University in St. Louis
St. Louis, Missouri

Brittany J. Blue, MD
Attending Neonatologist
Pediatrix Medical Group of Florida, Inc
Tampa, Florida

Kylie M. Bushroe, MD
Resident Physician
Department of Pediatrics
Washington University in St. Louis
St. Louis, Missouri

Cecelia L. Calhoun, MD, MPHS
Assistant Professor
Department of Pediatrics, Division of Hematology/Oncology
Department of Medicine, Division of Hematology
Washington University School of Medicine
St. Louis, Missouri

Shelley C. Choudhury, MD
Resident Physician
Department of Pediatrics
Washington University School of Medicine in St. Louis
Saint Louis, Missouri

Áine Cooke, MD
Los Angeles, California

Raja Dandamudi, MD
Assistant Professor
Department of Pediatrics
Division of Pediatric Nephrology
Washington University School of Medicine in St. Louis
Saint Louis, Missouri

Elizabeth A. Daniels, MD
Pediatric Resident
Department of Pediatrics
St. Louis Children's Hospital
St. Louis, Missouri

T. Keefe Davis, MD
Assistant Professor
Department of Pediatrics
University of Saskatchewan
Saskatoon, Canada

Nicholas W. DeKorver, MD, PhD
Resident Physician
Department of Pediatrics
Washington University St. Louis
Saint Louis, Missouri

Jenna N. Diaz, MD
Pediatric Gastroenterology Fellow
St. Louis Children's Hospital
Department of Pediatric Gastroenterology, Hepatology and Nutrition
Washington University in St. Louis
St. Louis, Missouri

Alexa Altman Doss, MD
Clinical Fellow, Allergy/Immunology
Department of Pediatrics
Washington University School of Medicine
Saint Louis, Missouri

Amanda Reis Dube, MD
Instructor
Department of Pediatrics
Washington University in St. Louis
St. Louis, Missouri

Laura A. Duckworth, MD
Clinical Fellow
Department of Pediatric Gastroenterology
Washington University in St. Louis
St. Louis, Missouri

Jennifer Martens Dunn, MD
Assistant Professor
Department of Clinical Pediatrics
Washington University Clinical Associates
St. Louis, Missouri

Adam Eaton, MD
Primary Care Pediatrician
Washington University Clinical Associates
Assistant Professor of Clinical Pediatrics
Department of Pediatrics
Washington University School of Medicine
St. Louis, Missouri

Miranda Edmunds, MD
Physician
Washington University in St. Louis
Saint Louis, Missouri

Farid Farkouh, BS
MD Candidate
Washington University School of Medicine
St. Louis, Missouri

Katherine Ferguson, MD
Child Neurology Resident, PGY3
Washington University in St. Louis
St. Louis, Missouri

Mary E. Fournier, MD, MPH
Assistant Professor
Department of Pediatrics
Washington University School of Medicine in St. Louis
St. Louis, Missouri

Francisco Javier Gortes, MD
Radiologist
Department of Radiology
Mallinckrodt Institute of Radiology
St. Louis, Missouri

Kevin W. Graepel, MD, PhD
Resident Physician
Department of Pediatrics
St. Louis Children's Hospital, Washington University in St. Louis
St. Louis, Missouri

Lauren Gregory, MD
Instructor
Department of Pediatrics
Washington University in St. Louis
St. Louis, Missouri

Jennifer Horst, MD
Assistant Professor of Pediatrics
Department of Pediatrics
Division of Pediatric Emergency Medicine
Washington University in St. Louis
St. Louis, Missouri

Julianne Ivy, MD
Resident Physician
Department of Pediatrics
Washington University in St. Louis
St. Louis, Missouri

Grace Ellen Kennedy, BA (mod.), MB, BCh, BAO
Senior Medical Officer
Health Protection Surveillance Centre
Dublin, Ireland

Lauren Littell, MD
Pediatric Resident Physician
Washington University in Saint Louis Children's Hospital
Saint Louis, Missouri

Audrey R. Odom John, MD, PhD
Chief, Division of Infectious Diseases
Department of Pediatrics
Children's Hospital of Philadelphia
Perelman School of Medicine, University of Pennsylvania
Philadelphia, Pennsylvania

Maleewan Kitcharoensakkul, MD, MSCI
Assistant Professor
Department of Pediatrics
Washington University in St. Louis
St. Louis, Missouri

Ray Kreienkamp, MD, PhD
House Physician
Department of Pediatrics
Washington University School of Medicine
St. Louis, Missouri

Natasha Lalos, MD
Resident Physician
Department of Pediatrics
Washington University in St. Louis
St. Louis, Missouri

Itay Marmor, MD
Clinical Fellow
Division of Rheumatology and Immunology
Department of Pediatrics
Washington University in St. Louis
St Louis, Missouri

Jennifer D. May, MD
Fellow Physician
Department of Pediatric Endocrinology
Washington University in St. Louis
St. Louis, Missouri

Kyle P. McNerney, MD
Assistant Professor
Department of Pediatrics
Division of Endocrinology & Diabetes
Washington University in St. Louis School of Medicine
St. Louis, Missouri

Ali Yusuf Mian, MD
Assistant Professor
Department of Radiology, Neuroradiology Section
Chief
Department of Pediatric Neuroradiology
Director
Department of Neuroradiology Residency Education
Mallinckrodt Institute of Radiology
Washington University School of Medicine
St. Louis, Missouri

Cory P. Miller, MD
Pediatric Resident Physician
Department of Pediatrics
Washington University in St. Louis
St. Louis, Missouri

Caroline Noel, MD
Pediatrician
Department of Pediatrics
Washington University in St. Louis
St. Louis, Missouri

Amir B. Orandi, MD
Consultant, Pediatric Rheumatology
Assistant Professor, Pediatric and Adolescent Medicine
Mayo Clinic
Rochester, Minnesota

William B. Orr, MD, FACC
Assistant Professor of Pediatrics
Division of Cardiology
Washington University School of Medicine
St. Louis, Missouri

Rachel C. Orscheln, MD
Associate Professor
Department of Pediatrics
Washington University in St. Louis
St. Louis, Missouri

Alex S. Plattner, MD, MBA
Resident Physician
Department of Pediatrics
Washington University in St. Louis
St. Louis, Missouri

Sara Procknow, MD, PhD
Clinical Fellow
Department of Pediatrics
Division of Genetics and Genomics Medicine
Washington University in St. Louis
St. Louis, Missouri

Peter Putnam, MD
Associate Professor
Department of Pediatrics
Washington University School of Medicine
St. Louis, Missouri

Patrick J. Reich, MD, MSCI
Associate Professor
Department of Pediatrics
Washington University School of Medicine
St. Louis, Missouri

Brian D. Reinholz, MD
Resident Physician
Department of Pediatrics
Washington University in St. Louis
St. Louis, Missouri

Shruti Sakhuja, MD
Fellow
Department of Pediatric Gastroenterology, Hepatology, and Nutrition
Texas Children's Hospital
Houston, Texas

Julie A. Steinberg, MD
Resident Physician
Mallinckrodt Institute of Radiology
Washington University in Saint Louis
Saint Louis, Missouri

Joshua W. M. Theisen, MD, PhD
Postdoctoral Fellow
Department of Pediatrics
The University of Chicago
Chicago, Illinois

Katherine Velicki, BA
Medical Student
Washington University School of Medicine
St. Louis, Missouri

Luke T. Viehl, MD
Newborn Medicine Fellow
Department of Newborn Medicine
Washington University School of Medicine
St. Louis, Missouri

Jennifer A. Wambach, MD, MS
Associate Professor
Department of Pediatrics
Washington University School of Medicine
St. Louis, Missouri

Julia T. Warren, MD, PhD
Fellow
Department of Pediatrics, Division of Hematology/Oncology
Washington University in St. Louis, School of Medicine
St. Louis, Missouri

Brian T. Wessman, MD, FACEP, FCCM
Associate Professor
Departments of Anesthesiology and Emergency Medicine
Washington University in Saint Louis, School of Medicine
St. Louis, Missouri

Alexander Weymann, MD
Assistant Professor of Clinical Pediatrics
Department of Pediatrics
The Ohio State University College of Medicine
Medical Director, Liver Center and Liver Transplantation
Division of Gastroenterology, Hepatology and Nutrition
Nationwide Children's Hospital
Columbus, Ohio

Andrew J. White, MD

James P. Keating, MD, Professor of Pediatrics
Washington University in St. Louis School of Medicine
St. Louis Children's Hospital
St. Louis, Missouri

Hannah C. B. White, BA

Research Technician II
Department of Neurology
Washington University in St. Louis
St. Louis, Missouri

Robert D. Williams, MD, MS

Pediatric Resident Physician
Department of Pediatrics
Washington University School of Medicine-St. Louis Children's Hospital
St. Louis, Missouri

David B. Wilson, MD, PhD

Professor
Department of Pediatrics and Developmental Biology
Washington University in St. Louis
St. Louis, Missouri

Kimberly Wiltrout, MD

Pediatric Epilepsy Fellow
Department of Neurology, Division of Pediatric Neurology
Washington University in St. Louis
St. Louis, Missouri

Roger D. Yusen, MD, MPH

Associate Professor of Medicine
Division of Pulmonary and Critical Care Medicine
Washington University School of Medicine
St. Louis, Missouri

Ana S. Solís Zavala, MD

Resident Physician
Department of Pediatrics
Washington University in St Louis
St. Louis, Missouri

Nicholas R. Zessis, MD

Instructor
Department of Pediatrics
Northwestern University
Chicago, Illinois

Rachel Zolno, MD

Resident Physician
Department of Pediatric Neurology
Washington University in St. Louis
St. Louis, Missouri

Foreword

This book epitomizes academic pediatrics. These case studies are teaching and learning exercises initiated by my mentor, friend, and colleague, James Peter Keating, at Washington University and St. Louis Children's Hospital (SLCH) during his 44 years as the Chief Resident, then Director of the General Pediatric Residency Program, and then Professor Emeritus. Following his blue collar upbringing in Pittsburgh, a football career, and medical school education at Harvard College and School of Medicine, Jim spent a year caring for Vietnamese civilians under the primitive conditions there. I believe this made him into the thorough, caring, and knowledgeable pediatrician that he became—literally the best physician I have ever known.

Dr. Keating joined SLCH as the Chief Resident in 1968—when I was a medical student—in the era when there were no in-house attending physicians. Learning through experience, including the process of care-related, independent, often urgent decision-making, was intense. Jim was the mentor, glue, teacher, and conscience for all of us—always present, always teaching, always pushing us to provide the best care, and always available during difficult situations and emergencies. During his 34-year-long tenure as Residency Director, Jim supervised about 1000 burgeoning pediatricians, directly and intensely. To those of us who worked closely with him—I as an attending intensivist and cardiologist with him for over 20 years—Jim was an incredible colleague, exhibiting in-depth knowledge and great judgment and always teaching and learning with others.

As part of the Residency Program, Dr. Keating developed the "Diagnostic Clinic" in 1992, to which problematic patients were referred by community and academic pediatricians puzzled by unusual and difficult symptoms and illnesses. As a required rotation for residents, this became an academic learning experience and the origin of these Patient of the Week (POW) case studies and write-ups. Jim required a detailed case description with attention to both historical symptoms and physical signs of impact to the differential diagnosis. Appropriate, relevant laboratory results were delineated. The next critical component was a detailed discussion of potential diagnoses and the essential features leading to the end diagnosis. Most essential then was a review of the literature and pertinent bibliography so that readers and learners could further delve into the subject. For now more than 30 years, these academic experiences have been distributed and read by thousands of interested clinicians, including me.

Dr. Andrew White, who succeeded Dr. Keating as Residency Director, has continued this academic pediatric learning work and has done a marvelous job in maintaining this educational format.

Many of us continue to learn from Drs. Keating and White's treasure trove of diagnostic dilemmas. We know that this tome of learning will serve academic pediatrics well.

Arnold W. Strauss, MD
SLCH '72

Preface

Case-based learning is the crux of medical education. Collecting and piecing together the various tidbits of information from different sources, while integral to the process, alone is not sufficient to provide the diagnosis. Understanding and knowing the symptoms and presentations of most diseases is requisite but also not enough to always synthesize a logical and coherent differential diagnosis. Thinking through these exemplary cases is akin to practicing scales for the musician or working on your form at the free throw line—it is training your diagnostic abilities.

These cases are modeled after the Patient of the Week series started in 1991 by Dr. James P. Keating as "a way of teaching odd bits of medicine, quickly, with a minimum amount of work required from the resident physicians for whom they were created." He hoped to sharpen the senses of the young physician to detect the nuggets of wisdom and diagnostic clues found in patients' narratives and to help them feel the pleasure that comes from providing an answer to a child's problem that comes only from the mind of a clinician. The original cases of the Patient of the Week series were shared by email, which in 1991 was a relatively new form of communication and which Jim used to expand the reach of his teaching from the dozen or so residents who were able to attend resident's report. The new format allowed him to teach without the essential, but intrusive, element of active participation. Jim, a master at eliciting active participation, did at times attempt to tamp down his "intrusiveness."

I have done my best to maintain adherence to Jim's unique vernacular, his disdain for and attempts at elimination of medical jargon, and his framework for thinking about each patient. Efforts to standardize various presentation styles and formats are intentionally left nonstandard, as the patients do not always follow templates, and the different style of the presenter is too varied, and often distracting. In these patient stories, however, the common theme of a diagnostic clue is what keeps the reader attuned.

All of the patients in these cases have signed HIPAA releases, but as additional protection of their identities, I have altered their ages, genders, family and past medical histories and geographic locations to further hide their identities, when possible, and when not directly relevant to the case.

Andrew J. White, MD
SLCH '97

Contents

Abbreviations

3D three-dimensional
ACE angiotensin-converting enzyme
ADEM acute disseminated encephalomyelitis
AGA appropriate for gestational age
aHUS atypical hemolytic uremic syndrome
ALL acute lymphoblastic leukemia
ALPS autoimmune lymphoproliferative syndrome
ALT alanine transaminase
ANA antinuclear antibody
ANC absolute neutrophil count
ANCA antineutrophil cytoplasmic antibody
AOS Adams-Oliver syndrome
APD afferent pupillary defect
ARB angiotensin II receptor blocker
ARFID avoidant/restrictive food intake disorder
AST aspartate aminotransferase
AVM arteriovenous malformation
BMI body mass index
BNP B-type natriuretic peptide
BP blood pressure
BRBNS blue rubber bleb nevus syndrome
CBC complete blood count
CBF cerebral blood flow
CCB calcium channel blocker
CDC Centers for Disease Control and Prevention
CDK congenital dislocation of the knee
CFB complement factor B
CFH complement regulatory protein factor H
CGD chronic granulomatous disease
CHS cannabis hyperemesis syndrome
CMA chromosome microarray analysis
CMP comprehensive metabolic panel
CMTC cutis marmorata telangiectatica congenita
CMV cytomegalovirus
CNS central nervous system
CPR cardiopulmonary resuscitation
CRP C-reactive protein
CRRT chronic renal replacement therapy
CSF cerebrospinal fluid
CT computed tomography
CXR chest x-ray
DBP vitamin D binding protein
DIC disseminated intravascular coagulation
DOL day of life
DVT deep vein thrombosis
EBV Epstein-Barr virus
ECG electrocardiogram
ECMO extracorporeal membrane oxygenation

ECT electroconvulsive therapy
EDAMS encephalo-duro-arterio-myo-synangiosis
ED emergency department
EEG electroencephalogram
EGA estimated gestational age
EIM extraintestinal manifestation
ELISA enzyme-linked immunosorbent assay
EMS emergency medical services
ERMS embryonal rhabdomyosarcomas
ESR erythrocyte sedimentation rate
ESRD end-stage renal disease
FDA Food and Drug Administration
FFP fresh frozen plasma
FLAIR fluid-attenuated inversion recovery
FMF familial Mediterranean fever
FSGS focal segmental glomerulosclerosis
FSH follicle-stimulating hormone
G6PD glucose-6-phosphate dehydrogenase
GBS Guillain-Barré syndrome
G-CSF granulocyte colony-stimulating factor
GERD gastroesophageal reflux
GI gastrointestinal
HAART highly active antiretroviral therapy
HHT hemorrhagic hereditary telangiectasia
HIE hypoxic-ischemic encephalopathy
HIV human immunodeficiency virus
HL Hodgkin lymphoma
HLH hemophagocytic lymphohistiocytosis
HR heart rate
HSV herpes simplex virus
HUS hemolytic uremic syndrome
HVA homovanillic acid
IBD inflammatory bowel disease
ICP intracranial pressure
ICU intensive care unit
IDSA Infectious Diseases Society of America
IE infective endocarditis
IFA immunofluorescence assay
Ig immunoglobulin
IGRA interferon gamma release assay
IHC immunohistochemistry
IIH idiopathic intracranial hypertension
IIHWOP idiopathic intracranial hypertension without papilledema
INR international normalized ratio
INSS International Neuroblastoma Staging System
IRIDA iron refractory iron deficiency anemia
ITP immune thrombocytopenic purpura
IUGR intrauterine growth restriction
IV intravenous
IVC inferior vena cava
IVDU intravenous drug use
IVF intravenous fluid
IVIG intravenous immunoglobin
LAD leukocyte adhesion deficiency
LCH Langerhans cell histiocytosis
LDH lactate dehydrogenase
LH luteinizing hormone
LHON Leber hereditary optic neuropathy

LLQ left lower quadrant
LMP last menstrual period
LP lumbar puncture
LVH left ventricular hypertrophy
MCP metacarpophalangeal/membrane cofactor protein
MCTD mixed connective tissue disease
MD Meckel diverticulum
MDEM multiphasic demyelinating encephalomyelitis
MIBG metaiodobenzylguanidine
MOG myelin oligodendrocyte glycoprotein
MRA magnetic resonance angiography
MRI magnetic resonance imaging
MRSA methicillin-resistant *Staphylococcus aureus*
MS multiple sclerosis
MSM men who have sex with men
MSSA methicillin-sensitive *Staphylococcus aureus*
MYH7 myosin heavy chain 7
NAIT neonatal autoimmune thrombocytopenia
NAT nonaccidental trauma
NEC necrotizing enterocolitis
NG nasogastric
NGD neonatal Graves disease
NGS next-generation sequencing
NK natural killer
NMO neuromyelitis optica
NS normal saline
NSAID nonsteroidal anti-inflammatory drug
OCP oral contraceptive pill
OR operating room
OSH outside hospital
PAVM pulmonary AVM
PC pheochromocytoma
PCP primary care physician
PCR polymerase chain reaction
PDA patent ductus arteriosus
PET positron emission tomography
PGF paternal grandfather
PICU pediatric intensive care unit
PID pelvic inflammatory disease
PIP proximal interphalangeal
POI primary ovarian insufficiency
PPI proton-pump inhibitor
PRBC packed red blood cell
PRP pityriasis rubra pilaris
PTH parathyroid hormone
PT prothrombin time
PTU propylthiouracil
PUV posterior urethral valve
RA rheumatoid arthritis
RBC red blood cell
RDS respiratory distress syndrome
RMSF Rocky Mountain spotted fever
RMS rhabdomyosarcomas
RNA ribonucleic acid
RNP ribonucleoprotein
ROHHAD rapid-onset obesity, hypoventilation, hypothalamic and autonomic dysfunction
RUL right upper lobe
RUQ right upper quadrant

RVH right ventricular hypertrophy
SCFE slipped-capped femoral epiphysis
SCJ sternoclavicular joint
SCN severe congenital neutropenia
sIL2R soluble IL2 receptor
SLE systemic lupus erythematosus
SNP single nucleotide polymorphism
SOB shortness of breath
SSRI selective serotonin reuptake inhibitor
SS serotonin syndrome
SSSS staphylococcal scalded skin syndrome
STIR short tau inversion recovery
SVC superior vena cava
SVD spontaneous vaginal delivery
TAAD thoracic aortic aneurysm and dissection
TB tuberculosis
TEE transesophageal echocardiogram
THC tetrahydrocannabinol
THI transient hyperphosphatasemia of infancy
TIBC total iron-binding capacity
TMA thrombotic microangiopathy
TNN13 troponin 13
TNSALP tissue-nonspecific alkaline phosphatase
TRAbs TSH receptor–stimulating antibodies
TRALI transfusion-related acute lung injury
TSH thyroid-stimulating hormone
TSI thyroid stiffness index
TTE transthoracic echocardiogram
tTG tissue transglutaminase
UA urinalysis
URI upper respiratory infection
UTI urinary tract infection
UV ultraviolet
VBDS vanishing bile duct syndrome
VHL syndrome von Hippel-Lindau syndrome
VMA vanillylmandelic acid
VSD ventricular septal defect
VUS variant of unknown significance
VZV varicella-zoster virus
WBC white blood cell

1

It's Just a Virus

Andrew J. White, Patrick J. Reich

CHIEF COMPLAINT

Fever and fatigue

HISTORY OF PRESENT ILLNESS

A 15-year-old girl presented with fevers and fatigue. One week ago she developed acute onset of fatigue, body aches, headache, and sore throat. This was followed by daily fevers ranging from 102 °F to 105 °F. Her symptoms were somewhat improved with ibuprofen, but they never fully resolved. She also complained of nausea and decreased oral intake, but she had no vomiting or diarrhea. She was seen in the emergency department (ED) 4 days prior to admission and discharged home with a diagnosis of a "viral illness." Two days later, she began feeling better and was starting to defervesce. She had more energy and was starting to eat more consistently. The following day she saw her pediatrician for a regularly scheduled appointment. He ordered a complete blood count (CBC), which was notable for WBC count 1.5k, hemoglobin 12, and platelets of 77k. She was directly admitted to evaluate the cytopenias with concern for malignancy.

PAST MEDICAL HISTORY

- Mild intermittent asthma, never hospitalized
- Menorrhagia, treated with Depo-Provera and improved
- Recent yeast infection, treated with fluconazole
- Seasonal allergies

Medications

- Cetirizine
- Albuterol prn
- Ibuprofen prn

Family/Social History

- She lives with her father, who smokes.
- She does not smoke or use illicit drugs.
- Sexually active with one male partner, always with condoms.
- No pets or animal exposures.
- No recent travel.

EXAMINATION

- Vitals: Temperature 37.5 °C, pulse 64, respiratory rate 16, blood pressure 109/66, saturating 98% on room air
- Gen: She is in no distress, appears comfortable, talkative
- HEENT: Tympanic membranes are clear, sclera anicteric, PERRL, EOMI, MMM, no oral lesions, oropharynx clear without exudates, no malar rash

- Neck: Supple, with a 1 cm nontender posterior cervical lymph node
- Pulm: Clear, no wheezing, or stridor
- CV: Regular rate and rhythm, no murmur
- Abd: Soft, NT/ND, no masses or HSM, normal bowel sounds
- Ext: Warm, well perfused, somewhat sweaty palms, no clubbing, cyanosis, or edema
- Neuro: Alert, symmetric 5/5 strength, sensation intact
- Skin: No rash

DIAGNOSTIC CONSIDERATIONS

- Leukemia was considered given the cytopenias, but the improvement in her symptoms was less supportive of this diagnosis.
- Infectious mononucleosis, which may cause leukopenia, thrombocytopenia, elevated AST/ALT, and lymphadenopathy, was thought likely.
- Systemic lupus erythematosus is well known to cause cytopenia.

Investigation

- CBC: WBC 1.4 > Hb 10.7 < Plt 88%, 4% bands, 32% neutrophils, 54% lymphocytes, 6% monocytes. No blasts were seen with direct examination of the blood smear
- CMP: Notable for AST 107, ALT 94
- TSH 2.07, free T4 1.27
- LDH 352, Uric Acid 1.8
- CMV IgM positive, IgG negative
- EBV IgM negative, IgG positive
- CXR: Normal lungs
- NP swab: Negative
- Rapid HIV: Negative

Results

- Blood CMV PCR: Negative
- ANA and dsDNA: Negative
- Hepatitis panel: Negative

DIAGNOSIS

As the results returned normal, and the leading diagnoses were excluded, repeat tests and more specific tests were considered. An HIV fourth-generation assay was sent and was **reactive**, leading to the diagnosis of **acute retroviral syndrome** from HIV infection.

Treatment/Follow-up

She attended the HIV clinic 5 days after discharge, and confirmatory HIV testing results were disclosed to her and her family. She had a viral load of >10,000,000 copies/mL with a K103N RT mutation. With more detailed questioning, she had a total of three lifetime male partners but still claimed consistent condom use with all. She was started on Bactrim prophylaxis. Within 2 weeks of her diagnosis, she was started on Stribild (tenofovir/emtricitabine/elvitegravir/cobicistat), a one-pill once-a-day, integrase inhibitor–based regimen.

TEACHING POINTS

1. **Updates in HIV testing.** The rapid HIV test performed in the ED was negative, but HIV testing done in house was positive. The ED test used was a rapid third-generation HIV ELISA that measures HIV 1 and 2 IgG and IgM. The third-generation test will generally be positive in most individuals 3 to 6 weeks after initial infection, after the body has had time to mount an immunologic response. However, individuals with acute HIV infection may present prior to that time, and this test may be negative during this window period.

The newest HIV test available is the fourth-generation HIV ELISA + p24 antigen test. This tests for HIV 1 and 2 antibodies like the third-generation test but also tests for p24 antigen, an early product of HIV replication that is detectable before the antibodies are and can be positive 10 days after infection. The fourth-generation assay is a better test for acute infection if this is suspected, but it is more expensive. If acute infection is suspected and the fourth-generation test is negative, it is appropriate to send an HIV RNA PCR (viral load). It is **not** typically indicated to send a Western blot (previous method of confirming a positive HIV ELISA) as the fourth-generation assays can be positive up to 3 weeks before the Western blot turns positive.

2. **HIV evaluation and treatment guidelines are updated annually.** Since 2016, US guidelines recommend starting highly active antiretroviral therapy (HAART) in all new diagnoses that are willing and capable because of evidence of better immune system restoration.

3. **Ongoing epidemic in US youth, especially those of color.** In the United States, **youths 13 to 24 years of age** represent a high-risk segment of the population with over 7800 new HIV infections in this age group in 2018, particularly in youth of color and men who have sex with men (MSM). Individuals who are acutely or recently infected disproportionately infect others due to their very high viral loads. Early diagnosis and treatment of a youth with acute HIV infection, therefore, has tremendous potential to decrease ongoing transmission in our community.

4. **Index of suspicion is key.** In an adult ED study looking retrospectively at specimens from patients diagnosed with a nonspecific viral syndrome, **1% of individuals had acute HIV infection!** Remember acute HIV infection can look exactly like mononucleosis, influenza, and other common viral illnesses. Laboratory findings can include leukopenia, atypical lymphocytosis, thrombocytopenia, and transaminase elevation. Youth will likely not be forthcoming with a stranger regarding their private lives, so they may not give history of sexual activity. In any teen with a viral illness severe enough to make them seek an outpatient evaluation, HIV should be on the differential!

Suggested Readings

Center for Disease Control and Prevention. HIV and Youth. Accessed 2019. https://www.cdc.gov/hiv/group/age/youth/index.html

Center for Disease Control and Prevention. HIV in the United States and Dependent Areas. Accessed 2019. https://www.cdc.gov/hiv/statistics/overview/ataglance.html

Hecht FM, Busch MP, Rawal B, et al. Use of laboratory tests and clinical symptoms for identification of primary HIV infection. *AIDS*. 2002;16(8):1119-1129.

Panel on Antiretroviral Guidelines for Adults and Adolescents. Guidelines for the use of antiretroviral agents in HIV-1-infected adults and adolescents. Department of Health and Human Services. Accessed 2019. http://www.aidsinfo.nih.gov/ContentFiles/AdultandAdolescentGL.pdf

Pilcher CD, Eron JJ Jr, Galvin S, Gay C, Cohen MS. Acute HIV revisited: new opportunities for treatment and prevention. *J Clin Invest*. 2004;113(7):937-945.

Rosenberg NE, Pilcher CD, Busch MP, Cohen MS. How can we better identify early HIV infections? *Curr Opin HIV AIDS*. 2015;10(1):61-68.

Routy JP, Cao W, Behraj V. Overcoming the challenge of diagnosis of early HIV infection: a stepping stone to optimal patient management. *Expert Rev Anti Infect Ther*. 2015;13(10):1189-1193.

Rutstein SE, Sellers CJ, Ananworanich J, Cohen MS. The HIV treatment cascade in acutely infected people: informing global guidelines. *Curr Opin HIV AIDS*. 2015;10(6):395-402.

Zetola NM, Pilcher CD. Diagnosis and management of acute HIV infection. *Infect Dis Clin North Am*. 2007;21(1):19-48, vii.

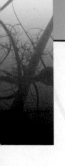

2 Lucky Break

David B. Wilson, Julie A. Steinberg

CHIEF COMPLAINT

"Fell out of bed"

HISTORY OF PRESENT ILLNESS

A 4-year-old boy with sickle cell disease (Hb SS) fell from a bunk bed 3 days PTA. On the DOA, he was taken to the emergency department for evaluation of worsening **arm pain and swelling**. He has had no fevers and no other symptoms whatsoever.

PAST MEDICAL HISTORY

- Prematurity
- G-tube placement/removal
- SVT, age 7 month, resolved
- One episode of sickle cell pain

Medications

- PCN VK 250 mg po BID
- Hydroxyurea 250 mg po qD
- Ibuprofen PRN
- Acetaminophen/hydrocodone PRN
- Miralax

Family/Social History

- **Diet**: Picky eater; diet lacks Fe-rich foods.
- **FH**: Sickle cell trait, both parents.
- **SH**: Lives with grandmother, mother, and sibling.

EXAMINATION

- Vitals: T = 37.6 °C; P = 126; R = 23; BP = 116/63.
- Head: Atraumatic and normocephalic.
- Eyes: Pupils equal, round, and reactive to light and conjunctiva clear.
- Nose: Clear, no discharge.
- Throat: Moist mucous membranes without erythema, exudates, or petechiae.
- Neck: Supple, no lymphadenopathy.
- Lungs: Clear to auscultation; no wheezing, crackles, or rhonchi; breathing unlabored.
- Heart: Normal PMI. RRR with a loud II/VI systolic murmur, normal S1 and S2.
- Abdomen: Soft, nontender. BS normal. No masses or organomegaly.
- Neuro: Face symmetric, moves right upper and bilateral lower extremities spontaneously against gravity.
- Musculoskeletal: The left arm is swollen and tender to palpation. No tenderness to palpation of right upper extremity or bilateral lower extremities.
- Skin: Warm, no rashes, no ecchymosis.

DIAGNOSTIC CONSIDERATIONS

A fracture of humerus was the main, and essentially only concern, although dislocation was thought possible. Sickle cell pain crises were thought plausible, and laboratory tests were sent.

Investigation

- WBC = 12.9, **Hb = 6.6**, Retic = 5%, Plt = 368. A review of serial CBCs showed progressive microcytosis (MCV = 66), suggesting concurrent Fe deficiency
- CMP normal
- **CRP = 146.1**
- **ESR = 32**
- Blood culture = negative
- **25-OH Vit D = 11 (nl > 20)**
- Ferritin = 345

Results

Radiograph depicting the fracture is given in Figure 2.1.

The radiograph prompted a skeletal survey, which then prompted a magnetic resonance imaging (MRI).

Skeletal survey:

- Partially visualized left humerus fracture with underlying moth-eaten appearance of the left humerus and overlying periosteal reaction. **Similar appearing findings are noted of the mid-to-distal right tibial diaphysis**, with possible **nondisplaced fracture through the right distal tibial diaphysis.**

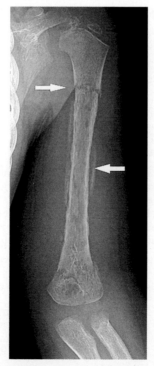

FIGURE 2.1 Radiograph of left arm showing a moth-eaten appearance of the left humerus with a periosteal reaction (lower white arrow) and fractures of the left humeral shaft (transverse fracture of the proximal shaft (upper white arrow). Mid-diaphyseal fracture and supracondylar fractures are also apparent.

- No additional acute or healing fractures are identified.

  MRI:

- Diffuse marrow signal loss of the left humerus, generalized periosteal reaction with moth-eaten cortex, axillary lymphadenopathy, and large fluid collection surrounding the distal humerus are concerning for osteomyelitis superimposed on bone infarction.
- Marrow heterogeneity, periosteal reaction, immediately distal to tibial diaphysis. There are no fluid collections in the lower extremity.

On the first hospital day, he was taken to the operating room (OR) for incision, drainage, and/or a biopsy of the left humerus. Purulence was evident immediately upon incision. Samples and cultures were sent, and in 48 hours, the **cultures grew Salmonella species**, sensitive to ampicillin, ceftriaxone, and ciprofloxacin.

DIAGNOSIS

1. Multifocal salmonella osteomyelitis
2. Traumatic fractures of left humerus; additional fracture of right tibia
3. Vitamin D deficiency
4. Possible Fe deficiency
5. Sickle cell disease

Treatment/Follow-up

He was given a simple blood transfusion of packed red blood cells prior to surgery. Antibiotic treatment was initiated upon his return from the OR with parenteral ceftriaxone. After several days of parental antibiotic, and return of the culture sensitivities, he was subsequently switched to oral therapy with amoxicillin and completed a 6-week course. Casts were applied to his left arm and right leg. He was started on vitamin D supplementation and empiric Fe supplementation.

TEACHING POINTS

Patients with sickle cell disease are at increased risk of salmonella infections.
Predisposing factors are thought to include the following:

- Intravascular sickling of gastrointestinal capillary vessels may permit salmonella invasion.
- Impaired function of the phagocytes in the liver and spleen.
- Abnormal opsonization and complement function.
- Sluggish blood flow leading to ischemic foci for bacterial localization.

The majority of salmonella infections in sickle cell patients involve bones (especially long bones) and joints and occur most frequently in early childhood (only 18% of cases occur after age 12 years). Typically, multiple sites are involved.

The most frequent clinical manifestations are persistent high fever and local pain in the affected bone(s), making this case unusual in terms of clinical presentation. It is fortuitous that this boy sustained a traumatic fracture, as it led to the identification of this serious infection.

Suggested Reading

Anand AJ, Glatt AE. *Salmonella* osteomyelitis and arthritis in sickle cell disease. *Semin Arthritis Rheum.* 1994;24:211-221.

3

Sleepy

Amanda Reis Dube

CHIEF COMPLAINT

Sleepy

HISTORY OF PRESENT ILLNESS

A 4-month-old girl presented to an emergency room with 1 day of decreased oral intake, decreased urine output, decreased energy, and tactile fevers. Over the last 12 to 16 hours, she had been sleepy and uninterested in feeding. She has had no sick contacts, no trauma, and no cold symptoms. She was exclusively breastfed and had not been given any other foods. Parents did comment that she had not stooled in 6 days, which was not typical for her.

PAST MEDICAL HISTORY

Born at 39 weeks via normal spontaneous vaginal delivery, with shoulder dystocia and nuchal cord but no resuscitation, Apgar scores were 8 and 9. At birth, her weight was 80th percentile but is now down to 25th percentile. She has not yet received her 4 month vaccines.

Family/Social History

An elder sister has ulcerative colitis. Two other sisters are healthy. No one in the family has any known genetic or metabolic disorders, nor any failure to thrive in infancy.
　　She lives at home with mother, father, and three sisters. She does not attend daycare.

EXAMINATION

- VS: T 36.6, HR 143, RR 30, SpO$_2$ 100%
- Gen: Listless, but with strong cry
- HEENT: Anterior fontanelle open, soft, and flat; tympanic membranes normal; mucous membranes moist; neck supple; **pupils large (8 mm)** but equal and reactive to light
- CV: Regular rate and rhythm; no murmurs
- Pulm: Breathing comfortably with symmetric breath sounds, no crackles, and no retractions
- Abd: Soft, normal bowel sounds, no masses
- GU: Normal external Tanner I female genitalia
- Neuro: Mildly hypotonic, decreased interaction

DIAGNOSTIC CONSIDERATIONS

- Sepsis
- Central nervous system infection
- Ingestion (eg, of an anticholinergic medication)
- Nonaccidental trauma (ie, child abuse)
- Guillain-Barré syndrome
- Myasthenia gravis, congenital
- Spinal muscular atrophy

- Poliomyelitis
- Inborn error of metabolism
- Infant botulism

Investigation

- CBC: WBC 10.7 (15% N, 77% L), Hgb 12.1, **Plt 562**
- CRP: 0.25
- BMP: Na 139, K 4.6, Cl 101, CO_2 19, BUN 11, Cr 0.2, **Glu 58**, Ca 10.3
- UA (specimen obtained via catheter): 2+ ketones, trace blood, negative nitrites/LE, 0 to 5 white blood cells, 0 to 5 red blood cells, trace bacteria
- Urine drug screen: negative
- Urine and blood cultures obtained and ultimately negative

Results

Initial management was focused on the hypoglycemia. After a D10 bolus, the hypotonia improved and she became more alert. She was diagnosed with a viral illness and admitted to a general pediatrics floor. Over the course of the day, however, she began exhibiting increased work of breathing, decreased tone, and decreased alertness. She was given a dose of antibiotics and transferred to the pediatric ICU, where she was started on 1 L oxygen via nasal cannula for tachypnea/shallow breathing. Her heart rate and blood pressures became labile during the transfer.

In the ICU, she became more lethargic with a weak cry, slight drooping of the right eyelid, a protruding tongue, poor suck, weak gag, and pooling secretions, suggestive of bulbar hypotonia.

Infantile botulism was raised as a possible diagnosis, given the bulbar weakness with mydriasis, constipation, and autonomic instability. Sepsis was thought less likely given normal WBC, CRP, and lack of fever. Further workup was initiated and included head CT (normal), LP (unremarkable), and metabolic studies (serum amino acids, urine organic acids, carnitine, and acylcarnitine—all normal).

Stool studies for botulism were sent, and botulinum immunoglobulin (BabyBIG) was ordered. Overnight, her respiratory status deteriorated, and she was intubated. She was given the BabyBIG the following day. Stool studies were ultimately positive for botulinum toxin. She gradually improved and was extubated 15 days later.

Upon further discussion, and with more specific questioning, the parents had been around several construction sites as they looked for a new home. They continued to deny any honey exposure.

DIAGNOSIS

Infant botulism

TEACHING POINTS

Clostridium botulinum is a gram-positive, spore-forming, anaerobic bacteria found in soil. When spores are ingested, toxin is released. In adults, intestinal flora and bile acid provide protection against the deleterious effects of the toxin. In infants, the toxin causes blockade of the cholinergic receptors at the neuromuscular junction, causing anything from mild weakness to complete flaccid paralysis. The first manifestation is often constipation from decreased intestinal motility, followed by central and extremity weakness including loss of reflexes. Diaphragmatic weakness can lead to respiratory failure. Autonomic dysfunction may also develop.

There are an estimated 250 cases of infant botulism per year. Fifty percent are in California. Ninety percent of patients present at less than 6 months of age. While honey is the classic culprit, dust and soil exposure are thought to be responsible in a majority (almost two third) of cases.

When infant botulism is suspected, a stool toxin neutralization bioassay at a state laboratory or the CDC can confirm diagnosis. EMG-nerve conduction studies may show characteristic findings in some but not all cases. Laboratory tests, cultures, EEG, and neuroimaging are generally normal.

Supportive care is the mainstay of treatment, especially when respiratory failure develops. In 2003, human botulism immune globulin (BabyBIG) was developed to decrease the morbidity and mortality of infant botulism. It has been shown to significantly decrease hospital length of stay, by an average of 3 weeks. Prior to botulism immunoglobulin, 50% to 77% of patients were intubated. Since the introduction of botulism immunoglobulin, this number has decreased, with one case series of 13 babies reporting approximately 25% intubation rate.

With early diagnosis and supportive management, prognosis is generally excellent with high rates of survival (as high as 99% of those treated in hospitals) and, if no complications develop, no neurologic sequelae. This patient was discharged after a 1-month hospital stay. She is currently doing very well, meeting all of her developmental milestones.

Suggested Readings

Arnon SS, Midura TF, Damus K, Thompson B, Wood RM, Chin J. Honey and other environmental risk factors for infant botulism. J Pediatr. 1979;94(2):331-336. doi:10.1016/S0022-3476(79)80863-X

Arnon SS, Schechter R, Maslanka SE, Jewell NP, Hatheway CL. Human botulism immune globulin for the treatment of infant botulism. N Engl J Med. 2006;354(5):462-471. doi:10.1056/NEJMoa051926

Cagan E, Peker E, Dogan M, Caksen H. Infant botulism. Eurasian J Med. 2010;42(2):92-94. doi:10.5152/eajm.2010.25

Cox LM, Yamanishi S, Sohn J, et al. Altering the intestinal microbiota during a critical developmental window has lasting metabolic consequences. Cell. 2014;158(4):705-721. doi:10.1016/j.cell.2014.05.052

Fox CK, Keet CA, Strober JB. Recent advances in infant botulism. Pediatr Neurol. 2005;32(3):149-154. doi:10.1016/j.pediatrneurol.2004.10.001

Rosow LK, Strober JB. Infant botulism: review and clinical update. Pediatr Neurol. 2015;52(5):487-492. doi:10.1016/j.pediatrneurol.2015.01.006

Schreiner MS, Field E, Ruddy R. Infant botulism: a review of 12 years' experience at the Children's Hospital of Philadelphia. Pediatrics. 1991;87(2):159-165.

Thompson JA, Filloux FM, Van Orman CB, et al. Infant botulism in the age of botulism immune globulin. Neurology. 2005;64(12):2029-2032. doi:10.1212/01.WNL.0000166950.35189.5E

No Iris? No!

Shannon C. Agner, Ali Yusuf Mian

CHIEF COMPLAINT

"Her skin graft is turning white."

HISTORY OF PRESENT ILLNESS

A 5-year-old girl with a complicated medical history was admitted to the pediatric intensive care unit immediately postoperation after having revision of a skin graft. She is 10 days status post encephalo-duro-arterio-myo-synangiosis, a revascularization procedure for moyamoya-like vasculopathy.

Seven months prior to this admission, she had an ischemic stroke in the right anterior cerebral artery territory, diagnosed after she began having left-sided weakness while playing tee-ball with dad. Brain imaging revealed cerebral vasculopathy as well as a right anterior cerebral artery distribution stroke (Figure 4.1). An explanation for the vasculopathy was not determined at that time.

During this current hospitalization, the patient had three separate attempts at skull flap engraftment; the third and final was successful.

Genetics was consulted to evaluate the poor wound healing episodes and some congenital abnormalities.

PAST MEDICAL HISTORY

- Congenital limb abnormalities
- Aniridia
- Cerebral vasculopathy, noted at 5 years of age, unexplained
- Right anterior cerebral artery territory stroke at 5 years of age

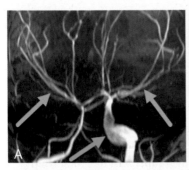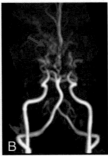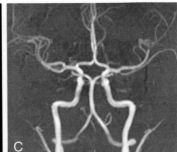

FIGURE 4.1 A, Magnetic resonance angiography (MRA) of the head of the patient with ACTA2 mutation described in the case. Note the straight course of the middle cerebral arteries and distal branches (yellow arrows). Marked ectasia is also noted in the internal carotid artery (green arrow). B, MRA of a patient with typical moyamoya vasculopathy. The "puff of smoke" sign (red arrow) is an indication of collateral blood supply to the circle of Willis. C, An MRA from a healthy child, demonstrating normal course and caliber of the arteries of the anterior circulation of the brain.

- Gut malrotation, repaired at 4 months of age
- Hypoplastic aortic arch, PDA, and ASD, repaired at 3 months of age

Family/Social History

Developmental history: Normal. Despite limb anomalies, she pulled to stand and walked on time. She speaks in full, complex sentences. She has no fine motor deficiencies. She is scheduled to attend kindergarten in the upcoming school year.

Parents and two siblings are in good health.

EXAMINATION

General examination highlights:

- 1/6 systolic murmur.
- Symphalangism of distal interphalangeal joints on digits 3 and 4 on the right hand.
- Right foot with nubbin-like toes without distinct toenails. On the left, posterior remnant of foot with a heel, but anterior portion of the foot is missing with five toelike nubbins at the end of foot remnant.
- Dusky appearance to skin flaps over right forehead, right clavicle, abdomen, and right thigh.

Neurologic examination highlights:

- **Pupils fixed and dilated**.
- Extraocular movements intact. Face symmetric.
- Tongue and uvula midline.
- Patient moving all extremities spontaneously.
- Reflexes 2+ at biceps, brachioradialis, patellar tendons bilaterally.

DIAGNOSTIC CONSIDERATIONS

Due to the limb abnormalities, cerebral vasculopathy, and poor wound healing, there was concern for a systemic vascular disease. Possible etiologies included the following:

- Adams-Oliver syndrome, an autosomal dominant disorder considered a vascular disruption sequence that causes vascular and connective tissue abnormalities as well as transverse limb anomalies
- Vasculopathy associated with thoracic aortic aneurysms (TAAD)

However, it was the "aniridia" that held the diagnostic clue. On careful physical examination and review of the prior eye examinations, the aniridia was actually congenital mydriasis.

Investigation

Chromosomal microarray showed a variant of unknown significance.

Additional investigations:

- MRI/MRA
  - Acute ischemia in medial right hemisphere consistent with right anterior cerebral artery territory stroke.
  - Atretic right internal carotid artery. Ectatic left internal carotid artery.
- Conventional angiogram:
  - Hypoplastic descending thoracic aorta.
  - Small, stretched, and straightened intracranial arterial branches.
  - Hypoplastic external carotid artery branches including superficial temporal arteries.
- Targeted genetic testing:
  - ACTA2 gene testing.

Results

An ACTA2 mutation was detected at position arginine 179. The parents were also tested and were negative. Thus, the patient had a de novo mutation.

DIAGNOSIS

ACTA2 mutation

TEACHING POINTS

The ACTA2 gene encodes for α-actin, an actin subtype found in smooth muscle. Mutations in ACTA2 lead to smooth muscle dysfunction. Since elastin is an inhibitor of actin, in arteries with elastin, there tends to be ectasia of the blood vessels. In arteries without elastin, there is an overproliferation of dysfunctional smooth muscle cells, causing narrowing of these blood vessels. ACTA2 mutations were first described in familial thoracic aortic aneurysms, but they have increasingly become a well-recognized genetic etiology of pediatric stroke. This mutation can also be associated with congenital mydriasis (due to absent contractility of the pupillary constrictor), gut malrotation, and bladder hypotonia.

The cerebral vasculopathy is notable due to postoperative complications that may arise from surgical intervention for these patients from dysfunctional blood vessels; they often have poor wound healing and ultimately fail to revascularize. The moyamoya-like cerebral vascular pattern is distinguishable due to lack of collateral "moyamoya"-like vessels to perfuse the brain.

Congenital mydriasis in a child with stroke is nearly pathognomonic for this disease. Although ACTA2 is found on the thoracic aortic aneurysm testing panel, targeted ACTA2 testing was performed for this patient because she had congenital mydriasis in addition to other characteristics typical of the phenotype.

Suggested Readings

Guo DC, Papke CL, Tran-Fadulu V, et al. Mutations in smooth muscle alpha-actin (ACTA2) cause coronary artery disease, stroke, and Moyamoya disease, along with thoracic aortic disease. *Am J Hum Genet A.* 2009;84(5):617-627. doi:10.1016/j.ajhg.2009.04.007

Khan N, Schinzel A, Shuknecht B, Baumann F, Østergaard JR, Yonekawa Y. Moyamoya angiopathy with dolichoectatic internal carotid arteries, patent ductus arteriosus and pupillary dysfunction: a new genetic syndrome? *Eur Neurol.* 2004;51:72-77. doi:10.1159/000076248

Meuwissen ME, Lequin MH, Bindels-de Heus K, et al. ACTA2 mutation with childhood cardiovascular, autonomic and brain anomalies and severe outcome. *Am J Med Genet A.* 2013;161A(6):1376-1380. doi:10.1002/ajmg.a.35858

Milewicz DM, Østergaard JR, Ala-Kokko LM, et al. De novo ACTA2 mutation causes a novel syndrome of multisystemic smooth muscle dysfunction. *Am J Med Genet A.* 2010;152A(10):2437-2443. doi:10.1002/ajmg.a.33657

Moller HU, Fledelius HC, Milewicz DM, Regalado ES, Ostergaard JR. Eye features in three Danish patients with multisystemic smooth muscle dysfunction syndrome. *Br J Ophthalmol.* 2012;96(9):1227-1231. doi:10.1136/bjophthalmol-2011-301462

Munot P, Saunders DE, Milewicz DM, et al. A novel distinctive cerebrovascular phenotype is associated with heterozygous Arg179 ACTA2 mutations. *Brain.* 2012;135(pt 8):2506-2514. doi:10.1093/brain/aws172

Reid AJ, Bhattacharjee MB, Regalado ES, et al. Diffuse and uncontrolled vascular smooth muscle cell proliferation in rapidly progressing pediatric Moyamoya disease. *J Neurosurg Pediatr.* 2010;6(3):244-249. doi:10.3171/2010.5.PEDS09505

Richer J, Milewicz DM, Gow R, et al. R179H mutation in ACTA2 expanding the phenotype to include prune-belly sequence and skin manifestations. *Am J Med Genet A.* 2012;158A(3):664-668. doi:10.1002/ajmg.a.35206

Roder C, Peters V, Kasuya H, et al. Analysis of ACTA2 in European Moyamoya disease patients. *Eur J Paediatr Neurol.* 2011;15(2):117-122. doi:10.1016/j.ejpn.2010.09.002

5

Riverbed Rales

Natasha Lalos

CHIEF COMPLAINT

Shortness of breath

HISTORY OF PRESENT ILLNESS

A 13-year-old boy was transferred from an outside facility for shortness of breath (SOB) and chest pain, which was worse when he was lying down. These symptoms had been present for about a week, and he had been admitted locally where a pulmonary embolus workup was negative. He was discharged home with a diagnosis of pleurisy. One week later, however, he had no improvement in symptoms and his pediatrician ordered an echocardiogram which was remarkable for a large pericardial effusion. At the outside hospital, he was given a normal saline bolus and was then transferred directly to the pediatric intensive care unit (PICU). He had no fevers.

PAST MEDICAL HISTORY

Obesity

Medications

None

Family/Social History

No early-onset heart failure

EXAMINATION

First admission:
- Vitals: T 37.2, HR 104, RR 24, Sao$_2$ 98% on RA
- General: Obese, generally well-developed, talkative
- HEENT: Normocephalic, atraumatic, R/L TM wnl, PERRL, EOMI, MMM, no oral lesions, oropharynx clear without exudates
- Pulm: **Tachypnea and SOB which improves when sitting up.** No wheezing, no respiratory distress, no chest wall tenderness.
- CV: Mild tachycardia, no murmur
- Abd: Soft, obese, normal bowel sounds
- Ext: Warm and well-perfused
- Neuro: A&Ox3

Second admission:
- Vitals: T 36.9 °C, HR 102, RR 22, BP 122/75, Sao$_2$ 96% on RA
- General: Increased WOB, diaphoretic

- HEENT: Normocephalic, atraumatic, PERRL, EOMI, MMM, no oral lesions, oropharynx clear without exudates
- **Pulm: Increased WOB, decreased breath sounds over LLL, LML**
- CVS: Regular rate and rhythm, no murmur, no rub
- Abd: Soft and nontender, obese, BS normal
- Ext: Warm, and well-perfused
- Neuro: A&Ox3
- Skin: No rash

DIAGNOSTIC CONSIDERATIONS

- Idiopathic pericardial effusion.
- Infectious pericardial effusion. Bacterial infection is possible, but the lack of fever and the chronicity of the complaints argued against this cause. More subtle infections such as tuberculosis or histoplasmosis were considered.
- Secondary pericardial effusion. Lupus, rheumatoid arthritis, and cancer were considered.

Investigation

- Imaging: CXR, echocardiography, EKG
- ID: NP swab, HIV, EBV, CMV, enterovirus, HHV-6, mycoplasma, adenovirus, Histoplasma Ag and Ab, PPD, blood culture
- Rheum: CRP, ESR, C3, C4, Anti-dsDNA, ENA, ANA, ANCA, IgG

Results

- Echo and CXR: Large pericardial effusion (see Figure 5.1); BNP 22, troponin <0.03; EKG: normal
- Pericardiocentesis: Drained 900 mL and sent for culture, drain left in place
- Repeat Echo: Pericarditis s/p pericardial drain placement
- ID labs: Negative, Histoplasma Ag negative, Histoplasma Ab (pending at discharge)
- Rheum labs: CRP 136, ESR 90, C3, C4 nl, Anti-dsDNA < 1.0; ANA, ENA, ANCA negative, IgG normal

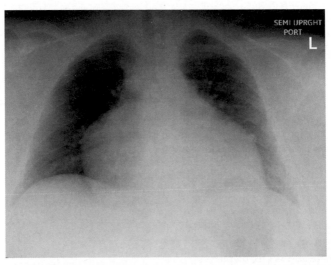

FIGURE 5.1 Pericardial effusion during the first admission to the pediatric intensive care unit (PICU).

One month follow-up: Rales are present on the left. A repeat CXR showed left-sided pleural effusion, with white out of 75% of left lung field (see Figure 5.2). Histoplasma antibody returned positive.

Diagnosis

1. **Histoplasmosis**, pulmonary
2. Pericarditis, secondary to #1
3. Pleural effusion, secondary to #1

Treatment/Follow-up

According to the Infectious Diseases Society of America's (IDSA's) Histoplasmosis Guidelines, nonsteroidal anti-inflammatory drugs (NSAIDs) alone are sufficient to treat mild cases of histoplasmosis-associated pericarditis. These were initiated, given that he had improved after the effusion was drained. However, after several weeks, he began to have new chest pain, repeat imaging showed reaccumulation of fluid, and he was admitted for further management. These symptoms prompted the initiation of itraconazole and steroids as listed in the IDSA Histoplasmosis Guidelines. He subsequently developed increased WOB, and repeat CXR showed a large tension pleural effusion with mediastinal shift. He underwent thoracentesis, draining 1250 mL of fluid. Repeat CXR a week later showed residual pleural effusion (see Figure 5.3). He was treated with steroids for 2 weeks and itraconazole for 12 weeks and eventually recovered. Evaluation for an underlying immune deficiency that did not reveal a detectable issue. The source of the infection was not identified (he did not keep chickens, eg), but he did live near the Mississippi River.

Teaching Points

- Histoplasmosis is a fungal infection that occurs mainly in the central United States, particularly around the Ohio and Mississippi river valleys. It may be encountered in soil that contains large amounts of bird droppings, and fungal spores are generally inhaled. Most people do not get sick at all, but some may have severe infections.
- Prednisone (0.5-1.0 mg/kg daily) is recommended for patients with histoplasmosis with evidence of hemodynamic compromise or unremitting symptoms after several days of therapy with nonsteroidal anti-inflammatory therapy.
- Removal of pericardial fluid is indicated in patients with hemodynamic compromise.

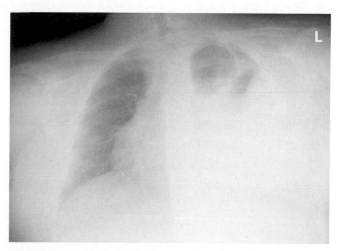

FIGURE 5.2 Chest x-ray demonstrating large tension pleural effusion during the second admission.

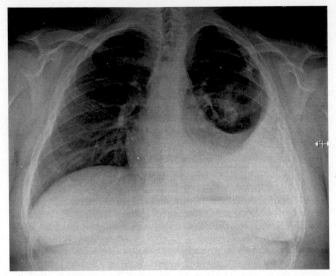

FIGURE 5.3 Chest x-ray (CXR) on the day of discharge, showing a residual pleural effusion but improved after thoracentesis (removal of 1250 mL).

- Itraconazole (200 mg TID for 3 days and then once or twice daily for 6-12 weeks) is recommended if corticosteroids are administered.
- Fungal burden is generally high in patients within 1 month of exposure who have diffuse infiltrates. Antigen and antibody testing is recommended to provide the highest sensitivity.
- Chronic sequelae of pulmonary histoplasmosis including chronic cavitary pulmonary histoplasmosis, granulomatous mediastinitis, fibrosing mediastinitis, broncholithiasis, and histoplasmomas (long-term pulmonary nodules).

Suggested Readings

Azar MM, Hage CA. Clinical perspectives in the diagnosis and management of histoplasmosis. *Clin Chest Med*. 2017;38(3):403-415. PMID: 28797485.

Wheat LJ, Azar MM, Bahr NC, Spec A, Relich RF, Hage C. Histoplasmosis. *Infect Dis Clin North Am*. 2016;30(1):207-227. PMID: 26897068.2019.

Wheat J, Freifeld AG, Kleiman MB, et al; Infectious Diseases Society of America. Clinical practice guidelines for the management of patients with histoplasmosis: 2007 update by the Infectious Diseases Society of America. *Clin Infect Dis*. 2007;45(7):807-825.

6

But I had No Injury

Natasha Lalos

CHIEF COMPLAINT

Fever and petechiae

HISTORY OF PRESENT ILLNESS

A 13-year-old boy presents with a diffuse petechial and pustular, pruritic rash. He also has a large purple-black bruise on his L upper thigh. He first noted the bruiselike mark on his thigh, a week or so ago, and the other rashes occurred a few days later. His school nurse diagnosed him with a bruise and told him that it would improve in a few days, although he denied any injury and was skeptical. He also had other symptoms, which included rhinorrhea, congestion, and a sore throat. Three days later, he became nauseous, and he began vomiting and developed a fever of 102 °F. On day 4, the thigh bruise became painful and that is when the petechial rash broke out all over his body. On day 5, he had a pustular outbreak on his forehead, back, and genitals. His skin is diffusely tender.

No recent travel history. No sick contacts. No contacts with similar rash. No known animal exposures. He has not noticed any ticks or pulled off a tick. He does have dogs at home, so he may have had unknown tick exposure.

PAST MEDICAL HISTORY

None

Medications

None

Family/Social History

Pet dog, who is allowed outdoors

EXAMINATION

- Vitals: T 37.4 °C, PR 90, RR 15, BP 110/68, Sao$_2$ 100% RA.
- **Constitutional: He appears distressed, in pain, and shaking.**
- HENT: Aphthous ulcers present on the tongue. PERRL, EOMI.
- CVS: Regular rate and rhythm, no murmur.
- Pulm: Effort normal, BS normal. No respiratory distress.
- Abdominal: SNT, BS present.
- **Genitourinary: Pustular rash present on the shaft of penis and scrotum.** No chancre.
- MSK: Normal range of motion. He exhibits no tenderness.
- LAD: He has cervical adenopathy, no other palpable LAD.
- Neurological: A&Ox3. He displays normal reflexes. He exhibits normal muscle tone.
- **Skin: Diffuse erythroderma that is flat and nonpalpable. Pustulosis of size 1 mm is present on the neck (Figure 6.1), back, and genitals. The thigh has 5 to 6 cm violaceous-black macule (Figures 6.2 and 6.3), with sparse blisters, which is painful to touch.**

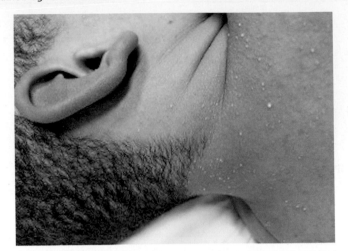

FIGURE 6.1   Pustulosis of the neck.

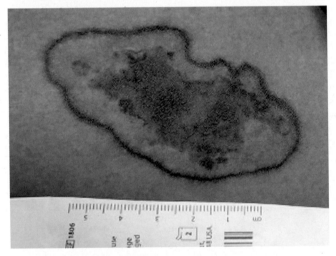

FIGURE 6.2   L thigh violaceous-black macule on admission.

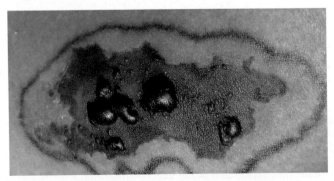

FIGURE 6.3   L thigh violaceous-black macule on admission day 4.

DIAGNOSTIC CONSIDERATIONS

Based on appearance alone, the differential diagnosis included loxoscelism. The painful skin and erythroderma suggest staphylococcal scalded skin syndrome. Other possibilities include tick-borne illness (Rocky Mountain spotted fever [RMSF], ehrlichiosis, anaplasmosis) and secondary syphilis. He denies any sexual activity or any presence in the past of a painless ulcer, making syphilis a less likely cause. Most houses in the Midwestern United States do harbor *Loxosceles reclusa*, and their presence was raised and confirmed with the father.

Investigation

- ID: Pustule swab, RMSF, ehrlichiosis, anaplasmosis studies, syphilis, HIV, blood culture
- CBC and RFP q12h, monitoring for hemolysis, rhabdomyolysis, and AKI
- aPTT, PT, INR
- ESR, CRP

Results

- Pustule swab: coagulase-negative staphylococci species; RMSF, *Ehrlichia*, *Anaplasma* negative, syphilis and HIV negative. Blood culture = No growth
- CBC 11.0, H/H 10.8/32.9, Plt 160
- aPTT, PT, INR nl
- ESR 28, CRP 76

DIAGNOSIS

Viscerocutaneous loxoscelism

Treatment/Follow-up

He was initially started on vancomycin, clindamycin, doxycycline, and ceftriaxone for coverage of the most likely etiologies. Vancomycin was discontinued, and he was maintained on once-daily ceftriaxone and clindamycin TID. He also started topical bacitracin for the eschar on L thigh. He developed worsening diffuse pruritus and orthostasis on day 2 of treatment with ceftriaxone, with eosinophilia, thought to be an allergic reaction and ceftriaxone was discontinued. The hemoglobin levels dropped from 10 g/dL on the admission to 7.1 g/dL on day 5, secondary to the known hemolytic complication of loxoscelism. He was given 1 U pRBCs with resolution of dizziness and light-headedness. After 7 days of clindamycin, he was discharged home.

TEACHING POINTS

- Loxoscelism is caused by the bite of the brown recluse spiders, *L. reclusa*, which live indoors in many homes in the world, and in particular in the Midwestern United States. Being shy creatures, they come out at night and often run for cover when discovered. They are often in basements, attics, behind shelving and storage bins, and dark, quiet, undisturbed areas. Clothing left on the floor is another prime location for them to be discovered. Symptoms are due to the venom and are usually local, causing a typically painless area of necrosis. Occasionally, the venom will have systemic consequences, causing the syndrome of viscerocutaneous loxoscelism. Antibiotics generally have no place in treatment, and while the necrotic wounds often appear infected, it is rare that this actually occurs.
- Viscerocutaneous reactions are generally more common with South American recluse spider bites.
- Both autoimmune and direct hemolysis are known to be delayed complications of a bite and should be kept in mind when seeing patients in follow-up. Often this presents 1 week after envenomation.

- Sphingomyelinase is thought to cause the necrotic eschar characteristic of recluse spider bites; it activates complement, neutrophil chemotaxis, apoptosis, and gelatinase expression.
- Bites typically occur when the spider is pinned between the person and an object (often clothing); thus, bites are commonly seen in covered areas such as upper arm, thorax, and inner thighs.
- A small case series suggests that loxoscelism in pediatric patients can be severe, with 65% of children developing major morbidity.

Suggested Readings

Hubbard JJ, James LP. Complications and outcomes of brown recluse spider bites in children. *Clin Pediatr.* 2011;50(3):252.

Mueller M, Doucette E, Freeman S, Williams A, Lindbloom E. Viscerocutaneous loxoscelism in an adult with acute generalized exanthematous pustulosis. *Mo Med.* 2014;111(2):139-142.

Tambourgi DV, Paixão-Cavalcante D, Gonçalves de Andrade RM, Fernandes-Pedrosa Mde F, Magnoli FC. *Loxosceles* sphingomyelinase induces complement-dependent dermonecrosis, neutrophil infiltration, and endogenous gelatinase expression. *J Invest Dermatol.* 2005;124(4):725-731.

7

Nonstandard Transmission

Kevin W. Graepel, Kevin T. Barton, Raja Dandamudi, Rachel C. Orscheln

CHIEF COMPLAINT

High creatinine and low sodium

HISTORY OF PRESENT ILLNESS

A 5-year-old boy presents 9 days after renal transplantation with abdominal pain, decreased oral intake, hyponatremia, and elevated creatinine. He was discharged from the hospital 3 days earlier with normal laboratory tests. He had some diffuse abdominal pain and loose stools but no florid diarrhea. His appetite was poor for solids, but he was drinking water. Gross hematuria was present, via the urethral stent that was in place as standard posttransplant practice. There was no drainage from the surgical site. No fever, cough, rhinorrhea, mucosal changes, rashes, headache, and neck stiffness.

His sister is COVID positive, but he has not had direct contact with her for 2 weeks. There are no healthcare workers in the family, no tuberculosis risk factors, no travel history, no animal or insect exposures, no recreational activities in wooded areas, and no standing water exposure.

Laboratory tests:

- Na = **123 mmol/L**
- HCO_3 = 18 mmol/L
- Anion gap = 10 mmol/L
- Creatinine = 0.69 mg/dL (0.35 mg/dL at discharge 3 days prior)
- WBC = 8.6 with 75% neutrophils (absolute neutrophils = 6.5)
- UA with 11 to 20 WBC, >50 RBC, 2+ leukocyte esterase, no nitrites
- Fractional excretion of sodium = 0.3%

PAST MEDICAL HISTORY

- End-stage kidney disease secondary to obstructive uropathy from posterior urethral valves.
- Hyperparathyroidism, due to renal insufficiency.
- Asthma.
- Deceased donor kidney transplant 9 days prior to admission. He and the donor had concordant EBV but discordant CMV (donor positive, patient negative) serologies. Induction immunosuppression included thymoglobulin 1.5 mg/kg × 3 doses and IV methylprednisolone 7 mg/kg once followed by 5 days of rapid prednisone taper.

Medications

- Immunosuppression: mycophenolate and tacrolimus
- Antimicrobial prophylaxis: trimethoprim-sulfamethoxazole, valganciclovir, nystatin
- Asthma: montelukast, fluticasone, albuterol
- Other: amlodipine, aspirin, potassium-sodium-phosphate supplement

Family/Social History

Lives with mother and five sisters in a single-family home in an urban area.

EXAMINATION

- Vitals: T 36.4 °C, HR 98/min, RR 24/min, BP 92/56 mm of Hg, Spo_2 99% on room air

Active, smiling child in mild pain. Normocephalic. PERRL, mild periorbital edema, MMM without lesions. Neck supple. Regular heart rate without murmur. Unlabored breathing and clear to auscultation. Abdomen soft and tender with palpable fluid collection in subcutaneous tissue overlying midline surgical incision. No drainage, warmth, or erythema of incision. Extremities were warm and well perfused without edema. He had no lymphadenopathy.

DIAGNOSTIC CONSIDERATIONS

Rejection of the new kidney was considered, complicated by GI loss from diarrhea.

He was admitted for dehydration and treated with IV fluids, and the creatinine normalized. He developed a fever to 38.3 °C on the day following admission and was started on ceftriaxone.

Investigation

After discussion with transplant surgery, the incisional fluid collection was explored and contained a large hematoma, but it was culture negative.

Additional infectious workup included blood cultures, urine cultures, SARS-CoV-2 RNA and IgG, and respiratory viral panel. He continued to have daily fevers despite broadening coverage to cefepime, and he developed pancytopenia (WBC = 1.7, Hgb = 6.5, PLT = 28). Infectious diseases were consulted for evaluation of persistent fever and pancytopenia. A workup was performed for infectious causes of pancytopenia including for viral, fungal, and tick-transmitted infections. He was also evaluated for MIS-C given his known family member with SARS-CoV-2 and the potential that other family members could have been infected and transmitted to him.

Results

The *Ehrlichia* polymerase chain reaction returned positive, and his laboratory evaluation was concerning for *Ehrlichia*-associated hemophagocytic lymphohistiocytosis (HLH). His ferritin peaked at 13,354 and triglycerides = 287 (normal = <99), but he did not meet the full criteria for HLH. He was started on doxycycline. He developed worsening respiratory distress and was transferred to the pediatric intensive care unit for bilevel positive airway pressure but was weaned to room air and returned to the floor 4 days later. He eventually recovered without long-term sequelae.

Discussion with transplant services revealed that the other patients who received organs from the same donor were also ill. Apparently, during acquisition of the organs, an engorged tick was seen embedded on the donor. *Ehrlichia* testing was therefore recommended on the other organ recipients and was positive on the other kidney recipient, who was also a pediatric patient.

DIAGNOSIS

1. **Ehrlichiosis**, kidney donor derived
2. **Ehrlichiosis-associated HLH**, partial

TEACHING POINTS

Ehrlichiosis is caused by *Ehrlichia* species including *Ehrlichia chaffeensis*, *Ehrlichia ewingii*, and *Ehrlichia muris eauclairensis*, with the former accounting for the majority of cases. *Ehrlichia* species are obligate intracellular (predominantly lymphocytes) bacteria transmitted primarily by tick bite from the lone star tick (*Amblyomma americanum*) and the black-legged tick (*Ixodes scapularis*). Ehrlichiosis was first recognized as a disease in the 1980s, but it was not a reportable disease until 1999. The incidence of ehrlichiosis has been steadily on the rise with 200 cases in 2000 and 1799 cases in 2018. Ehrlichiosis is most common in South Central and Southeastern states, with four states accounting for over half of reported cases: Arkansas, Missouri, Virginia, and New York. The peak months of infection are between May and August.

Symptoms of ehrlichiosis generally begin within 1 to 2 weeks after a tick bite and can include nonspecific symptoms such as fever, headache, muscle aches, gastrointestinal disturbances, and rash. A delay in administration of appropriate antibiotic therapy (doxycycline) increases the risk of development of severe illness. Severe manifestations can include acute respiratory distress syndrome, meningoencephalitis, multiorgan system dysfunction, and shock. Severe presentation of ehrlichiosis, including HLH, has been described in association with receipt of sulfonamide drugs.

Timely recognition of rickettsial disease in the early posttransplant period is uniquely challenging given the recent potent immunosuppression leading to severely suppressed immune function and blunted host response. Furthermore, most infections in the posttransplant period are due to reactivation of latent infections, so acquired infections may not be considered in the early postinfectious period. Most cases of ehrlichiosis in solid organ transplant recipients have occurred more than 6 months posttransplant so are especially difficult to diagnose in the early posttransplant period. Masterson and colleagues performed a review of all cases of ehrlichiosis from 1995 to present in solid organ transplant recipients. They found 103 cases in 102 patients, with most cases involving kidney transplantation. They found two donor-derived cases that both happened at 3 weeks posttransplant. The predominant clinical symptoms were fever and headache with some minor gastrointestinal complaints. The most common laboratory abnormalities were leukopenia, elevated transaminases, and thrombocytopenia. Hyponatremia was infrequently reported. Eighty-two percent of infections were due to *E. chaffeensis* and 18% due to *E. ewingii*. All patients in this series survived their infection.

Nonstandard transmission (donor-derived) of infections is rare but confers significant morbidity and mortality. The overall incidence of donor-derived infections is thought to be 0.2% but is ultimately unknown due to a lack of standardized reporting. Shingde and colleagues performed a review of the literature on this topic and found 207 recipient cases between 1948 and 2017. The most common transmitted infection was viral (116, 56%) with the human immunodeficiency virus being the most frequently transmitted (20, 9.7%). There was a relative tie between bacterial, fungal, and parasitic infections, all around 15%. The most frequent bacteria transmitted were *Mycobacterium tuberculosis* and *Pseudomonas aeruginosa*. *Candida* species and *Toxoplasma gondii* were the most frequent parasitic infections. Rabies conferred the highest probability for death at 90%, with a median time to death of 2.8 months posttransplant.

Suggested Readings

Masterson, Gupta S, Jakharia N, Peacock JE Jr. Ehrlichiosis in a recent kidney transplant recipient: the repellent that did not repel! A case report and literature review of ehrlichiosis in solid organ transplant recipients. *Transpl Infect Dis*. 2020;20:e13299.

Peters TR, Edwards KM, Standaert SM, et al. Severe ehrlichiosis in an adolescent taking trimethoprim-sulfamethoxazole. *Pediatr Infect Dis J*. 2000;19:(2):170-172.

Shingde RV, Reuter SE, Graham GG, et al. Unexpected donor-derived infectious transmissions by kidney transplantation: a systematic review. *Transpl Infect Dis*. 2018;20:e12851.

8 A Remote Consideration—But Always in Mind

Alexander Weymann

CHIEF COMPLAINT

Elevated liver function tests

HISTORY OF PRESENT ILLNESS

A 9-year-old girl was seen in her pediatrician's office twice in 1 week, initially for sore throat and low-grade fevers. Her temperatures ranged around 100 °F but increased to 102 the night prior to admission. She has now been febrile for 7 days, but intermittently, not daily. She had blisters in her mouth (lower lip, palate, oropharynx) which were initially painful, but less so once they ruptured, and most of them have now resolved. A few days later, she returned complaining of itching that was not responsive to diphenhydramine or cetirizine. The itching was worse at night and when taking a bath, and she has been unable to sleep the last two nights because of it. She developed right upper quadrant pain on the day of admission, and her pediatrician found her abdomen mildly tender on examination. He sent laboratory tests, and her bilirubin and transaminases were elevated.

She was admitted to the Hepatology service with infectious diseases consultation. Review of her chart revealed that her weight for age has decreased from 55% to 10% over the last 6 years. She has a loss of appetite, nausea, and early satiety.

PAST MEDICAL HISTORY

- Reflux
- Mild intermittent asthma
- No surgeries

Medications

- Albuterol MDI
- Fluticasone MDI

Family/Social History

She lives with her parents. No recent travel or sick contacts. Family history of asthma and allergies.

EXAMINATION

- Height: 141.8 cm (82%).
- Weight: 24.9 kg (9%).
- Vitals: Respiratory rate 24, heart rate 153, blood pressure 123/74, temperature 38.3 °C.
- General appearance: Alert, no acute distress, appears tired and ill, pale. Head/neck: Normocephalic, atraumatic; nontender, no focal lymphadenopathy.
- Eyes: No eyelid swelling, no conjunctival injection or exudate, no icterus.
- ENT: Nares patent, mucous membranes moist, no tonsillar enlargement, no tonsillar exudate; there are two ulcers on the mucosal surface of the lower lip—one is 2 mm in diameter

and the other is 4 to 5 mm; neither were painful when touched with tongue depressor; no gingivitis; no other oropharyngeal lesions.
- Lymph: No cervical, supraclavicular, axillary, or inguinal lymphadenopathy.
- Cardiovascular: Regular rate and rhythm, no murmur, brisk capillary refill.
- Chest/Respiratory: Breath sounds clear and equal bilaterally, no respiratory distress.
- Abdomen: Soft, not distended, no mass, no hepatomegaly or splenomegaly appreciated; tender in the right upper quadrant to light palpation with voluntary guarding and positive Murphy sign, no tenderness elsewhere.
- Extremities: No limb or joint swelling noted.
- Skin: Warm, dry, no rash.

DIAGNOSTIC CONSIDERATIONS

Problem list

1. Prolonged intermittent fever of at least 5 days, and likely 7 to 8 days
2. Oral ulcers
3. Transaminase elevation and direct hyperbilirubinemia
4. Nausea without vomiting
5. Microcytic anemia
6. Elevated inflammatory markers

Differential Diagnosis

- Acalculous cholecystitis
- Acute cholangitis
- Common bile duct stone
- Atypical Kawasaki disease
- Acute viral hepatitis (*EBV, CMV, HSV, enterovirus, parechovirus, adenovirus, hepatitis A, less likely hepatitis B or C*)
- Autoimmune hepatitis
- Wilson disease
- Malignant infiltration of the liver

Investigation

Laboratory: Serum electrolytes normal. Total bilirubin 2.6 mg/dL, direct 2.2 (0.1-1.0), alkaline phosphatase 489 U/L (151-342), **AST 257 U/L (15-50), ALT 315 U/L (<40)**, albumin 3.5 g/dL (3.4-5.3), total protein 7.4 g/dL (5.8-8.7), lipase 268 U/L (<202), WBC 7.1 × 10^3/μL (5-14.5), Hgb 9.4 g/dL (11.5-15.5), MCV 64.8 fL (77-95), RDW 17.1% (10-14.1), platelets 411 × 10^3/μL (140-440), ESR 125 mm/h (<13), CRP 13.3 mg/dL (<1.2), PT 15.4 seconds (12.4-14.7), and INR 1.2.

   More laboratory results: Hepatitis A, B, and C serologies negative. Enterovirus, adenovirus, parechovirus, EBV, CMV, HSV and histoplasma PCRs (blood) negative. ANA positive 1:320 (speckled/nucleolar); smooth muscle antibody and liver/kidney microsomal antibody negative; total serum IgG normal. Ceruloplasmin 56 mg/dL (21-53).

Results

Ultrasound

- Liver: Slightly hypoechoic with prominent portal triads. The right lobe extends below the kidney margin, suggesting mild hepatomegaly. No intrahepatic bile duct dilatation or focal mass.
- Common bile duct: Normal in caliber measuring 1.7 mm in diameter.
- Gall bladder: Bile-filled, without gallstone or gallbladder wall thickening. The bile is anechoic. No pericholecystic fluid.
- Ascites: None.

- Pancreas: Well visualized and sonographically normal in appearance. No pancreatic calcifications or peripancreatic fluid. There are a few small lymph nodes in the porta hepatis and adjacent to the head of the pancreas, with maximum short axis of 6 mm.
- Spleen: The spleen measures 9.7 cm in length and appears normal. There is a small splenule adjacent to the tip of the spleen, 0.9 cm in diameter.

Clinical Course

She was sent home without a diagnosis despite the laboratory testing and imaging. Four days after discharge from the initial hospitalization (48 hours), father called to report that she was not doing any better. She continued to have fevers, fatigue, and malaise. He (a physician) had noted that the ANA was positive and suggested systemic lupus erythematosus as a possibility.

A referral to Rheumatology was made, and because of persistent fevers now approaching 2 weeks, an echocardiogram was ordered to help exclude Kawasaki disease.

More Results

Echocardiogram: There is a posterior mediastinal mass approximately 6 by 4 cm that is compressing the left atrium. It does not appear to impact cardiac function. No valvular abnormalities. Normal biventricular size and systolic function. Normal coronary artery origins. No coronary dilation, ectasia, or aneurysms. Aortic root mildly dilated. No pericardial effusion.

CT chest with contrast: There is a large right mediastinal mass extending from the T1-T8 level. It demonstrates mass effect on the left brachiocephalic vein and the superior vena cava. The mass partially encases the brachiocephalic artery with mild mass effect. There is encasement and mass effect on the right upper, middle, and lower lobe bronchi with narrowing of the lumen.

A diagnostic procedure was performed, which was a lymph node biopsy.

DIAGNOSIS

Hodgkin lymphoma, mixed cellularity class.

TEACHING POINTS

This patient's clinical presentation was consistent with acute cholestatic hepatitis, cholangitis, cholecystitis, or biliary obstruction, and the differential mainly included infectious, less likely autoimmune or genetic/metabolic etiologies; malignancy was only a remote consideration.

However, hepatobiliary disease as the initial manifestation of Hodgkin lymphoma (HL) is well described.

Obstruction of the common bile duct by lymphadenopathy or infiltration, acute liver failure, cytomegalovirus (CMV) disease, "idiopathic cholestasis," primary sclerosing cholangitis, and autoimmune hepatitis associated with HL have all been reported.

Most publications on the subject are case reports of paraneoplastic vanishing bile duct syndrome (VBDS), a progressive destruction and eventual loss of intrahepatic bile ducts, leading to cholestasis. Acute cholestatic hepatitis as the initial presentation of HL is less commonly reported, but in one such case, the biopsy demonstrated prominent bile duct injury associated with a florid inflammatory reaction, and it has been speculated that this pattern precedes the eventual development of VBDS.

The pathogenetic mechanisms underlying either process are unknown; thus, therapeutic strategies are limited. For VBDS, rituximab, a chimeric monoclonal antibody against CD20 frequently expressed in HL, has been used with success in some patients. Another approach has been to use plasmapheresis in addition to chemotherapy and radiation. The data on treatment of cholestasis and pruritus with choleretic agents (ursodiol, rifampin) or bile acid binding resins (cholestyramine) are limited.

In this patient, the cholestatic hepatitis resolved promptly and completely after treatment was initiated. Whether the therapeutic response was entirely due to chemotherapy or whether ursodiol, which was given early in the course, played at least an adjunctive role, remains an open question.

This case illustrates that Hodgkin disease should be considered in the differential diagnosis of any child presenting with acute cholestatic hepatitis.

Suggested Readings

Bakhit M, McCarty TR, Park S, et al. Vanishing bile duct syndrome in Hodgkin's lymphoma: a case report and literature review. World J Gastroenterol. 2017;23(2):366-372.

Cervantes F, Briones J, Bruguera M, et al. Hodgkin's disease presenting as a cholestatic febrile illness: incidence and main characteristics in a series of 421 patients. Ann Hematol. 1996;72(6):357-360.

Das A, Mitra S, Ghosh D, et al. Vanishing bile duct syndrome following cytomegalovirus infection in a child with Hodgkin lymphoma. J Pediatr Hematol Oncol. 2018;40(1):83-84.

Gottrand F, Cullu F, Mazingue F, Nelken B, Lecomte-Houcke M, Farriaux JP. Intrahepatic cholestasis related to vanishing bile duct syndrome in Hodgkin's disease. *J Pediatr Gastroenterol Nutr*. 1997;24(4):430-433.

Gunasekaran TS, Hassall E, Dimmick JE, Chan KW. Hodgkin's disease presenting with fulminant liver disease. *J Pediatr Gastroenterol Nutr*. 1992;15(2):189-193.

Lefkowitch JH, Falkow S, Whitlock RT. Hepatic Hodgkin's disease simulating cholestatic hepatitis with liver failure. *Arch Pathol Lab Med*. 1985;109(5):424-426.

Liangpunsakul S, Kwo P, Koukoulis GK. Hodgkin's disease presenting as cholestatic hepatitis with prominent ductal injury. Eur J Gastroenterol Hepatol. 2002;14(3):323-327.

Marinone G, Lazzari R, Pellizzari F, Marinone MG. Acute cholestatic Hodgkin's lymphoma: an unusual clinical picture. Haematologica. 1989;74(3):293-296.

Mrzljak A, Gasparov S, Kardum-Skelin I, Colic-Cvrlje V, Ostojic-Kolonic S. Febrile cholestatic disease as an initial presentation of nodular lymphocyte-predominant Hodgkin lymphoma. World J Gastroenterol. 2010;16(35):4491-4493.

Yusuf MA, Elias E, Hübscher SG. Jaundice caused by the vanishing bile duct syndrome in a child with Hodgkin lymphoma. J Pediatr Hematol Oncol. 2000;22(2):154-157.

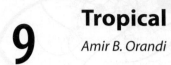

9 Tropical

Amir B. Orandi

CHIEF COMPLAINT

Fever and leg pain

HISTORY OF PRESENT ILLNESS

This 10-year-old boy's pain began abruptly 4 days ago and was located in the left midthigh. It was exacerbated with walking, knee extension, and palpation or pressure applied to the leg. It was improved with rest and when his knee was held slightly flexed and the leg laid out to the side. His symptoms have progressively worsened such that he is now barely able to bear weight or walk.

Other symptoms include fever with T-max 103 for the past 3 days and one episode of nonbloody, nonbilious vomiting. There is no rash, dyspnea, headache, or pain in other areas. There is no visible joint swelling. His symptoms first started when he was helping his family move boxes in their storage unit, but he does not recall a specific injury. The family had recently returned from a week-long trip to Florida.

PAST MEDICAL HISTORY

No chronic medical conditions, history of surgery, daily medications, or pertinent family history.

EXAMINATION

- Vitals: T 38.2, HR 100, RR 20, and BP 103/51.
- Well-appearing and friendly boy.
- Chest, abdominal, and neurologic examinations are normal.
- Musculoskeletal examination: Positioned at rest with his left leg slightly flexed at the knee and externally rotated. He has pain with any extension of the knee or internal rotation of the hip. He is tender to deep palpation along the medial thigh, but the skin is not warm, red, or tense. The knee joint has no effusion or warmth, and the lower leg, ankle, and foot are unremarkable.

Initial Testing

- Left femur x-ray: Normal
- Left hip ultrasound: No effusion
- WBC 6.6 (48%N, 34%L), Hb 13, Plt 267
- CMP: Normal. Creatine kinase 70
- ESR 25, CRP 59.6

DIAGNOSTIC CONSIDERATIONS

Infectious	Orthopedic/Trauma	Rheumatologic	Oncologic
Osteomyelitis	Slipped capital femoral epiphysis (SCFE)	Juvenile idiopathic arthritis	Ewing sarcoma
Pyomyositis	Hematoma	Idiopathic inflammatory myositis	Osteosarcoma
Septic arthritis	Myositis ossificans	Transient synovitis	

Investigations and Results

- Magnetic resonance imaging (MRI) with and without contrast left femur (Figure 9.1): T2/short tau inversion recovery (STIR) hyperintensity and enhancement centered in the left vastus medialis extending into the intermuscular fascia, abutting the posteromedial aspect of the femoral shaft. A small, nonenhancing T2 hyperintense lesion between the vastus medialis muscle and femoral cortex with diffusion restriction represents a nondrainable abscess.
- Blood culture: Methicillin-susceptible *Staphylococcus aureus* (MSSA) grew at 16 hours.

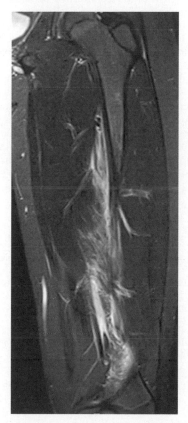

FIGURE 9.1   Magnetic resonance image depicting T2-weighted coronal view of the left thigh with purulent myositis in the left vastus medialis and intermuscular fascia.

DIAGNOSIS

1. **Pyomyositis** of the left thigh due to MSSA
2. MSSA bacteremia

TEACHING POINTS

Also known as "tropical myositis," pyomyositis is an acute intramuscular bacterial infection from hematogenous spread to skeletal muscle, neither derived from adjacent bone infection nor from penetrating trauma. First described by Scriba in Japan, ca 1885, it is known as tropical myositis, because in some tropical geographic regions, it occurs in a high frequency. It exhibits a 2:1 male predominance and up to 50% of cases occur in children and young adults. In the latter part of the 20th century, it became increasingly reported in more temperature regions but today still has a predilection to occur in southern regions of the United States. Although the majority of cases occur in previously healthy individuals, it is increasingly reported in immunocompromised patients, particularly those with HIV.

The pathogenesis is described in three stages: An early invasive stage where muscular symptoms of pain and swelling occur for up to 2 weeks, followed by a suppurative stage when systemic symptoms begin and local abscess formation develops (90% of patients present in this stage). A third, septicemic stage can follow if untreated. Leukocytosis and elevated inflammatory markers are commonly elevated in the second and third stages. Imaging is the most useful diagnostic tool with MRI being the preferred modality because of high sensitivity to identify abscesses and differentiate from necrotizing fasciitis. Disease can occur as single or multiple lesions with the pelvis and lower extremity musculature being the most common locations.

Staphylococcus aureus is the most common pathogen, but polymicrobial and sterile cases are published. Increasing incidence of community-acquired methicillin-resistant *Staphylococcus aureus* is also reported.

Although the left hip could not be completely examined due to pain, the symptoms localize to nonjoint areas of the leg which should raise suspicion for diagnoses independent of hip joint pathology. The presence of high fever, symptom progression, and examination findings suggest a deep-seated infection such as osteomyelitis, pyomyositis, or less likely septic arthritis. Any concern for these entities should encourage testing for bloodstream infection by culture.

Rheumatic disease would not be expected to present so acutely. Transient synovitis of the hip is a consideration; however, the symptoms do not localize to the hip joint, and high fever concurrent with the musculoskeletal symptoms would be inconsistent with transient synovitis, which typically is a postinfectious, reactive process.

Suggested Readings

Chou H, Teo HE, Dubey N, Peh WC. Tropical pyomyositis and necrotizing fasciitis. *Semin Musculoskelet Radiol*. 2011;15(5):489-505.

Christin L, Sarosi GA. Pyomyositis in North America: case reports and review. *Clin Infect Dis*. 1992;15(4):668-677.

Comegna L, Guidone PI, Prezioso G, et al. Pyomyositis is not only a tropical pathology: a case series. *J Med Case Rep*. 2016;10(1):372.

Lemonick DM. Non-tropical pyomyositis caused by methicillin-resistant Staphylococcus aureus: an unusual cause of bilateral leg pain. *J Emerg Med*. 2012;42(3):e55-e62.

Pannaraj PS, Hulten KG, Gonzalez BE, Mason EO Jr, Kaplan SL. Infective pyomyositis and myositis in children in the era of community-acquired, methicillin-resistant *Staphylococcus aureus* infection. *Clin Infect Dis*. 2006;43(8):953-960.

10

"It Hurts to Sit"

Ray Kreienkamp, Jenna N. Diaz

CHIEF COMPLAINT

"It hurts to sit."

HISTORY OF PRESENT ILLNESS

A 14-year-old girl presented to the emergency department with a 7-day history of increasing left gluteal pain. The pain markedly worsened over the prior week, such that the patient could no longer sit or bend over. She denied injury to the area, fever, nausea, vomiting, diarrhea, bloody stools, arthralgia, rashes, skin infections, family history of methicillin-resistant *Staphylococcus aureus* (MRSA) infection, or recent travel. She was noticeably small for her age. Weight: 21.9 kg ($z = -7.66$), height: 139 cm ($z = -3.39$), and body mass index (BMI) ($z = -6.49$). Her father reported she would eat three meals daily but had early satiety, estimating she finished <50% of what was offered to her. She has not gained weight well for the past several years and recently sustained a 20 lb weight loss. The patient and her father reported no problems with food security.

PAST MEDICAL HISTORY

At the age of 10 years, she underwent celiac testing because of poor growth. The tissue transglutaminase (tTG)-IgG was 14 U/mL (normal = <10 U/mL), while the tTG-IgA (<2 U/mL) and total IgA (207 mg/dL) were normal, and endomysial antibody IgA was negative. However, she was started on a gluten-free diet (with which she did not regularly comply) and an "appetite stimulant."

Family/Social History

FH: No systemic lupus erythematosus, celiac disease, inflammatory bowel disease (IBD), rheumatoid arthritis, or other autoimmune disorders. No early-onset malignancy. No known endocrine disorders.

SH: She has not seen a primary care provider for the past 2 years. She lives with father and is entering freshman year of high school.

EXAMINATION

- Vital signs: T 37.1, P 168, RR 36, BP 98/65, Spo2 96%
- General: alert, cooperative, in pain, severely malnourished, appears younger than stated age
- Eyes: conjunctivae clear, PERRL, EOMI
- Oropharynx: MMM, no lesions noted
- Nose: no drainage
- Neck: neck supple and no lymphadenopathy
- Lungs: clear to auscultation, normal work of breathing, and good air movement
- Heart: tachycardic, regular rhythm, normal S1 and S2, no murmur, rubs, or gallops
- Axillae: no axillary lymphadenopathy
- Abdomen: minimal adipose tissue, nontender, nondistended, bowel sounds present, no masses, no organomegaly

- GU: left buttock with a fluctuant, warm area along gluteal fold, 3 × 4 cm in area. There is spontaneously draining purulent material at superior aspect. Sensation intact
- Extremity: extremities warm and well perfused, no edema and no joint tenderness or swelling, no scratches
- Pulses: 2+ radial pulses, symmetric
- Skin: no rash, scattered fine hair, skin grafts on feet
- Neurologic: alert, face symmetric, PERRL, moves all extremities and normal tone

DIAGNOSTIC CONSIDERATIONS

- Crohn disease
- Abscess
- Anorexia
- Celiac disease
- *Helicobacter pylori*
- Malignancy
- Neglect

Investigation

- **Laboratory test results**:
  - CBC: WBC 15.1 K/mm^3, Hgb 8.4 g/dL, Hct 28.1%, Plt 620 K/mm^3, mcv 59.0 fL
  - CMP: Albumin 3.1 g/dL, Alk Phos 107 U/L, ALT <5 U/L, AST 12 U/L
  - ESR: 35 mm/h, CRP: 92.2 mg/L
  - TSH: 4.18 mc IU/mL, fT4 1.22 ng/dL
  - Phosphorus: 3.0 mg/dL
  - IgA 202 mg/dL, tTG-IgA < 0.5 U/mL
  - Iron 8 µg/dL, TIBC 186 µg/dL, transferrin saturation 4%
  - Vitamin D, 25-hydroxy 8 ng/mL
- **Imaging:**
  - Ultrasound of pelvis: Left buttock abscess measuring 3.4 × 3.1 × 3.1 cm^3.

Results

Surgical Procedures

Surgeon note: Under general anesthesia, the left gluteal abscess was incised and drained. A fistula tract was identified and traced from the abscess cavity into the anal canal and rectum, just distal to the dentate line. Approximately 20 mL of pus was drained. The wound was irrigated, and a seton was placed.

Additional Imaging

Magnetic resonance imaging (MRI) abdomen enterography: 10 cm segment of distal ileum and cecum with evidence of inflammation and surrounding phlegmonous change concerning for penetrating disease. Horseshoe-shaped intersphincteric diffusion restricting fluid collection with a left-sided drain in place.

DIAGNOSIS

Crohn disease, with perianal abscess and fistula

Treatment/Follow-up

- Prednisolone 1 mg/kg qD
- Ciprofloxacin 250 mg bid
- Metronidazole 220 mg tid
- Boost/Ensure two to three times per day in addition to meals to improve nutritional status

- Cholecalciferol 2000 IU qD
- Multivitamin with folic acid tablet qD
- Plan to start infliximab once infection/abscess has improved

TEACHING POINTS

Crohn disease is an immune-mediated IBD, notable for its transmural nature of inflammation. This transmural pattern leads to the development of fistulae and abscesses, as in this case, around the anus and in other locations along the gastrointestinal tract. Most patients present with intestinal manifestations, including abdominal pain, diarrhea, weight loss, and/or rectal bleeding.

This patient presented with perianal Crohn disease, which is defined as inflammation at or near the anus and includes tags, fissures, fistulae, abscesses, or stenosis. Patients may present with pain, itching, bleeding, purulent discharge, and/or incontinence of stool. Surgical drainage can be attempted, as in this case, to relieve pressure and pain, followed by antibiotics. Metronidazole has been used effectively but is often associated with high relapse rate after cessation. Metronidazole, ciprofloxacin, or combination are often used to treat patients, though further research is needed, particularly in pediatric patients, to determine the best regimen.

Crohn disease patients are at risk for multiple nutritional deficiencies. Vitamin D deficiency is common and may result in decreased bone density. Anemia is also common, often secondary to iron deficiency. However, in this setting, anemia might reflect chronic disease, with low total iron-binding capacity (TIBC), as in this case. Patients with Crohn disease involving the small bowel, especially those with disease affecting the terminal ileum, should be screened for serum vitamin B12 deficiency.

There are several instructive features of this case. Severe growth changes are becoming rarer as awareness in the community, early referrals, and the ease of colonoscopy have facilitated earlier diagnosis of Crohn disease. Furthermore, this patient's malnutrition was initially misattributed to celiac disease without further testing, thereby delaying the diagnosis of IBD.

Celiac disease is an immune-mediated disorder triggered by gluten and related prolamins in wheat, barley, and rye. Celiac disease testing should be considered in those with gastrointestinal symptoms such as chronic diarrhea, abdominal pain, distension, and/or weight loss without other identifiable cause, as in this case. The best test for celiac disease is tTG-IgA. With IgA deficiency, an IgG-based tTG, anti-endomysial antibody, or deamidated gliadin peptide assay is required to test for celiac disease. However, these tests are not recommended as an initial screening practice in IgA-competent individuals, since an isolated positive IgG-based test with negative IgA-based test in an IgA-competent individual is unlikely to be celiac disease. Abnormalities in these tests merely provide an indication for endoscopy with biopsy to confirm or exclude the diagnosis of celiac disease. In this case, the weight loss thought to be associated with celiac disease was most likely a manifestation of Crohn disease. In fact, there have been reports of positive celiac serologies in patients with poorly treated Crohn disease.

Suggested Readings

de Zoeten EF, Pasternak BA, Mattei P, et al. Diagnosis and treatment of perianal Crohn disease: NASPGHAN clinical report and consensus statement. *J Pediatr Gastroenterol Nutr.* 2013;57:401-412.

Di Tola M, Sabbatella L, Anania MC, et al. Anti-tissue transglutaminase antibodies in inflammatory bowel disease: new evidence. *Clin Chem Lab Med.* 2004;42:1092-1097.

Hill ID, Fasano A, Guandalini S, et al. NASPGHAN clinical report on the diagnosis and treatment of gluten-related disorders. *J Pediatr Gastroenterol Nutr.* 2016;63:156-165.

Husby S, Koletzko S, Korponay-Szabo I, et al. European society paediatric gastroenterology, hepatology and nutrition guidelines for diagnosing coeliac disease 2020. *J Pediatr Gastroenterol Nutr.* 2020;70:141-156.

Nitzan O, Elias M, Peretz A, et al. Role of antibiotics for treatment of inflammatory bowel disease. *World J Gastroenterol.* 2016;22:1078-1087.

Rufo PA, Denson LA, Sylvester FA, et al. Health supervision in the management of children and adolescents with IBD: NASPGHAN recommendations. *J Pediatr Gastroenterol Nutr.* 2012;55:93-108.

11

Gall

Audrey R. Odom John, Andrew J. White

CHIEF COMPLAINT

Itchy rash

HISTORY OF PRESENT ILLNESS

An 8-year-old girl was visiting a cabin in the woods, near a lake 1 hour west of St Louis, Missouri, during the first week of September. She had spent the day in and out of the lake, putting on her bathing suit that had been hung to dry on the back deck of the cabin. In the early evening, she removed her bathing suit and found scattered papules and small vesicles in a "bathing suit" distribution. They were intensely pruritic, highly distressing, and disruptive to her sleep. She had no fever, no rash elsewhere, and felt well.

PAST MEDICAL HISTORY

UTI at 6 weeks of age.

Medications

None.

Family/Social History

She has been sleeping in a cabin with obvious mouse cohabitation and has been hiking in the woods, swimming in a freshwater lake, and has received numerous mosquito bites. She has found some ticks crawling on her, although none were embedded. Two healthy dogs are in the home and accompanied the family to the cabin. Oak leaves are present on the cabin deck. No known exposure to chickenpox or shingles.

EXAMINATION

There are scattered papules over her chest, abdomen, groin, and back (Figure 11.1), sparing her face, neck, and extremities. All lesions were similar in appearance (no "crops of different ages"). Most were erythematous and 2 to 3 mm in diameter, and some lesions were vesicular.

DIAGNOSTIC CONSIDERATIONS

The initial thoughts in this case focused on the following:

1. Varicella in vaccinated child. This was considered unlikely given the simultaneous appearance of all lesions, prior vaccination, relative scarcity of vesicle, and lack of a known exposure.
2. Chigger bites (ie, insect bites from the family Trombiculidae, also known as berry bugs, harvest mites, red mites, and scrub-itch mites). This etiology was consistent with the intensity of pruritus observed in this case, and they may also be vesicular in appearance. However, chigger bites were considered unlikely given the distribution, as chigger dermatitis is most commonly observed on lower extremities where the insects come into contact with a patient who is often walking through tall grass.

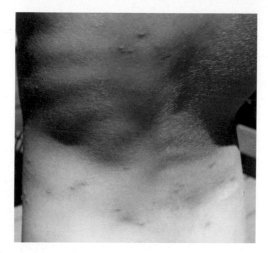

FIGURE 11.1   Rash.

3. Lake itch (also known as swimmer's itch or duck itch). Lake itch is a transient popular pruritus caused by the reaction to invading schistosome cercaria (flatworm larvae), which are present in many lakes in the United States. Humans are dead-end hosts for these zoonotic parasites, which are not to be confused with the causative agents of human schistosomiasis (*Schistosoma mansoni* and *Schistosoma haematobium*). Cercarial dermatitis tends to be widely distributed across water-exposed parts of the body, however, and is not consistent with the bathing suit rash distribution in this case.

However, the blatant bathing suit distribution, the bathing suit drying on the deck, and some additional thinking led to the diagnosis.

Diagnosis

Oak leaf gall mite dermatitis.

Teaching Points

Humans serve as accidental hosts for the tiny (smaller than the naked eye) mites that eat *oak leaf gall wasp midges*.

Gall wasps (of the family **Cynipidae, order Hymenoptera** [of which there are over 1300 species]) lay eggs on tree leaves, and when the eggs hatch, the larvae, called midges, feed upon the leaves. Initially, this causes a brown edge to the leaves but eventually the leaves form "galls" or abnormal growths, as seen in Figure 11.2.

Within these galls, there are numerous baby wasps (midges) and also a *second opportunistic insect*, the oak leaf gall mite **Pyemotes herfsi**, which feed on the wasp midges! (*P. herfsi* inject a potent neurotoxin that paralyzes the midge, allowing the mites to feed on the midges at leisure on their endolymph.)

These mites are very small, easily passing through screens in your window. They can be dispersed by the wind easily, and when they come into contact with humans, they are happy to bite them, causing an intensely pruritic rash. Thus, the ectoparasites are responsible for the human disease, not the gall wasps themselves. Treatment with topical or oral antihistamines is generally sufficient, and eliminating exposure to the mites is highly recommended.

Denouement: On the deck where the bathing suits were drying were numerous oak leaves with rampant gall.

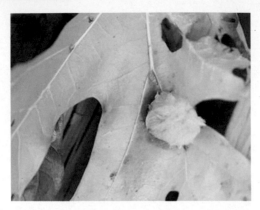

FIGURE 11.2   Oak leaf gall.

Suggested Readings

Broce AB, Zurek L, Kalisch JA, et al. Pyemotes herfsi (Acari: pyemotidae), a mite new to North America as the cause of bite outbreaks. *J Med Entomol*. 2006;43(3):610-613.
Hansen G, Taylor C, Goedeke J, et al. Outbreak of pruritic rashes associated with mites—Kansas, 2004. *MMWR (Morb Mortal Wkly Rep)*. 2005;54(38):952-955.

12

It's in the Genes

Lauren Littell, Grace Ellen Kennedy

CHIEF COMPLAINT

Abdominal pain

HISTORY OF PRESENT ILLNESS

A 13-year-old boy presented to an emergency department (ED) with 2 weeks of epigastric and right upper quadrant (RUQ) abdominal pain. The pain was constant and dull and worsened with movement. He had a few episodes of nonbloody nonbilious emesis. He had also grown weak, was fatigued, had a decreased appetite, and felt warm. He had trouble going up and down stairs and tired quickly when playing basketball.

In the ED his heart rate was 104 beats/min and his respiratory rate was 22 breaths/min. The evaluation there included:

- Epstein-Barr virus (EBV) IgM negative, EBV IgG positive.
- Complete metabolic panel: Protein 5.7 g/dL, **ALT 192 U/L, AST 127 U/L.**
- WBC 11.5 K/mm³, Hgb 12 g/dL.
- **Prothrombin time (PT) and international normalized ratio (INR) were elevated at 20.4 seconds and 1.8, respectively.**
- Viral hepatitis panel negative.
- Complete abdominal ultrasound was normal with the exception of small bilateral pleural effusions.
- A chest x-ray (Figure 12.1) showed mild cardiomegaly.

He was admitted to *the gastroenterology service* for the symptoms of vomiting and abdominal pain and the elevated serum transaminases with a presumed diagnosis of **hepatitis**.

PAST MEDICAL HISTORY

None

Family/Social History

Lives with parents. He had recently returned from a family vacation to Cancun, Mexico.

EXAMINATION

- HR 100 to 110 beats/min.
- General: An alert, but tired-appearing male.
- Eye: Pupils equal, round and reactive to light, no scleral icterus, or conjunctival erythema.
- Lungs: Clear without wheezing, rales, or rhonchi.
- Heart: Regular rate and rhythm, normal S1 and S2. No murmurs, rubs, or gallops. Normal precordium.
- Abdomen: Soft, nondistended. Mild diffuse tenderness to palpation with more severe tenderness in epigastrium and RUQ. Liver edge was 1 inch below the subcostal margin. No splenomegaly.

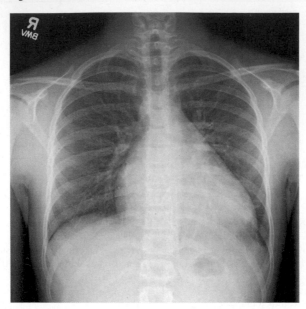

FIGURE 12.1 Chest x-ray.

DIAGNOSTIC CONSIDERATIONS

The combination of cardiomegaly, hepatomegaly, and fatigue with exertion led the admitting residents to consider heart failure as a possible etiology.

Investigation

Repeat laboratory test results showed slightly worsened transaminases but improving synthetic function with a lower INR.

B-type natriuretic peptide (BNP) was elevated at 1388 pg/mL (reference range 0-39 pg/mL).

Cardiology was consulted, and an echocardiogram was performed, which showed a dramatic reduction in biventricular systolic function with a shortening fraction of 7% and an ejection fraction of 19%.

DIAGNOSIS

Dilated cardiomyopathy

Treatment/Follow-up

He was transferred to the cardiac intensive care unit (ICU) and treated with a milrinone infusion and was diagnosed with dilated cardiomyopathy of (initially) unknown etiology.

He did not improve and was placed on the heart transplantation list and did subsequently received a heart transplant.

A chromosomal microarray showed mutations in myosin heavy chain 7 (MYH7) and troponin 13 (TNN13). Testing was then sent on the parents who were both positive for the TNN13 variant, and the mother was positive for the MYH7 variant.

TEACHING POINTS

Heart failure may result from either a structural (usually congenital) or functional (eg, cardiomyopathy) etiology. Congenital cardiac disease is a major cause of heart failure in infants, with an incidence of roughly eight in 1000 live births, 20% of whom develop heart failure. Clinical features of heart failure in infants are nonspecific and include poor feeding or sweating with feeds, respiratory distress, and poor weight gain. Older children may present with features that are similar to the classical adult presentation, such as exercise intolerance, dyspnea at rest, orthopnea, and edema or ascites but may not be recognized initially. While heart failure is a topic which is heavily emphasized at the extremes of age, pediatricians should learn to recognize the presentation in older children too.

Cardiomyopathy is present in about 12% to 15% of children with heart failure, and dilated cardiomyopathy accounts for about 90% of all pediatric cardiomyopathy. According to the Pediatric Cardiomyopathy Registry, in about two-thirds of cases of primary dilated cardiomyopathy, no cause is identified. Of those with a known cause, about half are due to myocarditis, and the remainder are due to neuromuscular diseases, mostly Duchenne and Becker muscular dystrophy, inborn errors of metabolism, or malformation syndromes. Secondary dilated cardiomyopathy, due to drug toxicity or endocrine disorders, may also occur.

Initially billed as a patient with a gastrointestinal illness, the admitting team considered cardiomyopathy based on the physical examination and the chest radiograph. The elevated transaminases were not particularly high, helping the team think outside the box (or outside the liver, as it were).

The existence of two mutations is interesting. The patient's parents were both heterozygous for TNN13 and the patient himself homozygous, which fits with the believed autosomal recessive pattern of inheritance in this form of cardiomyopathy. However, for the MYH7 gene, which is believed to be autosomal dominant, both the patient and his mother carried mutations, but only the patient was symptomatic. It was recommended that the mother be screened herself for cardiomyopathy with an electrocardiogram and echocardiogram.

The 5-year risk of death or cardiac transplantation is 50% for patients with dilated cardiomyopathy, but these percentages vary depending on the underlying cause. The patient in this case presented with risk factors known to have a worse outcome: older age, more advanced congestive cardiac failure, and poor ventricular function. Although heart transplantation was lifesaving for him, it still comes with its own risks and long-term issues.

Suggested Readings

Jayaprasad N. Heart failure in children. *Heart Views*. 2016;17(3):92-99.

OMIM Entry—# 611880—Cardiomyopathy, Dilated, 2A; CMD2A [Internet]. Omim.org; 2008. Accessed January 12, 2020. https://omim.org/entry/611880

OMIM Entry—#160760—Myosin, Heavy Chain 7, Cardiac Muscle, Beta; MYH7 [Internet]. Omim.org; 1986. Accessed January 12, 2020. https://www.omim.org/entry/160760

Rossano JW, Kim JJ, Decker JA, et al. Prevalence, morbidity, and mortality of heart failure-related hospitalizations in children in the United States: a population-based study. *J Card Fail*. 2012;18:459-470.

Taylor M, Carniel E, Mestroni L. Cardiomyopathy, familial dilated. *Orphanet J Rare Dis*. 2006;1(1):27.

Towbin JA, Lowe AM, Colan SD, et al. Incidence, causes, and outcomes of dilated cardiomyopathy in children. *J Am Med Assoc*. 2006;296(15):1867-1876.

13

Ben's Little Secret

Peter Putnam

CHIEF COMPLAINT

A 10-year-old boy "bringing up food" every day since the age of 3 to 4 years.

The mother and father were very good historians although the boy (Ben) provided much of the information himself.

HISTORY OF PRESENT ILLNESS

At 3 to 4 years of age, shortly after the family moved from the Midwest to the west coast (father is an engineer and the family has traveled often), the mother would notice a sour odor on Ben's breath toward the end of the day, which at times was associated with him rechewing food in the back of his mouth. Father admits that he is unaware of the behavior. Ben tells us that at least 20 times a day, he will "do it." He says he gets a "weird" feeling in his stomach, which goes away when he brings up some food or liquid. Sometimes he will swallow this back down immediately, and at other times, he will rechew the food and reswallow. He seldom ejects the food. This behavior seems not to cause him any discomfort.

He says that processed food such as hot dogs and school lunches, in contrast to food prepared by his mom, seem to make the problem worse. He also reports that milk products seem to make it worse. He has drunk "sweet acidophilus milk" for 3 years but with no change in his symptoms. I asked him if schoolmates have smelled vomit smell from him and moved their seats away from him. He said no, but mother says that she has smelled that odor.

This activity seems a part of his life, and he does not seem to be affected much by it. It does not interrupt his classes or social life because his friends and teachers do not know about it, as he is discrete about the activity. He does not complain of pain or burning sensation in his chest or epigastrium. He has never had fevers, dysphagia, or other symptoms of esophagitis. He also follows up regularly every 6 months with a dentist who has noted many problems. He does have a few fillings in his molars.

Mother is observant and is accepting of Ben's habit but has worried about the possibility of a price in the future and has encouraged him to try to reduce the frequency. She continues to note the foul smell on his breath toward the end of the day. She has suggested to him in the past that he try to inhibit the regurgitation every other time he has the urge to regurgitate. This has not seemed to decrease the habit because Ben fears that if he suppresses regurgitation, the funny feeling that he has in his stomach will last longer or get worse.

PAST MEDICAL HISTORY

He was a full-term baby who had no problems during infancy. He was breastfed for the first 6 months of life and then changed to formula and has eaten a balanced regular diet since that time. During the first 3 years of life, he had no problems with vomiting, diarrhea, constipation, or growth. He has always grown along the 50th percentile for height and weight.

DEVELOPMENTAL HISTORY

Ben has always done well in school. When talking with him and examining him today, he is a very bright boy for his age. He is very observant and verbalized his own thoughts, ideas, and questions about the discussion that went on about his habit. He, as his parents, did not seem overly concerned about the habit and seemed very well adjusted and a kid who enjoys many things in his life.

Family/Social History

He is in the fourth grade and participates in basketball and is active in other sports.

The family lives on a 30-acre plot of land. Ben is the older child and lives with his mother and dad and a six-year-old sister—all are well. Father is an engineer supervising oil drilling teams. It is work that he finds satisfying and provides them the financial security to allow them to live where they prefer, currently back here in the Midwest. He is away for 1 month and then at home for 1 month. Mother is at home.

EXAMINATION

- Vitals: Height 140.3 cm, weight 30 kg, both at the 50th percentile for his age
- General appearance: Well-grown, was quite talkative and observant for this age
- HEENT: Normal
- Oropharynx: Normal with no sores and the back of his teeth appeared normal (no pitting)
- Lungs: Clear bilaterally
- Heart: Regular rate and rhythm, normal S1/S2 without murmur or gallop
- Abdomen: Normal without masses or hepatosplenomegaly and without tenderness
- Extremity: Within normal limits
- Neurologic: Within normal limits

I thought I might have detected a hint of pride or bemusement in his voice and face when he was "center stage." He asserted himself in the interview, without me actually directing questions to him specifically; he answered most of them without looking at either parent, only at me. A distinctive behavior in a setting which is intimidating to many children his age. He projects self-confidence, a style which may reflect his intelligence and his father's frequent absence.

DIAGNOSTIC CONSIDERATIONS

- GERD
- Stimulus deprivation
- Self-stimulatory activity
- A "compensatory" behavior in response to a restrictive diet
- Propionic acidemia
- Achalasia

Investigation

Serum propionic acid, ammonia, and antigluten antibodies—all normal.

An upper GI was obtained and was interpreted as normal.

DIAGNOSIS

Rumination, benign

Treatment/Follow-up

1. Reassurance: Since children who ruminate may be teased by their peers about odor, we encouraged him that he should try to suppress it more and more. When asked, he says that if he tries to hold the food down, the funny feeling in his stomach continues and sometimes gets "worse." I encouraged him that that feeling would pass without bringing up food if he would take a series of deep breaths and relax his belly muscles.
2. Contingency: I told him and his parents that if his rumination continues, or if other symptoms appear, reassessment including upper endoscopy, manometry, biofeedback therapy, and/or behavioral modification should be considered.

TEACHING POINTS

With normal physical and psychological development, it is most likely that this rumination is a benign habit/behavior rather than a symptom of an underlying disease.

This case illustrates important lessons Dr Keating taught me relevant to my practice in general pediatrics. First, behavioral and social issues can mimic pathophysiology, and a careful, thorough history can uncover these diagnostic possibilities. Second, like a detective, Dr Keating's observations of the boy's behavior, not just his answers to Dr Keating's questions, helped "solve the case." Finally, though this case ended with a specific diagnosis, many patients who saw Dr Keating never received a diagnostic "answer." Often the physician's job is to identify normal and benign conditions and provide reassurance to patients and families, protecting children from the risk of further evaluation.

Suggested Readings

Amarnath RP, Abell TL, Malagelada JR. The rumination syndrome in adults. A characteristic manometric pattern. *Ann Intern Med.* 1986;105:513-518.

Alexander RC, Greenswag LR, Nowak AJ. Rumination and vomiting in Prader-Willi syndrome. *Am J Med Genet.* 1987;28:889-895.

Hillman RE, Keating JP, Williams JC. Biotin-responsive propionic acidemia presenting as the rumination syndrome. *J Pediatr.* 1978;92:439-441.

Levine DF, Wingate DL, Pfeffer JM, Butcher P. Habitual rumination: a benign disorder. *Br Med J (Clin Res Ed).* 1983;287:255-256.

Mackalski BA, Keate RF. Rumination in a patient with achalasia. *Am J Gastroenterol.* 1993;88:1803-1804.

Menking M, Wagnitz JG, Burton JJ, Coddington RD, Sotos JF. Rumination—a near fatal psychiatric disease of infancy. *N Eng J Med.* 1969;280:802-804.

Shay S, Johnson LF, Wong RK, et al. Rumination, heartburn, and daytime gastroesophageal reflux. A case study with mechanisms defined and successfully treated with biofeedback therapy. *J Clin Gastroenterol.* 1986;8:115-126.

14 Tales of Great Ulysses

Adam Eaton

CHIEF COMPLAINT

Seizure

HISTORY OF PRESENT ILLNESS

This 20-month-old boy has had seizures from DOL #1. On the day of admission, his eyes rolled up in his head and he was unaware of his surroundings briefly. Earlier imaging studies were interpreted as multicystic encephalomalacia, for which there was no known cause. From early on until the day of admission, he was treated with phenobarbital 3 mL bid (3 mg/kg/d). Today, he was assessed in a local emergency department (ED), and the seizures were stopped, but he was referred for a resulting abnormal laboratory test of concern.

PAST MEDICAL HISTORY

Laboratory results from the ED at the referring hospital

- Hgb 15.3
- WBC 16
- MCV 81
- Plt 550k
- Glucose 71
- BUN 10
- ALT 23
- AST 24
- **Alkaline phosphatase 4892 IU/L** (110-302)
- Alb 4.5
- Na 138
- K 4.9
- CO_2 22
- Ca 10.5

Family/Social History

Diet: Mixed diet including cow's milk with 400 U vitamin D/L. No one else with seizures.

EXAMINATION

- Weight 25%, Length 50%, OFC 25%.
- No pallor, jaundice, or cyanosis.
- No swollen wrists, bowed or knock-knees, no rachitic rosary, no frontal bossing, no abdominal mass. No dysmorphic features.

The serum enzymes were not ordered individually or specifically but came as part of a panel, in this case called a comprehensive metabolic panel (CMP). The primary goal of management in the ED was to improve seizure control which was achieved and accomplished by increasing the dose of phenobarbital.

The remaining problem was the markedly elevated alkaline phosphatase.

DIAGNOSTIC CONSIDERATIONS

- Occult tumor
- Rickets or another skeletal disease
- Obstruction of the biliary tree

Investigation

No additional studies were done at the time of admission.

DIAGNOSIS

The diagnosis of **transient hyperalkaline phosphatasemia** was entered, and the child was discharged home.

TREATMENT/FOLLOW-UP

The repeat serum alkaline phosphatase measured a month later was normal at **294 IU/L.**

FINAL DIAGNOSIS

Transient hyperphosphatasemia of infancy (THI), an insufficiently recognized and benign syndrome.

TEACHING POINTS

Transient hyperphosphatasemia has been described in more than 180 cases since 1980. This self-limited and benign condition has been called "**Ulysses syndrome**" because of the long, wandering, and sometimes dangerous searches for an underlying pathologic process that might explain the laboratory test. The elevations are often higher than those seen in pathologic processes which are associated with hyperphosphatasemia: biliary disease or rickets seldom give alkaline phosphatase above 3000, usually 600 to 1800. Children with THI are often 1500 to 12,000 IU/L.

The cause of THI remains uncertain. Isozyme studies show both liver- and bone-derived enzyme. It appears that the high serum level is due to delayed degradation of an abnormal (extrasialic acid) molecule rather than increased release of enzyme from tissue.

The level is usually back to normal within a month, but occasionally it increases before dropping to normal. It is often discovered when a panel is performed. The child usually has some unrelated disease process (commonly diarrhea), which led to the testing.

When a very high value for alkaline phosphatase is reported, usually you can suspect the nature of this benign problem immediately and reassure the parent and repeat the test in a month, rather than embark on the **Argo.**

Final Point

This case has always been interesting to me—not necessarily because of the elevation of alkaline phosphatase but because the nature of the case reminds us of the concept of pretest probability and its relation to the utility of a laboratory test. Perhaps the 1990s and 2000s were a time when laboratory "panels" were becoming commonplace, and now they are the norm. This increases the likelihood of any of us being distracted by an abnormal value. Pursuing additional testing or medical care can be expensive and meaningless to the patient, or worse, dangerous.

Additionally, the current state of medical care gives new meaning to this case. Follow-up testing was not pursued during the admission; instead, the alkaline phosphatase was repeated months later and was normal. This required coordination of effort between the hospital and the patient's primary doctor, to ensure the test was ordered, and to avoid additional or extra blood tests. As we have migrated toward hospitalist care and greater separation of inpatient and outpatient medicine, it may be tempting, but often unnecessary, to pursue additional workup while the patient is hospitalized. During this evolution of health care, we are all responsible for maintaining routines of appropriate physician to physician handoff, especially in these cases where time and appropriate follow-up may serve the patient better than additional testing.

Suggested Readings

Cohen MM, Baum BJ. Studies in Stomatology and Craniofacial Biology. IOS Press; 1996:245-273.

Crofton PM. What is the cause of benign transient hyperphosphatasemia. A study of 35 cases. *Clin Chem*. 1988;34:335-340.

Kraut JR, Merick M, Maxwell NR, Kaplan MM. Isoenzyme studies in transient hyperphosphatasemia of infancy. *Am J Dis Child*. 1985;139:736-740.

Kraut JR, Shah B. Simultaneous transient hyperphosphatasemia in a set of twins. *Am J Dis Child*. 1989;143:881-882.

Kruse K, Kurz N. Further evidence for infectious origin of isolated transient hyperphosphatasemia. *Eur J Pediatr*. 1989;148:453-454.

Oggero R, Mostert M, Spinello M, Iavarone A, Buffa J. Transient hyperphosphatasemia of infancy. Fifteen new cases. *Acta Paediatr Scand*. 1988;77(2):257-259.

Posen S, Lee C, Vines R, Kilham H, Latham S, Keefe JF. Transient hyperphosphatasemia of infancy—an insufficiently recognized syndrome. *Clin Chem*. 1977;23:292-294.

Rosalki SB, Foo AY. More on transient hyperphosphatasemia of infancy. *Clin Chem*. 1983;29:723.

Schmidt DE, Rosenblum JL, Rothbaum RJ, Keating JP. Transient isolated hyperphosphatasemia: a variant of the Ulysses syndrome. *Pediatr Res*. 1985;19:365-368.

Candy

Julianne Ivy

CHIEF COMPLAINT

Dark pee

HISTORY OF PRESENT ILLNESS

A 12-year-old boy was admitted for abdominal pain and dark urine. Three days prior to admission, he ate two or three mothballs because he "thought that they were candy." That night, he began having mild, watery diarrhea, and the next day he started experiencing waves of moderate right and left upper quadrant abdominal pain. Over the next 2 days, the abdominal pain became much more severe, he had two episodes of nonbloody, nonbilious emesis, and his urine turned reddish-brown. Primarily out of concern for the discolored urine, his mom took him to an outside emergency department (ED).

In the ED, he was jaundiced but was not in distress. On examination, he had moderate abdominal tenderness, particularly in the right upper quadrant. Laboratory results were notable for a hemoglobin of 11.3 g/dL, total bilirubin of 14.1 mg/dL with a direct component of 0.3 mg/dL, and normal transaminases and alkaline phosphatase. The urinalysis showed amber-colored urine, with no blood and no bilirubin. A methemoglobin level was 4.2%.

The patient was directly admitted as a transfer from the outside ED.

PAST MEDICAL HISTORY

He denied any past medical illnesses or hospitalizations.

Medications

None

Family/Social History

There are no family members with significant medical history. Patient and family moved from out of state a few months ago.

EXAMINATION

- Vitals: T-37.1, HR-104, RR-22
- General: Alert, well-appearing, conversational, in no acute distress
- Abdomen: Soft; nondistended; diffuse moderate tenderness to palpation, particularly in the right upper quadrant; no palpable masses or organomegaly
- Skin: Diffuse jaundice

DIAGNOSTIC CONSIDERATIONS

- Methemoglobinemia
- Hemolytic anemia
- Acute liver failure, idiopathic
- Acute viral hepatitis

Investigation and Results

Poison control was contacted, and they did not think that the patient's presentation was consistent with mothball-induced methemoglobinemia because his methemoglobin level was well below the treatment threshold of 20%. They did suggest that hemolytic anemia can be seen occasionally after mothball ingestion but only in patients with glucose-6-phosphate dehydrogenase (G6PD) deficiency. Additionally, the patient's hemoglobin in the ED was higher than would be expected in a true hemolytic crisis.

The patient's mother then arrived to the admitting hospital. On interview, she recalled that the patient had been admitted about 10 years ago to an out-of-state hospital. She could not remember any of the details of the admission except that "they gave him blood." Those records were obtained after some paperwork and faxing and showed that the patient had in fact been previously diagnosed with G6PD deficiency at the age of 21 months, after presenting in an acute hemolytic crisis precipitated by a viral upper respiratory infection. The family was completely unaware of this diagnosis.

Repeat laboratory tests obtained after admission showed a 2.4 g/dL drop in hemoglobin in the span of 6 hours. Lactic acid dehydrogenase (LDH) was 363 U/L.

DIAGNOSIS

* Hemolytic anemia, acute
* Naphthalene ingestion
* G6PD Deficiency

Treatment/Follow-up

He continued to have active hemolysis for the next 5 days. His lowest hemoglobin was 5.5 g/dL. He was given a total of four units of packed red blood cells during his hospital course. After nearly a week, the hemolysis ended, and he was discharged home in good condition. His family was taught about G6PD deficiency, and close follow-up was arranged with hematology and his primary care pediatrician.

TEACHING POINTS

G6PD is an enzyme involved in protecting cells, particularly red blood cells, against oxidative stress. Under normal circumstances, most G6PD-deficient individuals still have enough of this enzyme to prevent oxidants from accumulating to toxic levels. However, certain triggers, including some infections and medications, fava beans, and naphthalene in mothballs, are known to cause more oxidative stress than G6PD-deficient cells can handle. When these triggers are present, red blood cells rapidly hemolyze, and patients begin to show symptoms such as back or abdominal pain, jaundice, and dark urine. Laboratory tests reveal anemia with a high reticulocyte count, indirect hyperbilirubinemia, and elevated LDH.

The treatment for these acute episodes of hemolysis is primarily symptom based. Analgesics are given for pain. Red blood cells are transfused to preserve oxygen-carrying capacity. Hyperhydration may be used to prevent heme-induced acute kidney injury, and dialysis may be performed if the kidney injury becomes too severe. Once the hemolysis runs its course, patients typically recover well.

In the United States, the diagnosis of G6PD deficiency is often made only after a patient undergoes their first hemolytic crisis. However, it is possible that if patients were screened ahead of time, some of this morbidity could be prevented. Children and adults who know they have G6PD deficiency should be able to avoid many of the triggers of hemolytic crises, including known oxidative medications, fava beans, and, of course, mothballs. One study in Sardinia found that a robust program of education, newborn screening, and screening of anyone admitted to the hospital led to a 75% decrease in the incidence of favism, ie, hemolytic crises precipitated by fava bean ingestion.

In the United States, currently, Washington, DC and Pennsylvania are the only two regions that include G6PD on their newborn screen. The American Academy of Pediatrics recommends testing for G6PD only in neonates who require phototherapy and (1) are responding poorly to the phototherapy or (2) have a family history or ethnicity that places them at higher risk of G6PD deficiency. The World Health Organization guidelines, on the other hand, recommend screening in all populations where the prevalence is higher than 3% to 5% of males, which would include the United States' African-American population. As it stands, the debate on G6PD screening is still ongoing, and whether more states will expand their screening policies remains to be seen.

Suggested Readings

American Academy of Pediatrics Subcommittee on Hyperbilirubinemia. Management of hyperbilirubinemia in the newborn infant 35 or more weeks of gestation. *Pediatrics.* 2004;114(1):297-316.

Cappellini MD, Fiorelli G. Glucose-6-phosphate dehydrogenase deficiency. *Lancet.* 2008;371(9606):64-74.

Glucose-6-phosphate dehydrogenase deficiency. WHO Working Group. *Bull World Health Organ.* 1989;67(6):601-611.

Meloni T, Forteleoni G, Meloni GF. Marked decline of favism after neonatal glucose-6-phosphate dehydrogenase screening and health education: the northern Sardinian experience. *Acta Haematol.* 1992;87(1-2):29-31.

Watchko JF, Kaplan M, Stark AR, Stevenson DK, Bhutani VK. Should we screen newborns for glucose-6-phosphate dehydrogenase deficiency in the United States? *J Perinatol.* 2013;33(7):499-504.

16 One or the Other—Maybe Both

Caroline Noel

CHIEF COMPLAINT

"I had a seizure"

HISTORY OF PRESENT ILLNESS

A 16-year-old girl presented with two episodes of word-finding difficulty and a seizure. A week prior to presentation, she was working on a school paper and had a 10-minute long time period where she could not formulate words to write her paper. The day of presentation, she was speaking with a friend when she could not come up with words to use in midconversation. Later that day at school, she fell to the floor while walking and had a generalized tonic-clonic seizure that lasted 45 seconds. She was witnessed by several students to have full body shaking without any urinary or bowel incontinence. The seizure resolved without any medications, and she returned to her ordinary mental status 20 minutes later. She did seem to lose consciousness and had no recollection of the event. She did not have any other symptoms or recent illness.

PAST MEDICAL HISTORY

None

Family/Social History

No one in family has seizures or malignancy.

She was born and raised in Illinois. She had no pets or animal exposures. No tuberculosis (TB) exposures. She had visited India in early childhood, and her last visit to India was 2 years ago. She is a vegetarian with no recent meat consumption. No cave or construction exposure. No freshwater swimming. No alcohol, tobacco, or drug use.

EXAMINATION

- General: Alert and oriented, well appearing
- Head: Normocephalic, atraumatic
- Eyes: PERRL, EOMI, no injection
- Oropharynx: Clear with moist mucous membranes
- CV: Regular rate and rhythm with no murmur
- Lungs: Clear to auscultation bilaterally
- Abdomen: Soft, nondistended, nontender
- Skin: No rashes, ecchymosis
- Neuro: CN II-XII intact. 5/5 strength in upper and lower extremities. Gross sensation intact throughout. Normal gait. Normal coordination with finger to nose. Negative Babinski. Reflexes 2+ throughout

Initial Evaluation

- Head CT revealed small ring-enhancing lesions without calcification. No mass effect.
- Brain MRI revealed two well-defined rim-enhancing lesions (largest 1.3 × 0.8 cm) in the parietal lobe with perilesional vasogenic edema.

DIAGNOSTIC CONSIDERATIONS

- The leading diagnostic considerations for ring-enhancing lesions in the brain are infectious, such as neurocysticercosis, tuberculosis, fungal infections, or TORCH infections. Other causes might include inflammatory etiologies such as CNS vasculitis, CNS lymphoma, or a primary brain tumor.
- Neurocysticercosis commonly presents with a solitary intracranial lesion and new onset seizures; however, it is not endemic to the United States. CNS tuberculosis was thought less likely in this case given her lack of risk factors, although the remote history of travel to India kept this possibility on the list. Tuberculomas are usually larger in size, multiple, and posterior and are typically accompanied by infection elsewhere. A primary CNS lymphoma was less likely given her normal immune system.
- Imaging studies alone are generally suggestive of, but not purely diagnostic for, neurocysticercosis. While CT may detect calcifications or parenchymal cysticerci, MRI is more useful for detecting scolices, identifying edema, or degeneration of a cyst.
- A scolex was not visualized in this case, but the amount of edema was disproportionate to the lesion, which heightened the suspicion for neurocysticercosis.

Results

- CBC, CRP, and ESR normal.
- CXR and echocardiogram normal.
- CT chest/abdomen/pelvis to assess for other focuses of disease and lymphadenopathy consistent with lymphoma or TB was negative.
- Histoplasmosis serologies, blastomyces, cryptococcal Ag, galactomannan, toxoplasma, HIV, stool ova and parasite × 3, and blood culture all negative.
- CSF studies: Normal protein, glucose, gram stain. Anaerobic, aerobic, fungal cultures negative. AFB stain negative. Cryptococcal Ag negative.

Investigation

Infectious Disease, Neurology, Neurosurgery, and Oncology were consulted and concluded that a brain biopsy would best help to differentiate between possible diagnoses. Ophthalmology was consulted, and their examination showed no evidence of intraocular cysticercosis.

The patient's tuberculin skin test was positive with induration of 10 mm at 48 hours. An interferon gamma release assay (IGRA), however, was negative. She was diagnosed with latent TB.

While waiting for biopsy and serological test results, she began treatment for both neurocysticercosis and latent TB. The serum enzyme-linked immuno sorbent assay (ELISA) returned positive for detection of cysticercosis IgG.

DIAGNOSIS

1. **Neurocysticercosis**
2. **Tuberculosis**, latent

Treatment/Follow-up

Treatment

- Dexamethasone taper
- Albendazole × 14 days
- Keppra for a 6-month course
- Isoniazid and pyridoxine therapy × 9 months for latent TB infection

Follow-up

- Brain biopsy showed focal inflammation and necrotic debris of the cortex and a fibrous nodule containing granulomatous elements, suggesting a remote, resolving infection. There was no definitive evidence of infection or neoplasm.

- An MRI performed several months after completion of albendazole therapy showed decreasing size of lesions and resolution of edema.

TEACHING POINTS

- There is a set of absolute, major, minor, and epidemiological diagnostic criteria to determine the degree of certainty for diagnosing neurocysticercosis. These criteria are based on neuroimaging findings, clinical manifestations, epidemiological exposure, and exclusion of other etiologies.
- Negative serology results do not exclude neurocysticercosis as a diagnosis when clinical and radiology findings are consistent with disease. While serology is recommended, remember that serological testing may be negative in disease that involves a single cyst or only very few cysticerci.
- Seizures are one of the most common clinical presentations for intraparenchymal cysticerci. In extraparenchymal disease, patients are more likely to present with signs of increased intracranial pressure, headaches, nausea, vomiting, or focal neuro deficits.
- It is a misconception that neurocysticercosis disease must be acquired by eating undercooked, contaminated pork. Humans typically become *Taenia solium* tapeworm carriers by ingesting undercooked pork containing cysticerci. However, cysticercosis may occur after the ingestion of eggs shed in the feces of a human *T. solium* carrier. Therefore, transmission may include person-to-person contact with an asymptomatic carrier, autoinfection, or through contaminated food.
- Treatment consists of antihelminthic therapy and coadministration of corticosteroids. As cysts are killed by the antihelminthic therapy, an inflammatory response may increase risk for seizures and prevent lesion resolution. Corticosteroids that cross the blood-brain barrier (ie, dexamethasone) can regulate brain inflammation and its effects. Antiepileptic drugs are recommended in patients with seizures, although there is no clear recommendation for duration of antiepileptic therapy.

Suggested Readings

Bueno EC, Snege M, Vaz AJ, et al. Serodiagnosis of human cysticercosis by using antigens from vesicular fluid of *Taenia crassiceps* cysticerci. *Clin Diagn Lab Immunol.* 2001;8:1140-1144.

Cantey PT, Coyle CM, Sorvillo FJ, et al. Neglected parasitic infections in the United States: cysticercosis. *Am J Trop Med Hyg.* 2014;90:805-809.

Del Brutto OH, Nash TE, White AC, et al. Revised diagnostic criteria for neurocysticercosis. *J Neurol Sci.* 2017;372:202-210.

Gabriël S, Blocher J, Dorny P, et al. Added value of antigen ELISA in the diagnosis of neurocysticercosis in resource poor settings. *PLoS Negl Trop Dis.* 2012;6(10):e1851.

Schantz PM, Moore AC, Muñoz JL, et al. Neurocysticercosis in an Orthodox Jewish community in New York City. *N Engl J Med.* 1992;327:692-695.

White AC Jr, Coyle CM, Rajshekhar V, et al. Diagnosis and treatment of neurocysticercosis: 2017 clinical practice guidelines by the Infectious Diseases Society of America (IDSA) and the American Society of Tropical Medicine and Hygiene (ASTMII). *Clin Infect Dis.* 2018;66(8):e49-e75.

Zhao BC, Jiang HY, Ma WY, et al. Albendazole and corticosteroids for the treatment of solitary cysticercus tranuloma: a network meta-analysis. *PLoS Negl Trop Dis.* 2016;10:e0004418.

17

Chigger Bites

Kylie M. Bushroe

CHIEF COMPLAINT

A 13-year-old girl with high-risk pre-B cell acute lymphoblastic leukemia (ALL), currently on maintenance chemotherapy, presents with 10 days of right thigh pain.

HISTORY OF PRESENT ILLNESS

She mentioned the leg pain during an appointment in the oncology clinic where a lower extremity x-ray was negative for fracture and laboratory results included a stable mild neutropenia (ANC 1360). She was reassured with recommendations for continued over-the-counter pain management. But the pain persisted and worsened the day prior to admission. She presented to the emergency room with difficulty bearing weight on her right leg, as well as worsening pain which she now rated 10/10 in severity. Her examination was notable only for chigger bites which have been present for a week on the right lower leg. She reports that they initially appeared on the right foot after a visit to grandma's 2 weeks ago. She felt warm the last few days.

PAST MEDICAL HISTORY

Pre-B cell ALL diagnosed 2 years ago. Admitted 4 months ago for fever and neutropenia; diagnosed with left lower lobe pneumonia; treated with 10 days of IV antibiotics.

Medications

Oxycodone 5 mg every 4 hours as needed; mercaptopurine/methotrexate for chemotherapy at home.

Family/Social History

She lives at home with parents and one sister and is currently in the eighth grade. She does have recent exposures to dogs, hamsters, and parakeets. She does not recall a specific cat exposure, but she does like cats. Visited grandma 2 weeks ago, where she played outside and wore sandals in tall grass. After additional discussions with the primary and infectious disease teams, dad recalls that grandma had called sometime after the visit to report that she had just been diagnosed with shingles. Mother has anxiety and depression. Maternal grandmother has history of ovarian cancer.

EXAMINATION

- Vital Signs: T 38.4 °C, HR 105, RR 22, BP 91/57, Spo$_2$ 99%
- General: Alert, well-appearing
- Head: Normocephalic, atraumatic
- Eye: Conjunctivae clear, extraocular movements intact
- Nose: No drainage
- Oropharynx: Mucous membranes moist
- Chest: Central venous catheter intact, dry, and clean
- Lungs: Clear to auscultation bilaterally, normal work of breathing, and appropriate air movement bilaterally

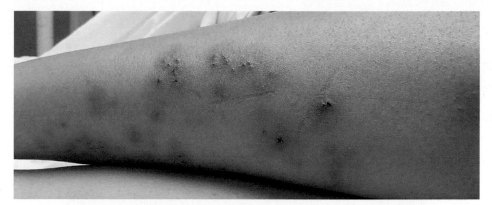

FIGURE 17.1 Photograph of the rash.

- Heart: Regular rate and rhythm, normal S1 and S2, no murmur, rubs, or gallops
- Abdomen: Soft, nontender, nondistended, bowel sounds present
- Extremity: Right lateral thigh pain worse with passive and active movement of right foot, knee, and hip; tenderness to palpation along right lateral thigh and hip with no obvious joint or extremity swelling, redness, or warmth
- Skin: Numerous small papules on right leg with mild surrounding erythema, some scabbed and a few with central eschar with no streaking or discharge; two pinpoint lesions on dorsum of left foot; one lesion on abdomen, few on lateral neck, two in scalp, and one lesion on left jaw (Figure 17.1)
- Neurologic: Alert, face symmetric, pupils equal, round and reactive to light, and moves all extremities

DIAGNOSTIC CONSIDERATIONS

Initial thoughts were focused on osteomyelitis, osteonecrosis, and recurrent malignancy. Cefepime was initiated, and her pain was treated with IV morphine. Vancomycin was added the next day. Clinical improvement was not seen on antibiotic therapy alone, and differential diagnosis is broadened to include viral and fungal etiologies. The additional history about grandma added varicella-zoster virus (VZV) to the differential. In addition, herpes simplex virus and disseminated fungal infections, such as aspergillosis, cryptococcosis, blastomycosis, and histoplasmosis, were considered, but thought less likely without more systemic symptoms.

Investigation

1. Repeat complete blood count and comprehensive metabolic panel were at baseline.
2. Daily blood cultures were negative.
3. An MRI of right hip, thigh, and knee was unremarkable.
4. An MRI of spine was obtained to exclude spinal metastases as source of pain.
5. Serum infectious testing was completed.
6. Open vesicles were swabbed and biopsied.

Results

1. Total spine MRI with and without contrast (Figure 17.2): Normal MRI of the total spine. Multiple bilateral areas of nodular pulmonary consolidation are incompletely evaluated. Findings are concerning for multifocal pneumonia in this immunocompromised patient. Chest CT is recommended.
2. Chest CT with contrast (Figure 17.3): Numerous bilateral pulmonary nodules, predominately in a peripheral distribution, surrounded by ground-glass opacity. Findings are concerning for multifocal fungal pneumonia.

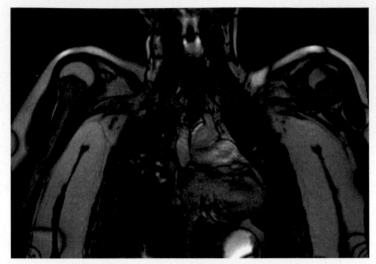

FIGURE 17.2 Magnetic resonance imagae (MRI) of spine detected pulmonary infiltrates.

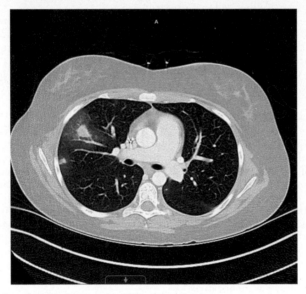

FIGURE 17.3 Computed tomography (CT) of the chest.

3. Serum testing.
   a. *Aspergillus* galactomannan antigen: Negative
   b. Enterovirus PCR: Negative
   c. Herpes simplex virus PCR: Negative
   d. VZV PCR: *Positive*
4. Vesicle testing
   a. Aerobic culture and Gram stain: Negative
   b. Mycobacteriology AFB culture and acid-fast stain: Negative
   c. Mycology culture and stain: Negative
   d. VZV PCR: *Positive*
5. Surgical pathology
   a. Punch biopsy of skin of right lower leg: *VZV infection*

Diagnosis

Disseminated varicella infection

Treatment/Follow-up

Acyclovir was started and continued once diagnosis was confirmed by PCR. IV acyclovir was changed to oral valacyclovir once she was clinically improving, for a total 10-day course of antiviral therapy. At clinical follow-up 2 weeks later, the lesions had crusted over and the pain had completely resolved.

Teaching Points

VZV may disseminate hematogenously to cause VZV pneumonia. Over 90% of varicella-zoster pneumonia is diagnosed in adults, patients with lymphoma, or those that are immunocompromised. Mortality rate can be as high as 20%. Generally lesions appear for 7 to 14 days with an average of 6 days before onset of pneumonia. Symptoms can include fever, cough, dyspnea, tachypnea, and chest pain. Risk of pneumonia development is related to absolute neutrophil count at time of infection. Histologic features involve interstitial mononuclear inflammatory infiltrate with protein exudate. Chest CT is generally significant for small nodules with surrounding ground-glass opacities.

   Introduction of the vaccine for varicella in the United States reduced the incidence of infection by 90%, mortality from varicella by 66%, and the rate of hospitalization for the virus by 80%. In 2006, the Centers for Disease Control and Prevention (CDC) expanded the recommendation to include a second dose of the vaccine to patients between 4 to 6 years of age and at least 3 months from the initial dose. This improved effectiveness to over 95%. Breakthrough infections, despite proper immunization, are more common in immunocompromised patients and generally result within 5 years of vaccination. In addition to pneumonia, complications from breakthrough varicella can include meningitis, encephalitis, keratitis, conjunctivitis, hepatomegaly, hepatitis, and sepsis.

   Treatment includes IV acyclovir 10 mg/kg/dose for 10 days. Studies have shown that anti-VZV hyperimmune immunoglobulin (VZV-Ig) and acyclovir have similar efficacy, though VZV-Ig can be both expensive and difficult to obtain. There is minimal risk of viral spread once the cutaneous lesions have crusted.

Suggested Readings

Bozzo J, Jorquera JI. Use of human immunoglobulins as an anti-infective treatment: the experience so far and their possible re-emerging role. *Expert Rev Anti Infect Ther.* 2017;15(6):585-604.
Feldman S. Varicella-zoster virus pneumonitis. *Chest.* 1994;106:22S-27S.
Kim JS, Ryu CW, Lee SI, Sung DW, Park CK. High-resolution CT findings of varicella-zoster pneumonia. *Am J Roentgenol.* 1999;72:113-116.
Leung J, Broder KR, Marin M. Severe varicella in persons vaccinated with varicella vaccine (breakthrough varicella): a systematic literature review. *Expert Rev Vaccines.* 2017;16(4):391-400.
Mangioni D, Grasselli G, Abbruzzese C, Muscatello A, Gori A, Bandera A. Adjuvant treatment of severe varicella pneumonia with IV varicella zoster virus-specific immunoglobulins. *Int J Infect Dis.* 2019;85:70-73.
Mirouse A, Vignon P, Piron P, et al. Severe varicella-zoster virus pneumonia: a multicenter cohort study. *Crit Care.* 2017;21:137.
Shapiro ED, Vazquez M, Esposito D, et al. Effectiveness of 2 doses of varicella vaccine in children. *J Infect Dis.* 2011;203:312-315.

18

A Fever a Day

Brian D. Reinholz

CHIEF COMPLAINT

Fever

HISTORY OF PRESENT ILLNESS

A 7-year-old girl presented with 3 months of low-grade fevers with intermittent spikes. At first, they occurred every 3 to 4 days and ranged between 100 °F and 102 °F. She initially experienced some watery, nonbloody diarrhea that resolved after a few days. She was seen by her pediatrician and diagnosed with *Mycoplasma pneumoniae* after a swab was sent and returned positive. She was treated with a course of azithromycin.

Despite the antibiotics, the fevers persisted. One month prior to admission, they became progressively more frequent, more predictable, and followed a routine. They occurred every night between 5 and 6 PM and ranged between 101 °F and 104 °F. Her parents would treat with acetaminophen or ibuprofen which seemed to curb the fevers enough so that by bedtime she was able to sleep. If they did not give her medication, she would have night sweats and was unable to sleep. When the fevers were present, she would become fatigued, developed a headache, and had an occasional rash on the inner portion of her left knee.

She was evaluated by rheumatology and had a number of tests obtained, including an elevated CRP and ESR, an indeterminate quantiFERON Gold, a mild normocytic anemia, a normal CMP, normal stool culture and O/P, and a negative ANA and RF.

She was admitted for more evaluation, although at the time of admission she was asymptomatic with no cough, vomiting, recent diarrhea, or abdominal pain, no rash, arthralgias, or myalgias. She had no sick contacts, travel, or animal exposures. She had not gained any weight over the last year.

PAST MEDICAL HISTORY

Healthy

Medications

Daily acetaminophen or ibuprofen for fever relief.

Family/Social History

All family members are healthy. Lives with mom, dad, and brother.

EXAMINATION

- Vitals: No fever
- General: Thin but well appearing, alert, cooperative, and no distress
- Head: Normocephalic, atraumatic
- Eye: Conjunctiva clear, PERRL, EOMI
- Nose: No drainage
- Oropharynx: MMM, no oral lesions, posterior pharynx clear, and no cavities

- Neck: Neck supple and no lymphadenopathy
- Lungs: Clear to auscultation bilaterally, normal WOB, and good air movement
- Heart: Regular rate and rhythm, normal S1 and S2, and no murmur, rubs, or gallops
- Abdomen: Soft, nontender, nondistended, bowel sounds present, no masses, and no organomegaly; no perianal abscess, tags, or fistulae
- Extremity: Extremities warm and well perfused, no edema, and no joint tenderness or swelling
- Lymph: No cervical, axillary, or inguinal lymphadenopathy
- Pulses: 2+ pulses and symmetric
- Skin: No rash or lesions and no jaundice
- Neurologic: Alert, face symmetric, PERRL, moves all extremities, and normal tone

DIAGNOSTIC CONSIDERATIONS

A wide differential was considered and grouped broadly into malignant, infectious, inflammatory, and gastrointestinal pathologies. Rheumatology considered the diagnoses of systemic JIA, Castleman syndrome, and periodic fever syndromes as likely possibilities.

Investigation

HIV, CMV, EBV, *Bartonella*, brucellosis, blastomycosis, and histoplasmosis tests were negative. Blood and urine cultures showed no growth. An echocardiogram and abdominal ultrasound were negative for endocarditis and intra-abdominal abscesses.

Results

GI workup included a negative fecal occult blood test and a pending fecal calprotectin on admission. She underwent an EGD/colonoscopy that showed one small erosion at the GE junction but was otherwise benign. Following EGD/colonoscopy, an MRE revealed evidence of active Crohn disease (30 cm of active colitis within the sigmoid and descending colon with associated ileal disease). Fecal calprotectin returned following MRE and was elevated at 463 µg/g of stool (normal <50).

DIAGNOSIS

Crohn disease

Treatment/Follow-up

She was started on oral prednisone. After starting the steroid therapy, she had no fever for the remainder of her hospital stay.

TEACHING POINTS

Crohn disease is an uncommon inflammatory bowel disease (IBD) that can present at any age with a wide variety of symptoms. While a majority of patients with Crohn disease experience primarily gastrointestinal symptoms such as long-standing diarrhea or vague abdominal pain, 25% of cases are discovered when a patient initially presents with nonspecific, extraintestinal manifestations (EIMs), independent of gastrointestinal symptoms. Common EIMs include weight loss (55%-80%), fever (38%), lethargy (13%-27%), anemia (69%), and osteopenia (8%-41%). Other common causes include musculoskeletal disease, oral ulcers, and skin involvement. Symptoms are protean and can present with involvement from essentially any organ system. Physicians may misdiagnose or fail to recognize these vague presenting EIMs, which are actually the beginning of IBD. EIMs tend to occur early in the disease course of IBD, an important point to remember when working with pediatric populations who represent some 25% of all cases of IBD. While fevers occur in approximately 38% of all cases, the extent and duration of fevers with Crohn disease are not well established. In this case, the patient had been experiencing fevers daily over the course of months, which was causing significant discomfort.

Suggested Readings

Jose FA, Heyman MB. Extraintestinal manifestations of inflammatory bowel disease. *J Pediatr Gastroenterol Nutr*. 2008;46(2):124-133.

Rosen MJ, Dhawan A, Saeed SA. Inflammatory bowel disease in children and adolescents. *JAMA Pediatr*. 2015;169(11):1053-1060.

Shapiro JM, Subedi S, LeLeiko NS. Inflammatory bowel disease. *Pediatr Rev*. 2016;37(8):337-347.

19 Another Video Game Complication

Kevin Baszis

CHIEF COMPLAINT

Rash on right leg for 3 months

HISTORY OF PRESENT ILLNESS

The 12-year-old boy's rash began without preceding trauma or illness. It is not pruritic, painful, swollen, or raised. It is pinkish-red and has not changed in color, but it is growing in size. He has never had anything like this before and has no rash on other parts of his body. He has not been applying any treatment or creams to the rash. He has had joint pain in the last few years and was diagnosed with both Sever disease and Osgood-Schlatter syndrome, but the pain is improving, and he now has only minimal intermittent knee pain after prolonged activity. He has no heel pain. He has not had fevers, weight loss, joint swelling, alopecia, oral ulcers, gastrointestinal (GI) symptoms, Raynaud disease, epistaxis, or difficulty urinating.

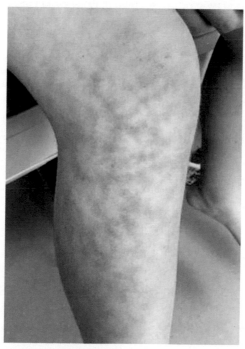

FIGURE 19.1   Rash on the patient's right leg.

PAST MEDICAL HISTORY

- Immunizations are up-to-date
- Never been hospitalized or had surgery
- Osgood-Schlatter syndrome
- Sever disease
- ADHD

Medications

- None

Family/Social History

- No one with rheumatoid arthritis, ankylosing spondylitis, scleroderma, Sjogren syndrome, dermatomyositis, vasculitis, SLE, psoriasis, thyroid disease, or IBD.
- Lives with parents and sister. He has two dogs and a rabbit.
- In seventh grade and plays in the band.
- He plays video games for hours in the basement with a nearby space heater to keep warm. The heater is located near his right leg.

EXAMINATION

- Height 161.3 cm and weight 51.6 kg.
- Temperature 6.7 °C (98.1 °F).
- Blood pressure 110/74 and pulse 78.
- Respiratory rate 16 and oxygen saturation 97% on room air.
- General: No distress, well-appearing, growth appropriate for age.
- HEENT: Pupils equal, round, reactive to light, sclera and conjunctiva noninjected, oropharynx without erythema, ulceration or exudate, and mucous membranes moist.
- Neck: Normal range of motion, no masses.
- Lymph: No lymphadenopathy.
- Lungs: Clear, without wheezes or rales.
- Cardiac: There are no murmurs, rubs, or gallops.
- Abdomen: Normal bowel sounds, soft, nondistended, no mass, no organomegaly.
- Skin: There is a blanching reticulated area of erythema on the lateral aspect of the right leg. The left leg has no rash. No nail fold telangiectases, no nail pits or ridging, no digital ulcerations, normal capillary refill, and no sclerodactyly.
- Neuro: Normal affect and cranial nerves intact, 2+ reflexes at knees.
- Musculoskeletal: Full range of motion of all joints without tenderness, erythema, warmth, or effusion.

DIAGNOSTIC CONSIDERATIONS

- Erythema ab igne
- Vasculitis
- Livedo reticularis
- Livedo racemosa

Investigation

- None

DIAGNOSIS

Erythema ab igne

TEACHING POINTS

The exposure to a heater near his right leg makes this diagnosis erythema ab igne. This is an asymptomatic cutaneous disorder resulting from chronic exposure to infrared radiation in the form of heat. The treatment involves removing the heat source. Hyperpigmentation may occur but will typically fade over months. Other diagnoses to be considered include livedo reticularis, which is typically symmetric/bilateral on the extremities, is reversible, not fixed, and is particularly noticeable with cold exposure. Livedo racemosa is a mottled, irregular hyperpigmentation that is fixed and partially blanchable. It is typically a violaceous, broken reticulated pattern and can be associated with underlying systemic disease. This patient is well-appearing and has no associated symptoms to suggest systemic autoimmunity or vasculitis, and given the well-documented and convincing exposure history, the diagnosis is erythema ab igne.

Suggested Readings

Arnold A, Itin P. Laptop computer-induced erythema ab igne in a child and review of the literature. *Pediatrics*. 2010;126(5):e1227-e1230. doi:10.1542/peds.2010-1390

Marie I. Erythema ab igne. *Arthritis Rheum*. 2018;70(11):1896. doi:10.1002/art.40561

Pincelli M. Livedo racemosa: clinical, laboratory, and histopathological findings in 33 patients. *Int J Low Extrem Wounds*. 2020:1534734619896938.

Sajjan V, Lunge S, Swamy MB, Pandit AM. Livedo reticularis: a review of the literature. *Indian Dermatol Online J*. 2015;6(5):315-321. doi:10.4103/2229-5178.164493

20 Not Your Grandmother's HUS

Amir B. Orandi, Joshua W. M. Theisen, T. Keefe Davis

CHIEF COMPLAINT

A 10-year-old boy with dark urine for 2 days

HISTORY OF PRESENT ILLNESS

He noticed his pee was dark 2 days ago. At first, he had no other symptoms, but he gradually started feeling warm, became nauseous, and had vomiting and abdominal pain. His urine output decreased. He had some loose stools without blood. His mom thought his eyes looked yellow. He had no headaches, bloody stools, upper respiratory symptoms, arthralgias, and no weight loss.

Three weeks earlier, he had developed multiple raised red skin lesions that were diagnosed as impetigo and treated with mupirocin, some of which improved, and others that now have a dark scab in the center (Figure 20.1).

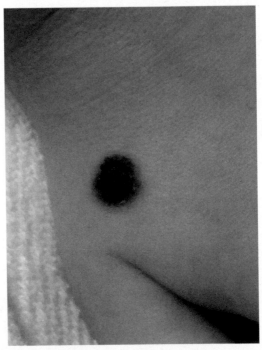

FIGURE 20.1   Photograph of patient hand showing bullous impetigo with secondary hemorrhage.

PAST MEDICAL HISTORY

No chronic medical conditions, surgery, or daily medications.

EXAMINATION

Vital signs: T 36.5, HR 93, RR 22, BP 114/99, SaO$_2$ 99% on room air.

Ill but nontoxic appearance. Scleral icterus is present. Diffusely inflamed oropharynx without tonsillar exudates. Soft abdomen, mild diffuse tenderness to palpation, and no hepatosplenomegaly. No peripheral edema and no joint effusions.

Skin examination: Mild jaundice on his torso. Minimal bruising. There are circumscribed crusted lesions of the left forearm and hand, posterior neck, forehead, bilateral inner thighs, left shin, scalp, and lower back that are each 2 to 3 cm raised erythematous lesions with central necrosis, in different stages of healing, without pus.

Initial Testing:

- WBC 7.4 (68%N, 26%L, 3%M), Hb 10.4, **Plt 3**, smear 1% to 10% schistocytes.
- CMP: Na 133, K hemolyzed, Cl 28, CO$_2$ 26, BUN 53, Cr 1.1, Glu 95, Ca 9.5.
- Total protein 7.1, Alb 3.7, Alk Phos 153, AST hemolyzed, ALT 28, total bilirubin 2.9.
- Coombs negative, haptoglobin < 10, **LDH > 2500**.
- Complement C3 141, complement C4 33.
- UA: 1.025, pH 6.0, **3+ protein, 3+ blood**, 3+ bilirubin, 2+ ketones, + nitrites, 2+ LE, neg glucose.
- Urine microscopy: No WBCs or RBCs. **1 to 5 coarse granular casts/LPF.**
- Rapid streptococcal throat swab negative. Nasopharyngeal PCR negative.

DIAGNOSTIC CONSIDERATIONS

- Sepsis with developing multiorgan involvement
- Infectious hepatitis
- Systemic lupus erythematosus
- Immune thrombocytopenic purpura (ITP)
- Evan syndrome (autoimmune hemolytic anemia and thrombocytopenia)
- Thrombotic microangiopathy (TMA) syndrome

Investigation

On hospital day #1, he was treated for ITP with a transfusion of platelets and IV immune globulin, but he only had transiently improved platelet counts. An infectious evaluation was initiated.

Dermatology consultation: Bullous impetigo with secondary hemorrhage. Biopsy of a lesion showed impetiginized scale-crust, purpura, and superficial microthrombi. Biopsy culture is positive for methicillin-sensitive *Staphylococcus aureus* (MSSA), sensitive to doxycycline.

On hospital day #2, he developed severe headaches and photophobia. Hemoglobin decreased to 6.7 g/dL, schistocytes increased to 11% to 30%, while BUN and creatinine increased to 60 and 1.3 mg/dL, respectively. He became critically ill with findings of volume overload and pleural effusions. He was treated with plasma exchange for two treatments with dramatic clinical improvement and gradual normalization of platelets, LDH, along with disappearance of schistocytes. He received a full course of doxycycline for MSSA skin infection.

Results

- Infectious testing: Negative for *Mycoplasma*, *Ehrlichia*, cytomegalovirus, Epstein-Barr virus, *Histoplasma*, and *Blastomyces*.
- Blood and stool cultures were negative.
- Streptococcal antibodies were negative.
- ADAMTS13 activity >115% (sent prior to plasma exchange).

- Genetic testing for thrombotic microangiopathies.
- Heterozygous for membrane cofactor protein (MCP) c.104G > A (p.C35Y).
- Heterozygous for complement factor B (CFB) c.724A > C (p.I242 L).

DIAGNOSIS

1. *Staphylococcus aureus* **bullous impetigo**
2. **Primary (genetic) complement-mediated TMA**, secondary to #1

Treatment/Follow-up

He responded swiftly to plasma exchange therapy returning to normal hematologic parameters and kidney function. These mutations individually offer distinctly different prognoses with the MCP loss of function mutation seen in 10% to 15% of cases imparting a low risk of recurrence and very low risk of death or end-stage renal disease (ESRD) within 1 year; whereas the CFB gain of function mutation is rare in prevalence (1%-4%), associated with a high risk of recurrence and higher risk of death or ESRD. It is unclear what the combination holds. Six months after hospitalization, he remained symptom free, off treatment, with normal laboratory monitoring.

TEACHING POINTS

Complement-mediated TMA, one of several related disorders and previously referred to as atypical hemolytic uremic syndrome (aHUS) is a rare disorder, with estimated incidence of two per million in the United States. It is gender indiscriminate in children and has higher prevalence in younger children, approximately 25% before 2 years of age, but still 50% in ages 1 to 7 years. The onset is usually sudden with constitutional symptoms predominant in the initial phase: malaise, anorexia, and pallor with or without edema. However, in 80% of cases, there is an antecedent infection, either upper respiratory or gastrointestinal with nearly 25% associated with diarrhea.

Complement-mediated TMA is a disorder of alternative complement pathway dysregulation with up to 60% of patients harboring mutations in genes that code for complement-regulating proteins making them more susceptible to developing TMA when challenged. Precipitating factors include, but are not limited to, viral or bacterial infections (commonly *Streptococcus pneumoniae* via neuraminidase and T-antigen exposure). Complement-mediated TMA can also be acquired, as in some cases when complement proteins are targeted by autoantibodies. More than 80% of mutations are considered sporadic and be either gain or loss of function with penetrance estimated at 50% of individuals. The most common mutations occur in the gene for complement regulatory protein factor H (CFH) at 20% to 30% followed by MCP at 5% to 15%, whereas the least reported mutation is in CFB at 1% to 4%. Prognosis for recurrence, progression to ESRD, possibility of renal transplant failure, and mortality all vary based on which mutation or combinations of mutations are present.

First-line treatment for complement-mediated TMA is plasma exchange followed by eculizumab. Eculizumab, a monoclonal antibody against C5, prevents terminal complement complex C5b-9 formation, and is indicated to treat refractory TMA, or those dependent on plasma exchange.

TMA syndromes are a heterogenous group of disorders that share pathophysiologic features of vascular damage from small vessel thrombosis and endothelial and vessel wall dysfunction. The presenting clinical triad of **microangiopathic hemolytic anemia, thrombocytopenia, and acute renal failure** has long been associated with hemolytic uremic syndrome (HUS) caused by Shiga toxin producing *Escherichia coli* 0157:H7 (ST-HUS). Patients with symptoms compatible with HUS, but without evidence of a Shiga producing infection, led to the use of the terms *atypical* HUS and "nondiarrheal HUS", both of which are no longer considered sufficiently accurate. When the triad of symptoms expands to include fever and neurologic symptoms, the pentad is recognized as thrombotic thrombocytopenic purpura, caused by absence or at least 90% deficient ADAMTS13 activity, a von Willebrand factor-cleavage protease (ADAMTS13-related TMA). Consistent with complement-mediated TMA syndromes,

ADAMTS13-related TMA can be hereditary (Upshaw-Schulman syndrome) or acquired as antibodies against the enzyme. Other causes of TMA include drug-related (dose toxicity or immune reaction), metabolic-related, and coagulation-related. TMA syndromes of any category can be precipitated by or occur independently from systemic infection, transplant, malignancy, pregnancy, or systemic autoimmune disease.

It is critical to promptly recognize the symptoms and representative clinical and laboratory findings of a microangiopathic process so that a stepwise evaluation and treatment can be implemented (Figure 20.2). This includes consideration of TMA when evaluating a patient with anemia and thrombocytopenia; assessment for hemolysis (ie, transaminase, bilirubin, and LDH elevations, consumption of haptoglobin), characterization of anemia (ie, Coombs positivity, analysis of peripheral smear for schistocytes), as well as detailed inventory of organ functions, primarily renal, hepatic, and neurologic. Assays for presence and activity of ADAMTS13 should be done early. Testing for *E. coli* should be done, as presence of Shiga toxin merits special treatment considerations. Subsequent testing for underlying disease processes or complement gene mutations should also be performed.

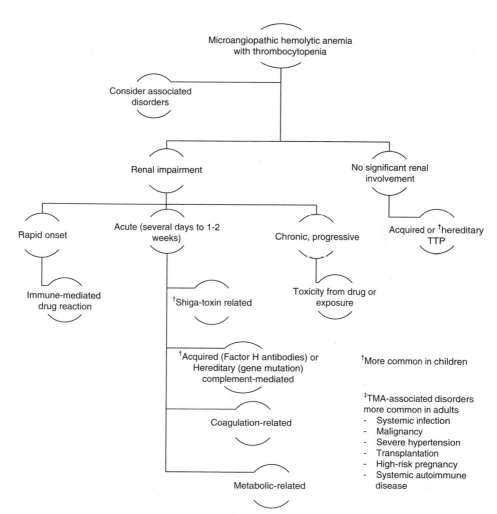

FIGURE 20.2 Algorithm of approach to the patient with microangiopathic hemolytic anemia. TMA, thrombotic microangiopathy. (Adapted from George JN, Nester CM. Syndromes of thrombotic microangiopathy. *N Engl J Med.* 2014;371(19):1847-1848.)

Suggested Readings

Davis TK, McKee R, Schnadower D, Tarr PI. Treatment of Shiga toxin-producing *Escherichia coli* infections. *Infect Dis Clin*. 2013;27(3):577-597.

Freedman SB, Xie J, Neufeld MS, et al. Shiga toxin-producing Escherichia coli infection, antibiotics, and risk of developing hemolytic uremic syndrome: a meta-analysis. *Clin Infect Dis*. 2016;62(10):1251-1258.

Geerdink LM, Westra D, van Wijk JA, et al. Atypical hemolytic uremic syndrome in children: complement mutations and clinical characteristics. *Pediatr Nephrol*. 2012;27(8):1283-1291.

George JN, Nester CM. Syndromes of thrombotic microangiopathy. *N Engl J Med*. 2014;371(19):1847-1848.

Hickey CA, Beattie TJ, Cowieson J, et al. Early volume expansion during diarrhea and relative nephroprotection during subsequent hemolytic uremic syndrome. *Arch Pediatr Adolesc Med*. 2011;165(10):884-889.

Kavanagh D, Goodship TH, Richards A. Atypical hemolytic uremic syndrome. *Semin Nephrol*. 2013;33(6):508-530.

Keating GM. Eculizumab: a review of its use in atypical haemolytic uraemic syndrome. *Drugs*. 2013;73(18):2053-2066.

Schindler EI, Sellenriek P, Storch GA, Tarr PI, Burnham CA. Shiga toxin-producing Escherichia coli: a single-center, 11-year pediatric experience. *J Clin Microbiol*. 2014;52(10):3647-3653.

Verhave JC, Wetzels JF, van de Kar NC. Novel aspects of atypical haemolytic uraemic syndrome and the role of eculizumab. *Nephrol Dial Transplant*. 2014;29(suppl 4):iv131-iv141.

21

"How'd It Get There?"

Amir B. Orandi

CHIEF COMPLAINT

A 14-year-old girl with abdominal pain, vomiting, and diarrhea for 3 days

HISTORY OF PRESENT ILLNESS

Three weeks ago, she awoke in the middle of the night with severe abdominal pain and vomiting. There was no blood or bile. She did not have fever, diarrhea, or skin rash. She was evaluated at a local emergency department with a computed tomography (CT) scan of her abdomen that showed a "ruptured ovarian cyst and some free fluid in the pelvis." Her pain improved with analgesia; she tolerated oral fluids and was sent home. She then developed high fevers and diarrhea for 3 to 4 days and was seen by her primary physician who obtained laboratory studies and stool cultures, which were normal. These symptoms continued for approximately 1 week before improving, but they never resolved. She returned to daily activities but had daily low-grade fevers and a poor appetite.

The patient then re-presented with 3 days of persistent vomiting, diarrhea, and abdominal pain. The emesis was frequent, large volume, and nonbloody but was occasionally bilious. Diarrhea was also frequent and nonbloody. Her abdominal pain was intermittent but sharp and located in the epigastrium with some radiation to the left side.

Other symptoms include a 20-pound weight loss over the past month and malaise. She had no easy bruising, bleeding, or headaches. Menarche was 6 months ago, and she has had irregular menses ever since. No recent travel, and no infectious exposures such as ill contacts, camping, freshwater exposure, or undercooked meats.

PAST MEDICAL HISTORY

Treacher Collins syndrome: Tracheostomy as a young child but was decannulated several years ago. Hearing loss status post several surgical interventions, most recently, 4 months ago. No history of abdominal surgeries. Immunizations are up-to-date.

Family/Social History

Her father has sarcoidosis; her mother has hypertension, and she has two healthy siblings. No history of other genetic disorders.

EXAMINATION

- Vital signs: Wt: 45 kg, Temp 38.5 °C, HR 120, RR 24, BP 104/53, O_2 97% on room air.
- General: Curled up in bed with rigors, responsive to examiner.
- HEENT: Microtia, downward slanting eyes, and micrognathia. Sclera is anicteric; mucous membranes are tacky.
- Neck: Supple with small, scattered lymphadenopathy.
- Chest: Clear lungs to auscultation. Heart has rapid rate but normal rhythm and no murmurs.
- Abdomen: No scars or discoloration, nondistended. Bowel sounds are absent. Diffusely tender to palpation, most in epigastrium and bilateral lower quadrants. There is some guarding but

no rebound. Negative Rovsing, obturator, and psoas signs. There is no hepatosplenomegaly but a fullness in the right lower abdomen.

- GU: Tanner 4. No inguinal lymphadenopathy. Pelvic examination reveals healthy mucosa and normal-appearing cervix. Bimanual examination reveals no cervical motion tenderness but an enlarged and palpable right adnexa.
- Extremities: Warm and well perfused with 2+ peripheral pulses and 2- to 3-second capillary refill.
- Skin: Warm to touch, dry with no rashes.

Initial Testing

- WBC 20.4 (85% N), Hgb 11.2, Hct 33.4, platelets 335, MCV 82
- Na 133, K 3.4, Cl 100, CO_2 20, BUN 12, Cr 0.7, Glu 103. Ca 8.5, Total protein 8.3, Albumin 2.8, Alk Phos 109, AST 13, ALT 5, total bilirubin 0.4
- Urinalysis: 1.040, pH 6.0, 2+ protein, 1+ LE, no cells
- Urine β-HCG: Negative
- Gonorrhea/chlamydia DNA urine probe and endocervical gonorrheal culture: Negative
- Urine, stool, and blood cultures: No growth
- Obstructive radiographic series: Multiple loops of gas-filled nondilated large bowel, with multiple mildly dilated loops of gas-filled small bowel, multiple air-fluid levels compatible with ileus or early partial small bowel obstruction

DIAGNOSTIC CONSIDERATIONS

Infectious	Gynecologic	Rheumatologic	Surgical
Gastroenteritis	Ovarian cyst with rupture and/or torsion	Inflammatory bowel disease	Congenital malrotation with volvulus
Appendicitis	Teratoma with hemorrhage and/or torsion	Mesenteric vasculitis	Adynamic ileus
Intra-abdominal abscess	Ectopic pregnancy		

Investigation

She was admitted with a diagnosis of dehydration and gastroenteritis. Over the ensuing 24 hours, she continued to have high fevers, rigors, and abdominal pain, but emesis and diarrhea resolved.

Abdominal and pelvic ultrasound: Appendix not visualized. Small area of fluid between the mesentery, which appears to contain several thin internal septations measuring up to 2.5 × 1.0 cm. The left ovary measures 2.6 × 3.6 × 1.9 for a volume of 9.4 mL. The right ovary is significantly larger measuring 5.7 × 4.7 × 5.2 for a volume of 72.7 mL. There is a large simple-appearing right ovarian cyst measuring up to 4.3 × 5.7 cm in diameter. There is blood flow to the right ovary on color Doppler imaging, which is abnormally located in the midline of the pelvis and abuts the uterus.

Evaluation by Pediatric Surgery and Pediatric Gynecology could not determine whether torsion was occurring, and a CT was suggested.

Results

CT of abdomen and pelvis with contrast: Complex heterogeneous ill-defined mass in the midline pelvis, abutting the uterus. A dominant fluid collection is present measuring up to 3.8 cm in diameter. The ovaries are not definitively identified. The proximal portion of the appendix is visualized; however, the appendix appears to course into the pelvis and is not well defined.

Further studies to evaluate the pelvic mass included the following:

- LDH: 268, Uric acid: 3.3
- Serum β-HCG: <5, alpha-fetoprotein: <3, CA 125 antigen: 11 (5-30), CEA antigen: <1

Anaerobic culture would remain sterile, but aerobic culture of the aspirated fluid grew **beta-hemolytic group A streptococcus**.

DIAGNOSIS

Primary intra-abdominal abscess, with *Streptococcus pyogenes*

TEACHING POINTS

Primary intra-abdominal infections are those that arise in the absence of any anatomical derangement in the viscera such as perforation or other loss of mucosal integrity. Thus, source control is not normally necessary as a significant localizing response in the peritoneum is absent. Conversely, secondary infections from perforation or hematogenous spread are usually intestinal flora that are more likely to cause sinus tracts or fistulas and thus would benefit from local source control.

The purported pathophysiology of primary intra-abdominal abscesses is migration of facultative pathogenic flora eventually being deposited in the abdomen, likely a reason this disease entity is more common in adolescent females. In males, this migration is thought to occur from oropharyngeal bacteria. The disruption leading to this imbalance can be related to hormonal or immunologic changes but also hygienic or iatrogenic. The result is a pre-dominance of facultative pathogenic flora of *Staphylococcus*, *Streptococcus*, and *Enterobacteriaceae* becoming dominant over the protective *Lactobacillus* species.

A study comparing vaginal and intra-abdominal abscess cultures in girls with pelvic inflammatory disease identified 33 cases of comparable cultures: 6 were both sterile, 11 had different isolates, and only 9 contained identical bacteria in both sites which were: *Escherichia coli*, *Bacteroides fragilis*, *Enterococcus faecalis*, *Peptostreptococcus*, *Haemophilus parainfluenzae*, and others.

In other case reports, hypotheses of the source of streptococcus positive cultures include a ruptured appendix, which could account for the biphasic presentation of symptoms, and an incompletely visualized appendix.

An acute presentation of fever, abdominal pain, and emesis in an adolescent female has a broad differential including infectious, surgical, and gynecologic etiologies. Evaluation for sexually transmitted infections and pregnancy should be considered even in the presence of a negative social history.

Also illustrated in this case is the utility of diagnostic imaging relative to a patient's symptom progression. A CT of the abdomen very early in the course of illness may not exclude a disease under development. Similarly, ultrasound was useful in identifying a mass and showing adequate blood supply to vital organs but lacked specificity. Although radiation should be minimized in children, repeat CT imaging in this case allowed for the nonsurgical intervention that was ultimately both diagnostic and therapeutic.

This case is consistent with the literature reports that primary intra-abdominal abscess in a surgically naive and nonsexually active female is an uncommon occurrence, but one with a variety of microbiologic culprits.

Suggested Readings

Algren SD, Strickland JL. Beta hemolytic streptococcus group f causing pelvic inflammatory disease in a 14-year-old girl. *J Pediatr Adolesc Gynecol*. 2005;18(2):117-119.

Brook I. Intra-abdominal, retroperitoneal, and visceral abscesses in children. *Eur J Pediatr Surg*. 2004;14(4):265-273.

Schindlbeck C, Dziura D, Mylonas I. Diagnosis of pelvic inflammatory disease (PID): intra-operative findings and comparison of vaginal and intra-abdominal cultures. *Arch Gynecol Obstet*. 2014;289(6):1263-1269.

Thompson AE, Marshall JC, Opal SM. Intraabdominal infections in infants and children: descriptions and definitions. *Pediatr Crit Care Med*. 2005;6(3 suppl):S30-S35.

22 Karma

Maleewan Kitcharoensakkul

CHIEF COMPLAINT

Hives and wheezing

HISTORY OF PRESENT ILLNESS

A 6-year-old boy presented to the emergency room with hives and wheezing. Three days earlier, he woke up with diffuse hives at 4 AM with no other symptoms. The hives resolved with one dose of diphenhydramine. He had eaten a cheeseburger for dinner, but there were no new foods or medication exposures. The next day he was doing well during the daytime, but again awoke at night with diffuse body hives. Mother gave him two doses of diphenhydramine. Later the following day, he was wheezing and had hives at his primary care provider's office. He was given prednisolone and albuterol, and started on scheduled diphenhydramine. On the day of admission, he again ate a cheeseburger around 1 PM and had more hives a few hours later. Around midnight, he woke up again with total body hives and wheezing. He did have some cold symptoms over the past 3 weeks, but otherwise he had no other symptoms. He has not had similar episodes of these symptoms in the past, except for an emergency room visit 1 year prior when he presented with fever and abdominal pain after having barbeque hamburger for dinner.

PAST MEDICAL HISTORY

- Attention-deficit hyperactivity
- Autistic spectrum disorder

Medications

Prednisolone and diphenhydramine

Family/Social History

No family history of chronic hives, or recurrent swelling. Mother with allergic rhinitis. He has a history of tick bites.

EXAMINATION

- Vital signs: Temperature 36.6 °C, blood pressure 96/42 mm Hg, heart rate 106/min, respiratory rate 19/min, and oxygen saturations 97% on room air.
- General appearance: Alert, itchy, but not in acute distress.
- Skin: Diffuse hives as shown in Figure 22.1.
- HEENT: Hives on face and neck. No facial or tongue swelling. Normal oropharyngeal examination.
- Pulmonary: Diffuse wheezing. No use of accessory muscles and no retractions.
- Cardiovascular: Regular rate and rhythm, no murmurs, rubs or gallops; normal S1 and S2; 2+ distal pulses.
- Abdomen: Soft, nondistended, nontender, normoactive bowel sounds.
- Neurologic: Awake and alert, answers questions appropriately for age.

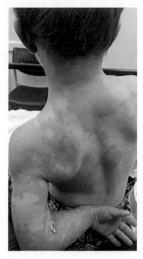

FIGURE 22.1 Photo of his rash.

DIAGNOSTIC CONSIDERATIONS

Problems:

1. Hives, recurrent
2. Wheezing, associated with #1
   - Alpha-gal syndrome (delayed red meat allergy)
   - Idiopathic anaphylaxis
   - Acute urticaria and angioedema associated with viral infection
   - Systemic mastocytosis

Investigation

Tryptase, alpha-gal IgEs, and viral studies including nasopharyngeal swab for respiratory viruses, and parvovirus, cytomegalovirus (CMV), and Epstein-Barr virus (EBV) IgMs were sent.

Results

Test	Reference	Results
Tryptase		
• At presentation	<11.5 ng/mL	29 ng/mL
• Repeat at 3 wk	<11.5 ng/mL	6 ng/mL
Alpha-gal IgE	<0.1 kU/L	0.82
• Beef IgE	<0.1 kU/L	0.64
• Lamb IgE	<0.1 kU/L	0.50
• Pork IgE	<0.1 kU/L	0.60
Respiratory pathogen multiplex PCRs	Negative	Negative
CMV, EBV, and parvovirus IgM	Negative	Negative

DIAGNOSIS

Based on clinical history of anaphylaxis and the elevated specific IgE to galactose-alpha-1,3-galactose (alpha-gal), an oligosaccharide of nonprimate mammals: **alpha-gal syndrome**.

Treatment/Follow-up

1. Avoid mammalian meat
2. Emergency action plan and prescription and teaching of an epinephrine autoinjector

TEACHING POINTS

Alpha-gal syndrome is a distinct form of red meat allergy. The prevalence of alpha-gal in the general population is unknown, although cases have been reported worldwide. The connection between alpha-gal IgE and delayed allergic reactions to red meat was established by Commins and colleagues in 2009. Patients with alpha-gal allergy react to eating red meat, internal organs, and other products derived from mammals. Alpha-gal allergy has several characteristics that differentiate it from typical food allergic reactions. The alpha-gal allergy can develop any time in life, and often in many patients who tolerated meat in the past. While common complaints in alpha-gal allergy include hives, swelling, gastrointestinal symptoms, and anaphylaxis, patients usually do not develop any symptoms until 3 to 6 hours after eating red meat. The reactions are intermittent and may not occur on every occasion that the patient eats red meat.

The mechanism of alpha-gal allergy is not completely understood; however, bites from certain ticks, particularly those who have fed on deers, are most likely the primary cause of alpha-gal sensitization. The occurrence of alpha-gal allergy in hunters, who are often in the woods and may suffer tick bites from the insects embedded in their prey, has led some to refer to this syndrome as Karma.

It is important to be aware that asymptomatic sensitization to meat is not uncommon, thus testing for alpha-gal allergy should be sent only in patients with consistent clinical history. Treatment consists of counseling patients on avoidance of red meat and providing patients with emergency plan including prescription of an epinephrine autoinjector. Patients can continue having milk and dairy products if they have previously tolerated these products. A minority of patients with alpha-gal allergy can react to gelatin-containing vaccines; thus caution should be used in parenteral administration of these products in alpha-gal patients. Long-term data from large case series are required to determine the prognosis of alpha-gal allergy; however, titers to alpha-gal usually diminish over time and many patients can tolerate reintroduction of red meat after a period of avoidance.

Suggested Readings

Commins SP, Satinover SM, Hosen J, et al. Delayed anaphylaxis, angioedema, or urticaria after consumption of red meat in patients with IgE antibodies specific for galactose-alpha-1,3-galactose. *J Allergy Clin Immunol*. 2009;123:426-433.

Platts-Mills TAE, Commins SP, Biedermann T, et al. On the cause and consequences of IgE to galactose-α-1,3-galactose: a report from the National Institute of Allergy and Infectious Diseases Workshop on understanding IgE-mediated mammalian meat allergy. *J Allergy Clin Immunol*. 2020;145:1061-1071.

Stone CA Jr, Commins SP, Choudhary S, et al. Anaphylaxis after vaccination in a pediatric patient: further implicating alpha-gal allergy. *J Allergy Clin Immunol Pract*. 2019;7:322-324.e2.

Wilson JM, Platts-Mills TAE. Red meat allergy in children and adults. *Curr Opin Allergy Clin Immunol*. 2019;19:229-235.

Wilson JM, Schuyler AJ, Workman L, et al. Investigation into the α-Gal syndrome: characteristics of 261 children and adults reporting red meat allergy. *J Allergy Clin Immunol Pract*. 2019;7:2348-2358.e4.

23

Tip of the Tongue

Maleewan Kitcharoensakkul

CHIEF COMPLAINT

White plaque on tongue and fever for 1 week

HISTORY OF PRESENT ILLNESS

An 18-month-old girl with recurrent otitis media since 4 months of age, presents with fever up to 102 °F and purulent discharge from one ear treated with topical antibiotic ear drops for 2 weeks. One week before presentation, parents noticed decreased appetite and a white plaque on the tip of her tongue. The plaque did not improve with topical nystatin. As she refused to eat and continued to have fever, her parents brought her to the emergency department.

PAST MEDICAL HISTORY

- Poor weight gain
- Recurrent otitis media status post bilateral myringotomy tube placement
- Gross motor delay

Medications

Oral nystatin

Family/Social History

No family history of recurrent infections, early childhood death, or autoimmunity. No history of consanguineous marriage in the family.

EXAMINATION

- Vital signs: T 38.1, HR 191/min, RR, 45/min, BP 85/49 mm Hg, and Spo$_2$ 98% room air
- General: Alert, irritable
- HEENT: Normocephalic, no dysmorphic features, intact myringotomy tubes bilaterally without drainage per tubes, no rhinorrhea, yellow and white plaque on her tongue, normal gum and buccal mucosa, normal tonsils, and clear oropharynx
- Cardiovascular: Tachycardia, normal S1 & S2, no murmurs, rubs, or gallops
- Pulmonary: No retractions, normal breath sounds, and clear to auscultations
- Abdomen: Soft, not tender, not distended, and no hepatosplenomegaly
- GU: Normal female genitalia
- Neuro: Normal tone, moves all extremities well
- Skin: No rash

DIAGNOSTIC CONSIDERATIONS

- Oral candidiasis
- Herpes simplex viral (HSV) infection
- Malignancy, oral

Investigation

- CBC: WBC 10,000 cells/mm³, 40% lymphocytes, 50% monocytes, Hgb 8 g/dL, and Plt 225,000/µL
- Peripheral blood smear: **Absent neutrophils**
- **ESR 90 mm/h and CRP 150 mg/dL**
- Cerebrospinal fluids: No cells, normal glucose and protein, and negative gram stain
- HIV testing by antibodies and PCR: Negative
- Lesion HSV PCR: Negative
- Tongue aerobic, acid-fast bacilli, and fungal cultures: Negative
- Blood cultures: No growth

Results

Additional studies to evaluate the remarkable neutropenia and mild anemia were sent.

- Iron studies: Low iron, total iron-binding capacities and transferrin saturations.
- Reticulocyte count: 0.4%.
- Bone marrow biopsy: Mildly hypocellular bone marrow with left-shifted myelopoiesis. No blasts on flow cytometry. Stains of bone marrow was negative for fungus and acid-fast bacilli.
- Severe congenital neutropenia genetic panel: Negative.
- Lymphocyte panel: CD3⁺ T cell 1050 cells/µL (reference 1400-3700), CD4⁺ T cell 720 cells/µL (reference 700-2200), CD8⁺ T cell 320 cells/µL (reference 490-1300), CD19⁺ B cells 2000 cells/µL (reference 390-1400), and CD16⁺/CD56⁺ NK cells 1000 cells/µL (reference 130-720).
- Lymphocyte proliferation to mitogen: Normal.
- Immunoglobulins: IgG 976 mg/dL (reference 424-1051), IgM 489 (reference 48-168), and IgA 73 (reference 14-123) mg/dL.
- Vaccine titers: Protective to tetanus, diphtheria, *Haemophilus influenzae* type b, and 6 of 12 serotypes of *Streptococcus pneumoniae* in Prevnar vaccine.

DIAGNOSIS

Tongue biopsy: extensive infiltration by **Actinomyces**, a gram-positive anaerobe.

Genetic panel sent for primary immunodeficiency revealed double heterozygous pathogenic variants of ataxia telangiectasia mutated (*ATM*) gene confirming the diagnosis of **ataxia telangiectasia**.

Treatment/Follow-up

For the *Actinomyces* infection, she was given 5 months of amoxicillin and had complete resolution of her symptoms. The neutropenia improved with granulocyte colony-stimulating factor (G-CSF). Alpha-fetoprotein was elevated at 90 ng/mL (reference 0.8-3). She was subsequently started on immunoglobulin replacement after another hospitalization, this time for pneumococcal bacteremia with a loss of protective titers to most serotypes in Prevnar. She later developed truncal ataxia at 2 years of age.

TEACHING POINTS

Ataxia-telangiectasia (A-T) is a rare autosomal recessive disorder characterized by progressive cerebellar impairment, oculocutaneous telangiectasia, immunodeficiency, radiation hypersensitivity, and predisposition to malignancy. The disease is caused by mutations in the *ATM* gene resulting in defects in cell cycle control and DNA repair. The prevalence of A-T is estimated to be <1 to 9/100,000. Classically, ataxia appears in the first 3 years of life. However, neurological and immunological manifestations of A-T are heterogenous, especially in the early stages, potentially leading to delays in diagnosis. Telangiectases involving conjunctivae and skin usually became noticeable around 3 to 6 years of age, but may not develop in all patients. Cutaneous granulomas are uncommon manifestations of immune dysregulation in A-T that may be extensive and refractory to treatment. Two-thirds of A-T patients have abnormal immune findings, including lymphopenia, hypogammaglobulinemia, impaired antibody responses, and impaired lymphoproliferative responses to mitogen and antigen. A small number of A-T patients have a hyper IgM phenotype (low IgG with normal or elevated IgM) as a result of class-switch recombination defects, and this finding is associated with a more severe disease course and probable increased frequency of lymphoproliferation and autoimmunity. Neutropenia is an infrequent finding in A-T, although this has been reported in the literature. A-T patients with immunodeficiency usually manifest with recurrent sinopulmonary infections starting early in life and can predate the onset of neurological symptoms. The opportunistic infection from *Pneumocystis jiroveci*, herpes simplex virus, human papillomavirus, molluscum contagiosum, and herpes zoster are uncommon but have been reported in A-T. Most likely, this patient's severe neutropenia contributed to the locally invasive infection from *Actinomyces*, a normal oropharyngeal flora. Elevated alpha-fetoprotein is seen in most A-T patients, permitting its use as a screening test in suspected patients aged 18 months and older. However, genetic testing is required to establish the diagnosis. There is no curative treatment for A-T, and patients usually die in the second-third decade of life from respiratory failure as a result of ineffective cough, aspiration, and immunodeficiency. Patients with A-T have an overall increased risk of developing at least one malignancy, most commonly lymphoma. Patients require long-term follow-up with a multidisciplinary team including neurology, immunology, hematology/oncology, pulmonology, endocrinology, and nutrition.

Suggested Readings

Amirifar P, Yazdani R, Moeini Shad T, et al. Cutaneous granulomatosis and class switching defect as a presenting sign in ataxia-telangiectasia: first case from the National Iranian Registry and review of the literature. *Immunol Invest*. 2020;49(6):597-610.

Chiam LY, Verhagen MM, Haraldsson A, et al. Cutaneous granulomas in ataxia telangiectasia and other primary immunodeficiencies: reflection of inappropriate immune regulation? *Dermatology*. 2011;223:13-19.

Davies EG. Update on the management of the immunodeficiency in ataxia-telangiectasia. *Expet Rev Clin Immunol*. 2009;5:565-575.

Nowak-Wegrzyn A, Crawford TO, Winkelstein JA, Carson KA, Lederman HM. Immunodeficiency and infections in ataxia-telangiectasia. *J Pediatr*. 2004;144:505-511.

Perreault S, Bernard G, Lortie A, Le Deist F, Decaluwe H. Ataxia-telangiectasia presenting with a novel immunodeficiency. *Pediatr Neurol*. 2012;46:322-324.

Rothblum-Oviatt C, Wright J, Lefton-Greif MA, McGrath-Morrow SA, Crawford TO, Lederman HM. Ataxia telangiectasia: a review. *Orphanet J Rare Dis*. 2016;11:159.

Stray-Pedersen A, Borresen-Dale AL, Paus E, Lindman CR, Burgers T, Abrahamsen TG. Alpha fetoprotein is increasing with age in ataxia-telangiectasia. *Eur J Paediatr Neurol*. 2007;11:375-380.

van Os NJH, Jansen AFM, van Deuren M, et al. Ataxia-telangiectasia: immunodeficiency and survival. *Clin Immunol*. 2017;178:45-55.

24

C Minus

Cecelia L. Calhoun, Brittany J. Blue

CHIEF COMPLAINT

Newborn with respiratory failure

HISTORY OF PRESENT ILLNESS

A 4-kg 36-week estimated gestational age (EGA) infant girl born via elective Cesarean section developed respiratory distress in the delivery room. A chest radiograph showed diffuse opacification of both lung fields. Respiratory failure progressed despite administration of surfactant, and she was placed on high-frequency oscillatory ventilation. Ampicillin and gentamicin were initiated for suspected sepsis. On day of life (DOL) 1, she developed areas of decreased perfusion to her feet and toes and began oozing blood from venipuncture sites. She was given several transfusion products including packed red blood cells (PRBCs), platelets, and fresh frozen plasma (FFP). Despite repeated administration of PRBCs, FFP, and platelet transfusions, her prothrombin time (PT) remained elevated. Imaging evaluation of her lower extremities for clot was negative. There were no signs of sepsis or a giant hemangioma as a cause of disseminated intravascular coagulation (DIC). By DOL 5, the infant developed oozing from the nose and new ecchymotic lesions on the scalp, trunk, and extremities. The older areas of poor perfusion on her toes and feet became ecchymotic and necrotic.

PAST MEDICAL HISTORY

She was delivered by elective Cesarean section to a 33-year-old gravida 4 para 3001→ 2 mother. Mother is A positive, with negative serology.

Family/Social History

The parents conceived four pregnancies together. Two of the pregnancies resulted in neonatal demise. The first infant died at 3 days of age following complications of intracerebral hemorrhage. Imaging findings also demonstrated cystic encephalomalacia suggesting these hemorrhages were both acute and chronic. She also had a unilateral absent red reflex. The second infant died in the delivery room at an hour of life from respiratory failure. Despite resuscitative measures, she was unable to be adequately ventilated, and chest x-ray (CXR) demonstrated no aeration of the lungs. Her laboratory test results demonstrated anemia (Hgb 6.1) and thrombocytopenia (4k). Whole genomic single nucleotide polymorphism (SNP) microarray and karyotype were negative.

The parents and surviving male sibling (third pregnancy) are healthy. Maternal and paternal grandmothers have a history of stroke. Maternal grandfather has a history of deep vein thrombosis (DVT). Evaluation for neonatal autoimmune thrombocytopenia (NAIT) was negative. Maternal protein-S activity was low, which may be due to pregnancy. Similarly, maternal protein-C activity was low, which cannot be explained by pregnancy.

EXAM

- VS: HR 136, T 37.9, and BP 67/38.
- Gen: Large for gestational age.

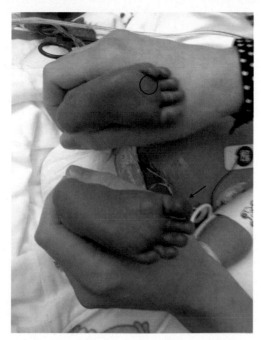

FIGURE 24.1 The feet demonstrate decreased perfusion of three toes on the left foot (arrow) and an area on the right sole (circle).

- HEENT: Normocephalic, AF soft and flat, sutures are overriding, ET tube in place, and ophthalmology examination demonstrated right retinal hemorrhage.
- Pulmonary: Pulmonary sounds obstructed by oscillator ventilator sounds.
- Abdomen: Full but compressible, no hepatosplenomegaly.
- Skin: Ecchymotic lesions on the scalp, trunk, and extremities. Oozing from venipuncture sites. Progressive areas of nonblanchable, decreased perfusion of the toes evolving to local tissues (Figures 24.1 and 24.2).

DIAGNOSTIC CONSIDERATIONS

- Sepsis
- Deficiency of vitamin K dependent clotting factor (II, VII, IX, X, protein C, and protein S)
- Thrombotic thrombocytopenic purpura
- Disseminated intravascular coagulation
- Vascular spasm from umbilical catheter

Investigation

At initial evaluation,

- CBC: WBC 24, Hgb 13.5, platelets 153
- PT: 17.1 (normal for age: 13.1)
- Factor II activity 48%
- Factor VII activity 60%
- Factor IX activity 51%
- Factor X activity 43%
- **Repeat laboratory results:** Hb 12.2, platelets 93, and PT 26.2 seconds
- Repeat laboratory tests following transfusion of red blood cells, FFP, and platelets
- Cranial ultrasound: Absent flow in the sagittal sinus consistent with thrombosis

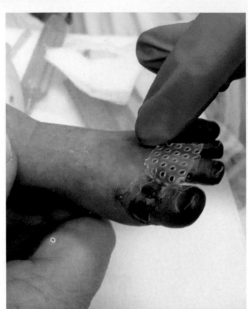

FIGURE 24.2 Necrosis of toes.

Results

Protein-C deficiency testing via PROC gene sequencing revealed the infant was heterozygous for two variants of uncertain significance, which explain her clinical presentation. A paternally inherited amino acid substitution (p.Gly403Arg) and a maternally inherited deletion (p.Ser119_Ser124del).

DIAGNOSIS

1. Neonatal purpura fulminans
2. Compound heterozygous protein-C deficiency

Treatment/Follow-up

Acute management consists of replacement of protein C as well as anticoagulation if thrombi are present. In this case, FFP was given every 12 hours initially, followed by Kcentra, a prothrombin complex concentrate product that contains all of the vitamin K-dependent factors. Protein C has the shortest half-life of all the vitamin K-dependent factors at 6 to 8 hours. A trough Protein-C level of >20% was achieved with q 8-hour dosing of Kcentra. Unfractionated heparin was initiated to treat the sagittal sinus thrombosis. A purified protein-C concentrate approved for this condition, Ceprotin, was initiated.

Long-term management consists of a combination of anticoagulation and protein-C replacement. Liver transplantation has been performed in some patients.

TEACHING POINTS

Homozygous protein-C deficiency is rare: there are an estimated <20 living individuals with this condition in North America. Given the carrier frequency of heterozygous protein-C deficiency of 0.2%, the estimated incidence of severe deficiency (typically compound heterozygous) should be 1 per million live births. As illustrated by this family, affected neonates may die without diagnosis. Protein C is a vitamin K–dependent factor that functions as an anticoagulant following activation by thrombin in the presence of the endothelial cofactor thrombomodulin. Activated protein-C degrades factors Va and VIIIa, thereby limiting further thrombin generation. The absence of protein-C leads to uncontrolled coagulation, manifest as DIC, thrombosis, and secondary hemorrhage. In newborns, this clinical picture, termed purpura fulminans, is easily mistaken for sepsis. Onset of clinical presentation typically occurs within 2 to 12 hours after birth. Affected infants may lack a red reflex if thrombosis occurs in the retina.

Suggested Readings

de Kort EH, Vrancken SL, van Heijst AF, Binkhorst M, Cuppen MP, Brons PP. Long-term subcutaneous protein C replacement in neonatal severe protein C deficiency. *Pediatrics*. 2011;127(5):e1338-e1342.

Goldenberg NA, Manco-Johnson MJ. Protein C deficiency. *Hemophilia*. 2008;14(6):1214-1221.

Minford A, Behnisch W, Brons P, et al. Subcutaneous protein C concentrate in the management of severe protein C deficiency—experience from 12 centres. *Br J Haematol*. 2014;164:414-421.

Price VE, Ledingham DL, Krumpel A, Chan AK. Diagnosis and management of neonatal purpura fulminans. *Semin Fetal Neonatal Med*. 2011;16(6):318-322.

25

Two Part Perf

Julia T. Warren

CHIEF COMPLAINT

"Big spleen"

HISTORY OF PRESENT ILLNESS

The patient is a 10-year-old girl with a 7-month history of a central nervous system (CNS) demyelinating disease, initially treated as multiphasic demyelinating encephalomyelitis (MDEM) or possibly CNS vasculitis, but with an inadequate response to steroids and rituximab. Due to her atypical and progressive clinical course, she underwent a computed tomography (CT) of chest/abdomen/pelvis to evaluate for possible alternative diagnoses—this revealed splenomegaly but no other findings. A follow-up positron emission tomography (PET) scan showed no metabolically active lesions. Her evaluations have included workup for autoimmune, infectious, neoplastic, and paraneoplastic processes. A brain biopsy showed a white matter–centered inflammatory demyelinating process including abundant CD3+ T-lymphocytes and CD68+ histiocytes in the perivascular and intraparenchymal regions, which were interpreted as nonspecific findings. She was referred to the hematology service for additional diagnostic evaluation of the splenomegaly.

PAST MEDICAL HISTORY

- Progressive CNS demyelinating disease (MDEM vs CNS vasculitis)
- Steroid-induced psychosis
- Seasonal allergies
- Recent left lower extremity traumatic sprain

Medications

- Prednisone
- Rituximab
- Acyclovir
- Keppra
- Famotidine
- Seroquel

Family/Social History

Parents are healthy; paternal cousin with epilepsy; no autoimmune diseases. Family not consanguineous.

EXAMINATION

- Vitals: T 36.8; HR 99; RR 18; BP 113/75; O_2Sat 100% on room air.
- General: Comfortable.
- HEENT: Normocephalic; **moon facies.** Conjunctiva clear, no scleral icterus. No drainage, no nasal masses. No oral lesions.

- Neck: Supple, full range of motion. No lymphadenopathy.
- Pulmonary/CV: Clear to auscultation, nonlabored. Regular rate and rhythm, normal peripheral pulses, good capillary refill.
- Abdomen: Soft, nontender, nondistended. **Splenomegaly palpable to 2 cm below the left costal margin,** no hepatomegaly, no masses. No inguinal lymphadenopathy.
- Extremities/MSK/skin: No edema, full range of motion, no contractures, no joint swelling. No rashes, bruises, pallor.
- Neurologic: Mental status appropriate. Cranial nerve examination notable for **horizontal nystagmus,** otherwise cranial nerves intact; strength 5/5 throughout, sensation intact; **dysmetria L > R on finger-nose-finger; heel-shin tests.** Gait assessment limited by left lower extremity cast but no obvious ataxia.

DIAGNOSTIC CONSIDERATIONS

- Autoimmune lymphoproliferative syndrome (ALPS). There are some case reports of this entity with CNS involvement.
- ALPS-like syndromes such as *CTLA4* or *LRBA* deficiency, also supported by a handful of cases with anecdotal CNS involvement.
- Isolated CNS hemophagocytic lymphohistiocytosis (HLH), supported by a few case reports.
- Other primary CNS processes, such as atypical for MDEM or CNS vasculitis. Previously had multiple CSF studies negative and brain biopsy analysis negative for a clonally expanded population, making CNS lymphoma unlikely. Biopsy findings and the clinical course were not consistent with neurosarcoidosis.

Investigation

1. CBC, CMP, LDH, fasting triglycerides, ferritin, PT/PTT, fibrinogen all normal
2. ALPS panel by flow cytometry uninterpretable due to chronic steroid use and absent B-cells from recent rituximab administration
3. ALPS next-generation sequencing (NGS) exome panel and targeted gene testing of *STAT3*, *CTLA4*, and *LRBA* normal
4. **HLH next generation sequencing (NGS) exome panel with heterozygous variant of unknown significance (VUS) in** *PRF1* **c.973T > C (p.Tyr325His)**

Results

The VUS in *PRF1* was in a highly conserved large, bulky hydrophobic amino acid present at an intermonomer interface and was predicted to be deleterious by multiple in silico prediction algorithms, raising the intriguing possibility that this heterozygous variant could act in a dominant fashion to affect perforin production or multimer stability. To confirm that the patient did indeed have a functional perforin deficiency, flow cytometric analysis of natural killer (NK) and cytotoxic CD8+ T-cells was sent, revealing **complete absence of perforin expression** on the cell surface. NK-cell activity was low, though challenging to interpret given the recent steroid administration. Soluble IL2 receptor (sIL2R) was normal. Parent-specific genetic analysis was undertaken showing that this missense mutation was inherited from her asymptomatic father. However, it also revealed that the patient and her mother carry a second VUS, c.1326_1328del (p.Phe443del), also predicted to be deleterious. This variant was not initially detected in the patient due to poor depth of sequencing coverage on the original NGS.

DIAGNOSIS

Familial hemophagocytic lymphohistiocytosis type 2/isolated CNS HLH secondary to compound heterozygous mutations in *PRF1*.

Treatment/Follow-up

She was started on HLH therapy with etoposide, intrathecal methotrexate, and high-dose dexamethasone as a bridge to a matched unrelated donor hematopoietic stem cell transplant.

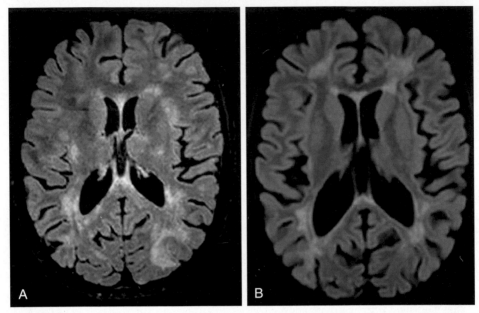

FIGURE 25.1 Brain MRI showing numerous T2 intense white matter lesions at the time of CNS HLH diagnosis (A) and improvement 1-year post-hematopoietic stem cell transplant (B). CNS, central nervous system; HLH, hemophagocytic lymphohistiocytosis; MRI, magnetic resonance image.

She achieved neuroinflammatory disease stabilization prior to transplant. She tolerated transplant extraordinarily well and 15 months post-transplant remained off immunosuppression without evidence of graft-versus-host disease. Her neurologic symptoms have resolved, and her brain magnetic resonance image (MRI) has greatly improved (Figure 25.1).

TEACHING POINTS

Isolated CNS HLH is an extraordinarily rare entity that requires a high index of suspicion and may have features overlapping with other CNS inflammatory disorders such as MDEM, CNS vasculitis, or Chronic Lymphocytic Inflammation with Pontine Perivascular Enhancement Responsive to Steroids. In case reports, serum markers (sIL2R, ferritin, triglycerides, CBC, CMP) and hemophagocytosis in the bone marrow, traditional diagnostic criteria for HLH, are normal or do not meet established cutoffs. Therefore, normal evaluations of systemic HLH manifestations should not preclude consideration of this diagnosis. Many of these patients may be currently taking, or have recent exposure to, immune-modulating drugs such as steroids; therefore, interpretation of NK-cell or CD8+ cytotoxic T-cell activity is particularly challenging. In this case, a bone marrow biopsy was not initially pursued as part of the diagnostic evaluation because (1) hemophagocytes in the bone marrow have limited specificity and would have been the only other positive diagnostic criteria besides splenomegaly, not permitting us to definitively confirm the diagnosis and (2) there is no clear criteria for what is considered "increased" numbers of hemophagocytes in the bone marrow, limiting the value of invasive bone marrow testing in this case. Though not currently included in the diagnostic criteria for HLH, flow cytometric testing for cell surface perforin and CD107a (and SAP, XIAP for males) is a straightforward way to help identify a potential case of familial HLH and should not necessarily be influenced by recent immune-modulatory therapy (with the exception of severe lymphopenia precluding adequate cell numbers for analysis).

 Genetic testing should be considered early in the diagnostic evaluation to avoid prolonged delays in diagnosis and to facilitate targeted treatment. However, this case also highlights an important point that NGS-based techniques are only as good as the depth of coverage in areas of interest. The only reason that the maternally inherited variant was identified is that parent-specific testing was performed using Sanger sequencing, and by chance, the maternal variant was in close proximity to the paternal variant of interest, allowing it to be identified. When clinical suspicion for an entity is high, functional testing should be performed whenever possible (in this case, cell surface expression of perforin by flow cytometry). Additionally, sometimes clinicians can request sequencing alignment files to perform a manual review for areas of low coverage or for missed variant calling. It is also worth noting that patients with CNS HLH likely will not have hemophagocytes on brain biopsy, as seen in this patient. A recent small histopathology case series has identified scattered perivascular inflammatory infiltrates in the brain biopsies of familial HLH patients with CNS involvement, a nonspecific finding that can also be observed with other inflammatory demyelinating processes. Finally, bone marrow transplant is the treatment of choice for familial HLH given the otherwise high likelihood of disease recurrence with immune modulation alone. A small series reported good outcomes for four pediatric patients with isolated CNS HLH who underwent hematopoietic stem cell transplantation.

Suggested Readings

Benson LA, Li H, Henderson LA, et al. Pediatric CNS-isolated hemophagocytic lymphohistiocytosis. *Neurol Neuroimmunol Neuroinflamm.* 2019;6(3):e560.

Dias C, McDonald A, Sincan M, et al. Recurrent subacute post-viral onset of ataxia associated with a PRF1 mutation. *Eur J Hum Genet.* 2013;21(11):1232-1239.

Feldmann J, Ménasché G, Callebaut I, et al. Severe and progressive encephalitis as a presenting manifestation of a novel missense perforin mutation and impaired cytolytic activity. *Blood.* 2005;105(7):2658-2663.

Gars E, Purington N, Scott G, et al. Bone marrow histomorphological criteria can accurately diagnose hemophagocytic lymphohistiocytosis. *Haematologica.* 2018;103(10):1635-1641.

Li H, Benson LA, Henderson LA, et al. Central nervous system—restricted familial hemophagocytic lymphohistiocytosis responds to hematopoietic cell transplantation. *Blood Adv.* 2019;3(4):503-507.

Marsh RA, Haddad E. How I treat primary haemophagocytic lymphohistiocytosis. *Br J Haematol.* 2018;182(2):185-199.

Moshous D, Feyen O, Lankisch P, et al. Primary necrotizing lymphocytic central nervous system vasculitis due to perforin deficiency in a four-year-old girl. *Arthritis Rheum.* 2007;56(3):995-999.

Pastula DM, Burish M, Reis GF, et al. Adult-onset central nervous system hemophagocytic lymphohistiocytosis: a case report. *BMC Neurol.* 2015;15(1):203.

Solomon IH, Li H, Benson LA, et al. Histopathologic correlates of familial hemophagocytic lymphohistiocytosis isolated to the central nervous system. *J Neuropathol Exp Neurol.* 2018;77(12):1079-1084.

26

Stumped
David B. Wilson

CHIEF COMPLAINT

"He has an infected belly button."

HISTORY OF PRESENT ILLNESS

A 10-week-old boy was seen for an infected belly button. He was born at 42 weeks by induced vaginal delivery without any pregnancy or delivery complications. The umbilical cord stump fell off at 17 days of age, but after it separated, the area became increasingly red, but without any drainage or bleeding. He was treated with oral antibiotics (cefalexin and clindamycin) without improvement. He developed a fever after his 2-month well-child check that was thought to be due to vaccination, but in light of persistent induration at the umbilicus, he was admitted to an outside hospital. He also had some left eye redness around the lacrimal duct with some scant drainage.

PAST MEDICAL HISTORY

- 42-week infant
- Omphalitis

Family/Social History

He has no siblings and lives with his parents, a dog, and two cats.

EXAMINATION

- Vitals: T = 37.3 °C, P = 148, R = 56, BP = 83/48, SpO_2 = 99%, Wt = 6.2 kg
- General: Alert, well nourished
- HEENT: Normocephalic, atraumatic, AFOF, PERRL, red reflex present bilaterally, redness around left lacrimal sac, TMs normal, MMM, and neck without adenopathy
- Lungs: Clear to auscultation, normal WOB, and good air movement
- Heart: Regular rate and rhythm, normal S1 and S2, and no murmur, rubs, or gallops
- Abdomen: Bowel sounds present, no masses, no organomegaly, and soft
- GU: Normal penis, testes present bilaterally, testes nontender, Tanner 1, and not circumcised
- Extremity: Extremities warm and well perfused, hips stable, and capillary refill 2 seconds
- Skin: Erythema around umbilicus particular on the left side (Figure 26.1)
- Neurologic: Alert, face symmetric, EOMI, moves all extremities, normal tone, positive Moro, and positive suck
- Back: Spine straight and no sacral abnormality

DIAGNOSTIC CONSIDERATIONS

- Omphalitis
- Leukocyte adhesion deficiency

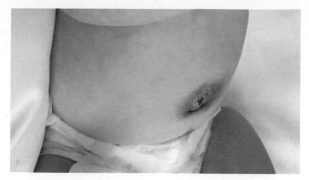

FIGURE 26.1 Photo of the umbilicus.

Investigation and Results

- Laboratory test results: WBC = 34.2, 90% neutrophils, Hb = 10.4, Hct = 30.4, and Plt = 604.
- CMP normal.
- DHR (detects defects in phagocyte oxidative burst) was normal.
- Flow cytometry of peripheral blood showed absent expression of CD18, CD11a, and CD11b.
- ITGB2 mutation analysis is pending.

DIAGNOSIS

1. Leukocyte adhesion deficiency (LAD), type 1
2. Delayed umbilical cord separation due to #1
3. Omphalitis due to #1

TEACHING POINTS

This is a textbook presentation of LAD. While exceedingly rare in real life, this clinical scenario is common on Pediatric Board examinations and is commonly discussed on rounds and consultations.

Omphalitis is a red flag for severely compromised phagocyte function and merits further testing. If the absolute neutrophil count (ANC) is low, the likely diagnosis is severe congenital neutropenia (SCN). If the ANC is high, the likely diagnosis is LAD.

Delayed umbilical cord separation is another hallmark of LAD.

The ITGB2 gene encodes the beta2-integrin subunit CD18. Integrins, cell-surface receptors that mediated binding to extracellular matrix, are composed of alpha and beta chains. A given alpha chain may combine with multiple beta chain partners, resulting in an array of functionally distinct integrins. The known binding partners of CD18 are CD11a, CD11b, CD11c, and CD11d.

Neutrophil adhesion and extravasation require intact function of beta2-integrins.

Lack of functional CD18 causes LAD, a condition characterized by a lack of leukocyte extravasation from blood into tissues and hence a markedly elevated circulating WBC.

The treatment is prompt hematopoietic stem cell transplantation. Donor selection (matched unrelated vs haploidentical) is underway.

Suggested Reading

van de Vijver E, van den Berg TK, Kuijpers TW. Leukocyte adhesion deficiencies. *Hematol Oncol Clin North Am.* 2013;27(1):101-116. doi:10.1016/j.hoc.2012.10.001

27

A Lot of O in TORCH

Miranda Edmunds

CHIEF COMPLAINT

Newborn with a blueberry muffin rash (Figure 27.1)

HISTORY OF PRESENT ILLNESS

The patient was born at 34 weeks via repeat Cesarean delivery to a now G4P3 mother. The pregnancy was complicated by rupture of membranes 10 days prior to delivery. Serologic testing of the patient's mother showed that she did not have immunity to rubella. There was no history of herpes infection, and group B strep testing was negative. Delivery was uncomplicated, the birth weight was 1.6 kg, and APGAR scores were 8 and 8. The infant was immediately noted to have a rash with diffuse lesions, some of which were ulcerative, and some of which resembled a blueberry muffin rash.

Medications

No maternal medications were taken during pregnancy.

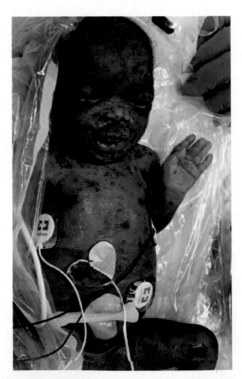

FIGURE 27.1   Diffuse ulcerative lesions with multiple sites of blue discoloration.

Family/Social History

No recent viral infections in mother or other family members

EXAMINATION

- Vitals on arrival: T 37.5, HR 153, RR 47, BP 56/25.
- General appearance: Preterm infant with features appropriate for gestational age.
- Head: Anterior fontanelle open soft and flat, diffuse rash over face and scalp.
- Eyes: Initially unable to examine eyes due to edema; however, absent red reflex bilaterally.
- Ears/nose/throat/palate: No ear pits or tags, nares appear patent, palate intact.
- Respiratory: Clear to auscultation bilaterally, no retractions, good aeration.
- Cardiovascular: Regular rate and rhythm, no murmur, femoral pulses 2+ bilaterally, brisk l capillary refill.
- Abdomen: Soft, nontender, nondistended, no hepatosplenomegaly.
- Skin: Diffuse, ulcerative skin lesions at different stages of healing, most prevalent on face, trunk, and extremities; also present on palms and soles. Areas of bluish discoloration, most prevalent on the trunk and face. No vesicles or bullae.
- Genitalia: Female—Tanner I.
- Anus: Appears patent.
- Spine: Straight, no sacral dimple or tuft.
- Extremities: No clavicular crepitus, hips stable without clicks or clunks.
- Neurologic: Asleep, arouses easily with examination; axial and appendicular tone is consistent with gestational age.

DIAGNOSTIC CONSIDERATIONS

Differential for bluish macules and papules and ulcerative lesions:

Infection	Neoplasm	Primary Skin Conditions
TORCH infections	Congenital leukemia cutis	Seborrheic dermatitis
Toxoplasmosis	Neuroblastoma	Impetigo
Other infections	Rhabdomyosarcoma	Erythema toxicum neonatorum
Syphilis	Langerhans cell histiocytosis	Transient neonatal pustular
Enterovirus	Primitive neuroectodermal	melanosis
Varicella-zoster virus	tumor	Neonatal erythropoiesis
Parvovirus B19		Disseminated neonatal
Zika		hemangiomatosis
Rubella		Infantile acropustulosis
Cytomegalovirus		
Herpes simplex virus		

Investigation

- Laboratory tests
  - CBC, CMP, PT/INR/PTT, serum varicella, serum HSV, RPR, rubella, toxoplasmosis, parvovirus B19, enterovirus, ANA/ENA, CMV
- Cultures
  - Blood
- Swabs
  - HSV, VZV, enterovirus
  - Fungal
- Consults
  - Infectious Disease, Dermatology, Ophthalmology
- Procedures
  - Eye examination, skin punch biopsies

Results

- Laboratory test results
  - CBC: Hbg 18.5, WBC 4.7, Plt 124; CMP and PT/INR/PTT: unremarkable
  - Serologies: Negative
  - Swabs: Negative
  - Cultures: Negative
- Procedures
  - Skin biopsy: Cells stained positive for CD1a and S100
  - Eye examination: Bilateral abnormal irides and cataracts

DIAGNOSIS

Langerhans cell histiocytosis (LCH) was diagnosed based on skin biopsy BRAF V600E positivity.

Treatment/Follow-up

1. Skeletal survey to determine the extent of disease involvement
2. Consultation with Hematology/Oncology
3. Isolated skin lesions: No treatment versus topical steroids
4. Systemic involvement: Chemotherapy versus immunotherapy

TEACHING POINTS

Although TORCH infections are an important diagnostic consideration in a neonate with a congenital rash and bilateral cataracts, primary neoplastic conditions should also be considered. LCH is a rare disease characterized by dysregulation of histiocytes, a cell in the dendritic cell lineage, infiltrating one or more organ systems. Penetrance of any organ system is possible with LCH but most often include the pituitary gland, liver, spleen, lungs, skin, and bone. The diverse presentation and heterogeneous organ involvement often lead to delayed diagnosis. The majority of patients present with cutaneous lesions, although lesion characteristics are extremely variable and do not confer any prognostic information regarding multisystem disease. While neonatal LCH is rare (1 per million neonates), full-term infants commonly present with limited cutaneous lesions that regress and are not associated with systemic disease. In contrast, premature infants are more likely to have severe systemic disease. Infants with LCH should undergo screening to assess for multiorgan disease, including a thorough physical examination, complete blood cell count, coagulation studies, liver function tests, urine osmolality, chest radiograph, and skeletal survey. The degree of organ involvement determines treatment approach, which may range from minimal therapy for lesions confined to the skin to chemotherapeutic or immunotherapeutic agents for significant systemic disease. This patient had no definite systemic involvement but was eventually treated with immunotherapy directed toward BRAF-positive LCH cells because of worsening clinical status, which included respiratory failure, bloody stools, and sepsis.

Suggested Readings

Allen CE, Merad M, Mcclain KL. Langerhans-cell histiocytosis. *N Engl J Med.* 2018;379:856-868. doi:10.1056/nejmra1607548

Inoue M, Tomita Y, Egawa T, Ioroi T, Kugo M, Imashuku S. A fatal case of congenital Langerhans cell histiocytosis with disseminated cutaneous lesions in a premature neonate. *Case Rep Pediatr.* 2016;2016:1-4. doi:10.1155/2016/4972180

Krooks J, Minkov M, Weatherall AG. Langerhans cell histiocytosis in children. *J Am Acad Dermatol.* 2018;78(6):1047-1056.

Poompuen S, Chaiyarit J, Techasatian L. Diverse cutaneous manifestation of Langerhans cell histiocytosis: a 10-year retrospective cohort study. *Eur J Pediatr.* 2019;178(5):771-776. doi:10.1007/s00431-019-03356-1

Satter EK, High WA. Langerhans cell histiocytosis: a review of the current recommendations of the Histiocyte Society. *Pediatr Dermatol.* 2008;25(3):291-295. doi:10.1111/j.1525-1470.2008.00669.x

Singh A, Mandal A, Singh L, Mishra S, Patel A. Delayed treatment response in a neonate with multisystem Langerhans cell histiocytosis: case report and review of literature. *Sultan Qaboos Univ Med J.* 2017;17:e225-e228. doi:10.18295/squmj.2016.17.02.016

28

Pod Problems

Cory P. Miller

CHIEF COMPLAINT

Weight loss, nausea, vomiting, and shortness of breath

HISTORY OF PRESENT ILLNESS

A 17-year-old boy presented to the emergency department (ED) with 42 lb of unintentional weight loss over the past 4 to 5 months. He was also nauseous and had been vomiting after meals for the past 3 to 4 weeks. In the last 2 weeks, he has had gradually worsening shortness of breath. Five days prior to presentation, he went to a different ED for these same symptoms, where an abdominal computed tomography (CT) scan showed mild splenomegaly and changes read as "bronchitis" in the lower lung fields. Blood work was largely normal, including AST and ALT and a total bilirubin of 1.2. He was prescribed azithromycin and discharged home. Due to lack of improvement, he presented to a third ED.

In addition to weight loss, nausea, vomiting, and shortness of breath, he was also having night sweats, intermittent chest pain that worsened with deep inspiration, muscle aches, fatigue, and generalized abdominal pain. He had no fevers, rash, diarrhea, bowel movement changes, dysuria, hematuria, or polydipsia.

PAST MEDICAL HISTORY

Healthy

Family/Social History

No leukemia, lymphoma, liver malignancies, or autoimmune diseases such as rheumatoid arthritis, systemic lupus erythematosus (SLE), diabetes, or autoimmune hepatitis.

He lives with his mother. He denies any outdoor expeditions, camping, or cave spelunking. He has four dogs and one cat. He has no exposure to farm animals or reptiles.

He admitted to using marijuana "once in a blue moon," most recently 1.5 weeks ago. With more conversation and questioning, he admits to smoking tetrahydrocannabinol (THC) daily. He primarily takes THC via inhalation of **THC wax** with the use of a vaping pen. In addition to his THC use, he smokes one JUUL pod per day. He has done this for the past 1.5 years. He buys his JUUL pods from a local store, not online. He says he quit smoking the pods 5 days ago.

EXAMINATION

- Vitals: T 99.7, P 133, RR 28, BP 114/71, 91% O_2.
- General: He is thin and malnourished with jaundiced skin and yellow eyes.
- Eyes: Pupils are equally reactive and round to light. He has scleral icterus bilaterally. Extraocular movements intact.
- Ears: External ears and tympanic membranes appear normal.
- Nose: No drainage.
- Mouth: Oral mucosa is pink and moist. Posterior pharynx nonerythematous.
- Neck: Supple. No cervical lymphadenopathy.

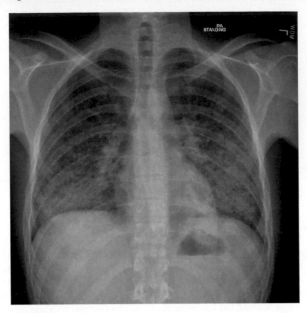

FIGURE 28.1 Chest x-ray.

- Lungs/chest: Diffuse crackles in the lower lung fields. No wheezes or rales. No subcostal or intercostal retractions.
- Heart: Regular rate and rhythm. No murmur. S1 and S2 present.
- Abdomen: Thin abdomen. Normal active bowel sounds. No distention. Mild tenderness to deep palpation over epigastric region. No masses or organomegaly.
- Skin: Jaundiced. Cap refill 2 to 3 seconds.
- Neuro: Alert and interactive. No altered mental status. Cranial nerves intact. Strength 5/5 in all four extremities. No sensory deficits.

Diagnostic Considerations

Weight loss, vomiting, cachexia, and crackles suggest either a chronic lung infection such as tuberculosis or an autoimmune disease such as granulomatosis with polyangiitis. Other considerations include malignancy, human immunodeficiency virus (HIV), viral hepatitis, Epstein-Barr virus (EBV), cytomegalovirus (CMV), or histoplasmosis.

Investigation

1. CBC, complete metabolic panel, GGT, ESR, CRP, coagulation studies, total/direct bilirubin, ferritin
2. Respiratory viral panel, HIV PCR, hepatitis viral panel, EBV PCR, CMV PCR, HSV PCR, histoplasmosis antibodies, T-spot
3. LDH, aldolase, haptoglobin, uric acid, peripheral blood smear
4. CXR (Figure 28.1) followed by chest/abdomen/pelvis CT (Figure 28.2)
5. Liver failure laboratory tests: Anti–smooth muscle antibody, copper, ceruloplasmin, liver/kidney microsome type 1 antibody, acylcarnitine, ammonia, AFP tumor marker, CK, and acetaminophen level

Results

Complete blood count showed WBC 17.2/mm³ (90% neutrophils), hemoglobin 11.9 g/dL, and platelets 330/mm³. Complete metabolic panel showed unremarkable electrolytes but elevated levels of total bilirubin 3.7 mg/dL, direct bilirubin 2.8 mg/dL, ALT 286 U/L,

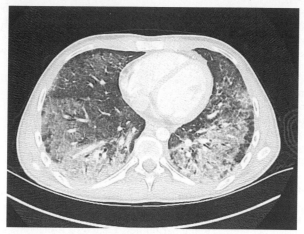

FIGURE 28.2 Chest computed tomography (CT).

AST 382 U/L, and GGT 102 U/L. Ferritin was high at 1010 ng/mL. C-reactive protein (CRP) and ESR were both elevated at 395 mg/L and 87 mm/h, respectively. Coagulation studies were prolonged with PTT of 42.5 seconds and PT of 24.3 seconds. These results combined with the elevated liver enzymes were suggested the possibility of acute liver failure. In response to these laboratory test results, acute liver failure laboratory tests were ordered (listed above) and came back negative.

The chest x-ray (Figure 28.1) showed "bilateral, mid-lower hazy airspace opacities suspicious for multifocal pneumonia." In response to these findings and the patient's overall clinical picture, a chest/abdomen/pelvic CT was done (Figure 28.2) which showed "diffuse ground-glass opacity involving the lungs in a noncardiogenic edema pattern with areas of tree-in-bud nodularity as well as diffuse bilateral hilar and mediastinal lymphadenopathy."

Malignancy screening laboratory tests were done which were normal. Lactate dehydrogenase, haptoglobin, and aldolase were only slightly elevated. Peripheral blood smear was examined and no blasts were present.

Infectious workup including a respiratory viral panel, hepatitis panel, HSV, HIV, EBV, and CMV PCRs were all negative. *Histoplasma*, *Blastomyces*, and *Bartonella* antibodies were negative.

DIAGNOSIS

E-cigarette or vaping product use–associated lung injury, aka **EVALI**

Treatment/Follow-up

He was admitted and several services were consulted, including infectious diseases, pulmonary, GI, toxicology, rheumatology, and hematology. No unifying diagnosis was identified, and EVALI was thought most likely based on the burgeoning story of drug use. On hospitalization day 7, he underwent a lung and lymph node biopsy which demonstrated signs of pulmonary hypertension, multifocal organizing pneumonia, and parenchymal necrosis. He was prescribed prednisone at 2 mg/kg/d. His laboratory tests and clinical symptoms improved throughout the hospitalization, and he was discharged home with firm instructions to avoid vaping.

TEACHING POINTS

E-cigarette use has become epidemic in the United States, and its usage is skyrocketing throughout the nation. According to the Monitoring the Future survey, a national survey polling 12th, 10th, and 8th graders about their vaping nicotine usage, E-cigarette usage has nearly doubled in all three populations from 2017 to 2019. With increased usage of E-cigarettes in young populations, medical professionals are starting to see side effects and complications from these products at increasing rates. As of December 3, 2019, there have been 2291 E-cigarette or vaping product use–associated lung injury hospitalizations (EVALI is a term that now describes this syndrome) from the 50 states, the District of Columbia, and two US territories. The risk of bronchitis-like symptoms is almost doubled in youth who use E-cigarettes compared to never users. As with pulmonary symptoms, gastrointestinal symptoms are also very common, occurring in 81% of patients from Illinois and Wisconsin in a preliminary report on EVALI cases in those states.

The alarming increase in hospitalizations for EVALI highlights the difficulty physicians face when it comes to educating youth against the harm of what is widely considered a benign habit. The specific lesson in this case is the importance of taking a thorough history, including specifically asking about the frequency of vaping, the names of products and brands used, and the mode of acquisition of these products.

Suggested Readings

Berry KM, Fetterman JL, Benjamin EJ, et al. Association of electronic cigarette use with subsequent initiation of tobacco cigarettes in US youths. *JAMA Netw Open*. 2019;2(2):e187794.

Layden JE, Ghinai I, Pray I, et al. Pulmonary illness related to E-cigarette use in Illinois and Wisconsin—final report. *N Engl J Med*. 2020;382(10):903-916. PMID: 31491072.

McConnell R, Barrington-Trimis JL, Wang K, et al. Electronic cigarette use and respiratory symptoms in adolescents. *Am J Respir Crit Care Med*. 2017;195(8):1043-1049.

Outbreak of Lung Injury Associated With the Use of E-Cigarette, or Vaping, Products. Centers for Disease Control and Prevention; 2019.

29

Murphy's Sign of the Times

Andrew J. White, Francisco Javier Gortes

Chief Complaint

Belly pain

History of Present Illness

A 14-year-old girl presented to an outside hospital emergency department (OSH ED) with 1 day of right-sided abdominal pain with bilious emesis and dizziness. In the ED, she vomited again and was given Toradol and a normal saline (NS) bolus. Physical examination was notable for some mild abdominal pain but no guarding. Lungs were clear, and she did not appear dehydrated. HR was 125, and BP was 120/80. Glucose was 122, ALT 66, and lipase 361. WBC 11.9, Hgb 9.4, and platelets 181. Abdominal x-ray was normal, except for a small metallic foreign body in the transverse colon.

She was admitted to the gastroenterology (GI) service for possible bowel obstruction.

On admission, she was afebrile and HR was 110 with normal blood pressure. An abdominal ultrasound showed a moderate amount of free fluid in the pelvis, which prompted a computer tomography (CT) scan.

Past Medical History

Unremarkable

Medications

None

Family/Social History

Lives with mother, father, sister, and a step-brother.

Examination

- Vitals: BP = 120/77, pulse = 137, Temp = 36.2 °C, Resp = 20, Spo_2 96%, Ht = 163 cm, Wt = 60.3 kg, and BMI 22.7 kg/m^2.
- General: No acute distress.
- HEENT: Normocephalic, atraumatic, pupils equal, EOMs grossly intact, neck supple, and trachea midline.
- RESP: Clear to auscultation bilaterally, normal effort.
- CARDIO: RRR, no murmur, rub, or gallop.
- ABDOMEN: Soft, nondistended, but tender with palpation throughout all quadrants, but worse in **RLQ with rebound tenderness.** A small crusted abrasion is present on the flank, 0.5 × 0.5 cm^2.
- GU: Normal genitalia, no hernias, no masses, no discharge or signs of infection.
- Ext: No cyanosis, clubbing, or edema. Warm and well perfused.
- Musculoskeletal: Grossly normal range of motion.
- Lymphatic: No cervical, supraclavicular, axillary, or inguinal lymphadenopathy.

- Neuro: Alert and oriented × 3.
- Psych: Appropriate mood and affect.

DIAGNOSTIC CONSIDERATIONS

- Obstruction from foreign body ingestion
- Appendicitis, with Murphy sign
- Loxoscelism (*long shot*) with hemolysis (perhaps the flank lesion could be a spider bite?)

Investigation

A CT of the abdomen and pelvis was performed to exclude or confirm obstruction or appendicitis (Figures 29.1 and 29.2).

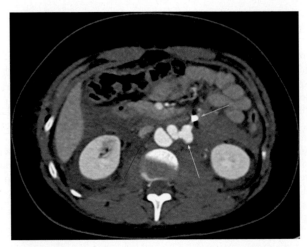

FIGURE 29.1 Bullet fragment (green arrow) is noted in the midabdomen. There is a large pseudoaneurysm of the infrarenal abdominal aorta (yellow arrow) with surrounding massive retroperitoneal and intraperitoneal hemorrhage. Thrombus in the inferior vena cava (blue arrow) is secondary to penetrating injury.

Results

Evidence of a **gunshot wound** is apparent to hepatic segment 6 (grade 4 with active extravasation), and the second portion of the duodenum, and the pancreatic head with massive hemoperitoneum and pneumoperitoneum. Active extravasation is apparent, most likely emanating from the aorta.

DIAGNOSIS

Gunshot wound, abdomen, unrecognized

Treatment/Follow-up

She underwent immediate exploratory laparotomy, with duodenal perforation repair, and repair of the injured infrarenal abdominal aorta using cryopreserved aortic graft as conduit, as well as primary repair of the infrarenal inferior vena cava (IVC). The intracolonic foreign body was confirmed as a bullet. She remained hospitalized for 28 days but was eventually discharged home in good condition.

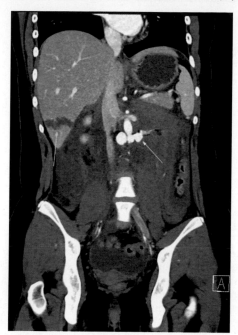

FIGURE 29.2 There is a large pseudoaneurysm of the infrarenal abdominal aorta (yellow arrow) with surrounding massive retroperitoneal and intraperitoneal hemorrhage. Also noted is a laceration through hepatic segment six (green arrow).

TEACHING POINTS

The patient did not disclose to medical providers that she suspected she had been shot until directly questioned by the surgery resident (post-CT scan). The patient's step-brother has been involved with gangs, and the family's home has been struck by gunfire several times over the past year. In hindsight, the parents heard a loud noise the night prior to admission, which may have been a gunshot outside the house that hit the patient. Police/Department of Forensic Science (DFS) were subsequently engaged to investigate the incident.

Gun violence accounts for 18,000 murders and 35,000 suicides annually. Approximately 67,000 people survive gun injuries annually according to the National Center for Injury Prevention and Control. We are currently experiencing higher than our (already high) typical amount of gun violence this year.

US homicide rates are 6.9 times higher than rates in the other high-income countries, driven in part by firearm homicide rates that are 19.5 times higher. For 15- to 24-year-olds, firearm homicide rates in the United States are 42.7 times higher than in the other countries.

It is unclear how she was able to survive the active bleeding from her injured aorta.

Suggested Readings

Hofmann LJ, Keric N, Cestero RF, et al. Trauma surgeons' perspective on gun violence and a review of the literature. *Cureus*. 2018;10:e3599.

Lewiecki EM, Miller SA. Suicide, guns, and public policy. *Am J Public Health*. 2013;103:27-31.

Richardson EG, Hemenway D. Homicide, suicide, and unintentional firearm fatality: comparing the United States with other high-income countries, 2003. *J Trauma*. 2011;70:238-243.

30

Spurge

Roger D. Yusen, Andrew J. White

CHIEF COMPLAINT

"Swollen eyes"

HISTORY OF PRESENT ILLNESS

An 11-year-old girl woke up and noticed her right eyelid was swollen and her face and ears were red. She did not take her daily cetirizine yesterday, and so she took 25 mg diphenhydramine at 0730 hours. It did not seem to help much. The day before the rash, she did not notice any swelling but had been experiencing increasing allergy symptoms such as rhinorrhea over the past week. She has had no new foods or medications and has no new pets and no new animal exposures. She has no pain when she moves her eyes around, and no blurry vision or double vision. She has not had any fevers, shortness of breath, cough, or rash. She also denies any recent trauma, injuries, or falls.

She had a similar episode a few years ago that was treated with diphenhydramine and resolved in a matter of days. No one in her family or circle of friends has been sick recently. She went to the local emergency department to seek treatment.

- ROS:
  - Yes: Clear nasal discharge
  - No: Fever, red/pink eyes, discharge from eyes, no discharge from ears, sore throat, no cough, SOB, vomiting, diarrhea, abdominal pain, blood in stools, decreased urination, pain with urination, low energy, bleeding, extremity swelling\tenderness, or swollen glands

PAST MEDICAL HISTORY

Environmental allergies

Medications

Cetirizine

Family/Social History

FH: No asthma, atopy, or recurrent infections.
SH: Lives with her family without secondhand smoke exposure.

EXAMINATION

Well-nourished, alert, attentive, but in **obvious discomfort from her swollen face** and eyelids.

- Vitals: T – 36.7, and RR – 24.
- Head: **Obvious swelling of the entire face and eyelids. Erythematous rash on cheeks and ears.**
- Eyes: PERRL, EOMI, and conjunctiva clear. **No tenderness on eye movement or pain to eye palpation.**
- Ears: TMs gray and translucent, normal landmarks bilateral, insufflation not done.

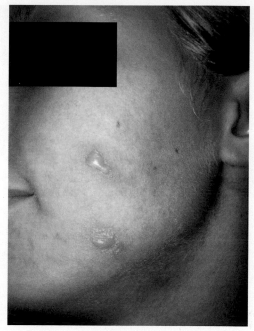

FIGURE 30.1 Bullae and erythema on the cheeks.

- Nose: No nasal flaring, no nasal discharge.
- Mouth: No decreased moisture.
- Throat: No tonsillar inflammation or exudate, no uvula deviation.
- Neck: Supple, no neck tenderness, no adenopathy.
- Chest wall: No tenderness. No chest wall retractions, no deformity.
- Lungs: No stridor, no wheezing, no rales, no rhonchi, no grunting, no accessory muscle use. Good air exchange.
- Heart: Normal rate, normal rhythm, no murmur, no rub.
- Abdomen: Soft, nontender, no guarding, no rebound, no organomegaly, no masses.
- Extremities: No swelling\tenderness, good pulses all extremities, capillary refill <2 seconds
- Skin: Warm, dry, good color, no rash.
- Neuro: Motor intact, sensory intact.

DIAGNOSTIC CONSIDERATIONS

Notes from the ED physician; "Edema from **environmental allergies**. Less likely **anaphylaxis** or **cellulitis**. Will treat with cetirizine and diphenhydramine 1 mg/kg. Will call PMD for close follow-up tomorrow to ensure this is not an early cellulitis and that the edema is improving." She was sent home on antihistamines.

Investigation and Results

The following day, the rash became **vesicular** (Figure 30.1), and she went back to the ED.

New diagnostic considerations:

- Impetigo
- Zoster
- Rhus dermatitis (aka poison ivy)
- Contact dermatitis

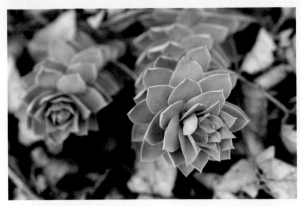

FIGURE 30.2 Myrtle spurge (*Euphorbia myrsinites*). (Photo courtesy photos-public-domain.com.)

While sitting in the ED waiting room, the patient's friend texted her saying that she had developed a weird rash on her cheeks and eyelids and was on her way to the ED at that very moment.

Upon further questioning, the girls had been playing together in the neighbor's yard and garden and had taken some leaves and berries from various plants to make "**potions**" including the one pictured below. They did not drink the potions but did apply them to their cheeks and eyelids like makeup.

The culprit is myrtle spurge (*Euphorbia myrsinites*) (Figure 30.2). It is well described (*in the gardening literature at least*) that the milky white sap causes severe cutaneous reactions.

DIAGNOSIS

Spurge dermatitis (contact dermatitis from the spurge plant)

Treatment/Follow-up

Topical steroids and antihistamines

TEACHING POINTS

Contact dermatitis from plants is relatively common. Most physicians are very familiar with poison ivy, oak, and sumac, but there are a number of other plants that can cause similar reactions. These syndromes may be broken down into categories according to the specific mechanism of reaction, as well as timing onset and duration of rash. They include contact dermatitis (onset of minutes to hours, duration of hours to days), a nonimmunologic contact urticaria (onset within minutes to an hour, duration of hours to 1 day), allergic contact dermatitis (onset of 24-48 hours, duration of up to a week), and a phytophotodermatitis (onset within 8-48 hours and duration of years in some cases) caused by photosensitizing agents like psoralens present in some plants.

In this case, the girls themselves held the key to the diagnosis; the doctors, however, failed to uncover enough history.

Suggested Reading

Modi GM, Doherty CB, Katta R, Orengo IF. Irritant contact dermatitis from plants. *Dermatitis.* 2009;20(2):63-78.

31

Under Pressure

Áine Cooke

CHIEF COMPLAINT

Shortness of breath

HISTORY OF PRESENT ILLNESS

A 16-year-old girl with a history of mild intermittent asthma presents to the emergency room complaining of 3 days of shortness of breath. She denies any sick symptoms or exposure to her known asthma triggers; indeed, her asthma is usually exacerbated by allergies in the Spring, and this visit occurs in November.

In triage, she is in mild respiratory distress and tells the nurse "my inhaler isn't helping like it usually does." The experienced triage nurse categorizes her presentation as *mild asthma exacerbation*, and she is given oral steroids and initiated on albuterol treatments.

When the physician staffing the emergency room is eventually able to examine the lower acuity patients, he is surprised to find that the young woman here with a *mild asthma exacerbation* is now demonstrating severe work of breathing and grunting and is unable to talk in complete sentences. The bedside registered nurse commented "she's just got worse and worse since she got here." While examining the patient, the physician notes that the blood pressure cuff is far too big and asks the nurse to obtain an appropriate size cuff (the patient care technician had upsized the cuff multiple times before obtaining a "good reading"). Plans to obtain vascular access and perform expedient laboratory and imaging diagnostics along with transfer to the intensive care unit are established while the following information is obtained from family: She does not use oral contraceptives and has not experienced chest pain, leg swelling, orthopnea, recent travel, or exercise intolerance.

PAST MEDICAL HISTORY

- Mild intermittent asthma.
- Presented to an urgent care center 6 months earlier with abdominal pain. On that visit, a blood pressure of 195/110 mm Hg was documented, she was prescribed carvedilol, which was never filled because of cost, and no follow-up evaluation for hypertension was pursued.

Medications

- Albuterol MDI PRN

Family/Social History

- No hypertension, cardiac disease, or blood clots.
- She has never been sexually active and has never used illicit substances.

EXAMINATION

- Vitals: T 37.0, HR 165, RR 35, **blood pressure 200/130**, pulse oximetry 91%.
- General: Thin teenage girl sitting up in bed, sweaty and in distress.
- HEENT: Oral mucosa is moist, PERRL, EOMI, conjunctiva and sclera are white.

- Pulmonary: Diminished breath sounds over lung bases with bibasilar crackles; no wheezing. Severely increased work of breathing along with sustained tachypnea, unable to speak in full sentences.
- Cardiovascular: Tachycardic; S1, S2, S3, and S4 are present; prominent jugular venous pulsation, peripheral pulses are bounding; hands and feet are cool with a central capillary refill time of 4 seconds.
- Abdomen: Soft, nontender, liver edge is palpable 8 cm below the right costal margin. No masses are present.
- Skin: No rashes, cyanosis, or lesions.
- Extremities: No joint deformities or edema.
- Neurological: Awake and alert, answers questions and follows commands appropriately, moving all four extremities.

DIAGNOSTIC CONSIDERATIONS

Causes of a hypertensive emergency include the following:

- Renovascular disease, such as renal artery stenosis
- Ingestion (PCP, cocaine)
- Serotonin syndrome
- Thyrotoxicosis
- Acute intermittent porphyria
- Eclampsia
- Myocarditis
- Dissection of the aorta

Investigation

- Labs:
  - CBC: WNL
  - CMP normal except for *glucose 152 mg/dL*
  - Free T4 and TSH WNL
  - D-dimer = WNL
  - *BNP = 2968 (nl 0-39)*
  - Troponin I = 0.08 (nl < 0.03)
  - Tumor markers: Blood metanephrines = 0.83 nM (nl < 0.5), *blood normetanephrines = 77 nM (nl < 0.9)*
- Imaging:
  - Chest x-ray: *Pulmonary edema*
  - Echocardiogram: *Mildly dilated LV with severely decreased systolic function. A 3-cm diameter intra-abdominal mass was noticed during the echocardiogram, prompting additional imaging*
  - CT (chest/abdomen/pelvis with contrast): *Bilateral suprarenal masses (3 cm on the right and 5 cm on the left)*

DIAGNOSES

1. **Pheochromocytoma (PC) crisis**, due to
2. **Bilateral PC**, causing
3. **Left ventricular systolic dysfunction**

Treatment/Follow-up

She was in a hypertensive crisis, with secondary heart failure, due to bilateral PC discovered fortuitously on echocardiogram and later confirmed on CT. Administration of albuterol may have exacerbated the heart failure due to tachycardia.

She was intubated to offset cardiac afterload and treat respiratory failure. Nicardipine was initiated, but her cardiac function deteriorated. She progressed to acute renal failure and was treated with chronic renal replacement therapy (CRRT) and, eventually, extracorporeal membrane oxygenation (ECMO) to augment cardiac pump function.

Prior to surgical resection, blood pressure control was maintained for 4 weeks. She underwent right-sided complete adrenalectomy and left partial adrenalectomy, which was tolerated well; subsequently, she was able to be extubated and taken off ECMO and CRRT.

Follow-up imaging showed no evidence of tumor recurrence and blood levels of both metanephrines and normetanephrines normalized after surgery.

Genetic testing showed a germline pathogenic variant in *MAX*, a variant that has been reported in several unrelated individuals with PCs.

Physical therapy, voice rehabilitation, and appointments with cardiology (heart function), endocrinology (adrenal hormone level management post adrenalectomy), and heme-oncology (surveillance of tumor markers) were prescribed after she was discharged from the hospital. Her systolic function recovered over time and her kidney function has returned to normal.

TEACHING POINTS

PCs are catecholamine (epinephrine, norepinephrine, and dopamine) secreting tumors arising from the chromaffin cells of the adrenal medulla. PCs are rare tumors with an estimated annual incidence of approximately 0.8 per 100,000 person-years, which may be an underestimate as autopsy series have shown that many cases are missed. Most PCs are sporadic tumors that occur in middle adulthood, but approximately 40% occur as a part of a familial disorder.

Hereditary PCs are more likely to present during childhood and are also more likely to be bilateral with concomitant paragangliomas (catecholamine secreting tumors arising from sympathetic ganglia that are histologically identical to PCs but are more apt to metastasize than the intra-adrenal PC). There are several familial disorders associated with adrenal PC, all of which have autosomal dominant inheritance: von Hippel-Lindau syndrome, multiple endocrine neoplasia type 2, and less commonly, neurofibromatosis type 1.

The presentation of PCs can range from an incidental finding on imaging in an asymptomatic individual to a PC crisis. The classic triad of symptoms for PC are headache, sweating, and tachycardia; although most patients do not present with all three symptoms. Other common complaints are anxiety, abdominal pain, palpitations, and headache. PCs should be on the differential for a child suffering from treatment-resistant hypertension or for paroxysmal hypertension (often precipitated by an invasive procedure). Patients with familial disorders that are associated with PCs or family history of PC should also be intermittently screened.

A PC crisis is a dreaded and rare sequela of PC, categorized by afterload-induced cardiomyopathy, which leads to pulmonary edema and eventual total circulatory collapse. Treatment of PC is surgical resection of the tumor. However, due to the catecholamines secreted by the tumor, alpha receptors on blood vessels are activated, leading to constriction and the hallmark hypertension. During resection of the tumor, the source of excess catecholamine secretion is abruptly removed, which can lead to life-threatening blood pressure fluctuations during surgery. Therefore, it is imperative that prior to resection of the tumor, patients are administered drugs that confer alpha blockade (prazosin, phenoxybenzamine). A minimum duration of 2 weeks is suggested.

While PCs are a rare cause of hypertension in general, this case illustrates a known clinical blind spot: the poor recognition of hypertension in children. One large cohort study found that 3.6% of children and adolescents met criteria for hypertension, but only 26% of those who met criteria had been diagnosed. Blood pressure should be taken from 3 years of age at well-child checks *with an appropriately sized cuff*. The cuff should not be upsized to obtain a "normal value." Blood pressure measurements should be checked against normalized values for children and adolescents based on age, sex, and height, and these are available in standardized tables (Table 31.1). Hypertension in a child should always warrant concern.

TABLE 31.1 Updated Definitions of BP Categories and Stages

For Children Aged 1-13 y	For Children Aged 13 y and older
Normal BP: <90th percentile	Normal BP: <120/<80 mm Hg
Elevated BP: ≥90th percentile to <95th percentile or 120/80 mm Hg to <95th percentile (whichever is lower)	Elevated BP: 120/<80-129/<80 mm Hg
Stage 1 HTN: ≥95th percentile to <95th percentile + 12 mm Hg or 130/80-139/89 mm Hg (whichever is lower)	Stage 1 HTN: 130/80-139/89 mm Hg
Stage 2 HTN: ≥95th percentile + 12 mm Hg or ≥140/90 mm Hg (whichever is lower)	Stage 2 HTN: ≥140/90 mm Hg

BP, blood pressure; HNT, hypertension.
Reprinted from Flynn JT, Kaelber DC, Baker-Smith CM, et al; Subcommittee on Screening and Management of High Blood Pressure in Children. Clinical practice guideline for screening and management of high blood pressure in children and adolescents. *Pediatrics.* 2017;140(3):e20171904.

Suggested Readings

Beard CM, Sheps SG, Kurland LT, Carney JA, Lie JT. Occurrence of pheochromocytoma in Rochester, Minnesota, 1950 through 1979. *Mayo Clin Proc.* 1983;58(12):802.

Chao A, Yeh YC, Yen TS, Chen YS. Phaeochromocytoma crisis—A rare indication for extracorporeal membrane oxygenation. *Anaesthesia.* 2008;63(1):86-88.

Flynn JT, Kaelber DC, Baker-Smith CM, Blowey D, Carroll AE. Clinical practice guideline for screening and management of high blood pressure in children and adolescents. *Pediatrics.* 2017;140(3):e20171904.

Hansen ML, Gunn PW, Kaelber DC. Underdiagnosis of hypertension in children and adolescents. *J Am Med Assoc.* 2007;298(8):874-879.

Mercado-Asis LB, Wolf KI, Jochmanova I, Taïeb D. Pheochromocytoma: a genetic and diagnostic update. *Endocr Pract.* 2018;24:78-90.

Rednam SP, Erez A, Druker H, et al. Von Hippel-Lindau and hereditary pheochromocytoma/paraganglioma syndromes: clinical features, genetics, and surveillance recommendations in childhood. *Clin Cancer Res.* 2017;23:e68-e75.

Sutton MG, Sheps SG, Lie J. Prevalence of clinically unsuspected pheochromocytoma. Review of a 50-year autopsy series. *Mayo Clin Proc.* 1981;56(6):354-360.

Taïeb D, Jha A, Guerin C, et al. 18F-FDOPA PET/CT imaging of MAX-related pheochromocytoma. *J Clin Endocrinol Metab.* 2018;103:1574-1582.

32

Don't Give Me Any Lip

Katherine Ferguson

CHIEF COMPLAINT

"Breathing hard"

HISTORY OF PRESENT ILLNESS

A 7-week-old presents with 6 days of cough, rhinorrhea, and noisy breathing. She was taken to her pediatrician 5 days ago who diagnosed bronchiolitis. Two days ago, she was taken to the emergency department (ED) where she was diagnosed with a viral illness and nasal suction was recommended. The noisy breathing worsened, and she looked like she was working harder to breathe, so she was taken back to the ED. She has not had fever. Recently, mom has been having to wake her to feed and has been giving her smaller volumes.

PAST MEDICAL HISTORY

She was born at 38 weeks via Cesarean section due to maternal preeclampsia. Mom was group B streptococcus positive. The infant has received two hepatitis B vaccinations. Her newborn screen was normal aside from sickle cell trait. Her growth has been appropriate.

Family/Social History

Lives with mom and dad. No other children in the home. Does not attend daycare.

EXAMINATION

- Vitals: T 36.7, HR 144, RR 60, BP 80/50, Spo$_2$ 100% on RA.
- General: Awake, alert, strong cry, breathing quickly and forcefully.
- HEENT: Normocephalic, anterior fontanelle soft and flat. Conjunctivae clear, no drainage or injection. Ears with clear and intact TMs, patent EAC. Clear nasal drainage, nares patent. Moist mucous membranes, palate intact.
- Neck: Supple, no lymphadenopathy, no masses
- Pulm: High-pitched inspiratory and expiratory stridor at rest, coarse breath sounds throughout. Subcostal and supraclavicular retractions are prominent.
- CV: Tachycardia, regular rhythm, no murmur/rub/gallop. Femoral pulses palpable and symmetric.
- Abdomen: Soft, nontender, nondistended, no masses, or organomegaly.
- Neuro: Alert, face symmetric, EOMI. Moves all extremities spontaneously, normal tone.
- Skin: Warm and dry. No rash, capillary refill 3 to 4 seconds.
- Extremities: No edema or deformity.

DIAGNOSTIC CONSIDERATIONS

- Viral bronchiolitis
- Laryngomalacia
- Tracheomalacia
- Laryngeal atresia, cyst, or web

- Subglottic stenosis
- Vascular ring
- Foreign body aspiration, doubt at this age
- Anaphylaxis, unlikely given chronicity
- Epiglottitis

Investigation

1. She was treated with 6 L high-flow nasal cannula for the work of breathing (not hypoxemia), which seemed to help her distress.
2. A respiratory viral multiplex swab was negative. CXR was normal.
3. Electrolytes and CBC were unremarkable.
4. CRP <1 mg/L, BNP 23 pg/mL, and EKG with normal sinus rhythm.
5. ENT was consulted due to continued stridor. On their examination, a 1 cm diameter thin red vascular plaque was present on right lower lip extending into lower gingiva (Figure 32.1).

The infant was taken for direct laryngoscopy and rigid bronchoscopy.

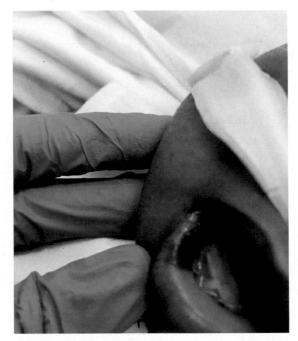

FIGURE 32.1   Right lower lip hemangioma.

Results

A circumferential subglottic hemangioma approximately 1 cm in length was discovered and is shown in Figure 32.2, resulting in Grade 3 subglottic stenosis.

DIAGNOSIS

Hemangioma, subglottic

Treatment/Follow-up

1. Dexamethasone × 48 hours.
2. Propranolol at 2 mg/kg/d divided TID until at least 10 to 12 months of age.
3. Dermatology consult to evaluate for additional hemangiomas.

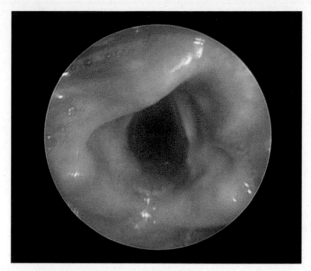

FIGURE 32.2   Circumferential subglottic hemangioma.

TEACHING POINTS

- Subglottic hemangiomas are congenital vascular lesions that grow rapidly in the first 1 to 3 months of life and stabilize in size at approximately 12 to 18 months of age. Ultimately, they involute, with 50% completely resolving by the age of 5 years and the remainder by the age of 12 years. They often present with recurrent croup and biphasic stridor, worse with crying and or upper respiratory infection. Diagnosis is confirmed with laryngoscopy.
- Subglottic hemangiomas are sometimes associated with PHACE syndrome (posterior fossa brain malformation, hemangiomas of the face, arterial anomalies, cardiac anomalies, and eye abnormalities).
- Propranolol therapy is the most common first-line treatment. Most patients have improvement of symptoms within 24 hours of initiation, although rebound growth does occur in approximately 10% of patients when the dose of propranolol is decreased. Other treatment options include systemic or intralesionally injected corticosteroids, laser ablation, surgical excision, and rarely tracheostomy.
- Approximately 50% of infants with subglottic hemangiomas also have cutaneous hemangiomas, particularly near the mouth, and the presence of the small lip hemangioma was the clue that led to the diagnosis in this case.

Suggested Readings

Ahmad SM, Soliman AMS. Congenital anomalies of the larynx. *Otolaryngol Clin North Am.* 2007;40(1):177-191.

Rahbar R, Nicollas R, Roger G. The biology and management of subglottic hemangioma: past, present, future. *Laryngoscope.* 2004;114(11):1880-1891.

Schwartz T, Faria J, Pawar S, Siegel D, Chun R. Efficacy and rebound rates in propanolol-treated subglottic hemangioma: a literature review. *Laryngoscope.* 2017;127(11):2665-2672.

33

The Kicker
Andrew J. White

CHIEF COMPLAINT

A 14-year-old boy with 3 weeks of groin pain

HISTORY OF PRESENT ILLNESS

A 14-year-old football player developed groin pain 3 weeks ago, located at the left upper thigh and which spread to involve scrotal pain/swelling. It then spread to the right side of his groin. He was evaluated twice by a urologist, both times with a scrotal ultrasound, and was reassured that he did not have a testicular torsion.

A week later he was seen by a Sports Medicine physician, who obtained plain radiographs which were read as a widened pubic symphysis but were otherwise normal. A noncontrast magnetic resonance image (MRI) was subsequently obtained and read as "edema of the parapubic symphysis musculature and pubic symphysis." He was diagnosed with osteitis pubis and treated with a course of nonsteroidal anti-inflammatory drugs (NSAIDs).

Despite the NSAIDs, the pain persisted and he began having trouble walking. He was prescribed narcotics, which did seem to help but only for a short while. He started developing low-grade fevers, and his mother took him to the emergency room. Physical examination there included pain at the pubic symphysis, but no other findings. He was admitted for possible osteomyelitis, but orchitis and epididymitis were considered high on the differential diagnosis.

During his 3-day admission, he had no fevers, and a bone scan was normal, excluding osteomyelitis. He was not treated with antibiotics, but with anti-inflammatory medications.

- WBC 10.3k, 65% polys 22% lymph, Hgb 13 mg/dL, Plt 396k, ESR 44 mm/h, CRP 92 (<3 mg/dL)
- Bone scan: Normal
- Diagnosis: Osteitis pubis, refractory, due to repetitive kicking at football camp
- Rx: NSAIDs

He was sent home on NSAIDs with a confirmed diagnosis of osteitis pubis and told to refrain from kicking. However, 5 days later, he went back to the emergency department with worsening pain.

Family/Social History

He had started football camp 1 week prior to pain onset, where he was the punter and kicker for the team. While at camp, he had accumulated a large number of bug bites, mostly mosquitos but perhaps a few ticks, he was not sure. He denies sexual intercourse, but confirms regular (daily) oral sex, but not during football camp.

EXAMINATION

He had a slow, plodding, wide-based gait and grimaced when asked to walk. He was exquisitely tender in the area of the pubic symphysis, but there was no visible swelling, erythema, or rash. Testes were nontender, and cremasteric reflex was intact. No ulceration, vesicles, or urethral discharge. No hernia was present, but he was unable to Valsalva due to pain.

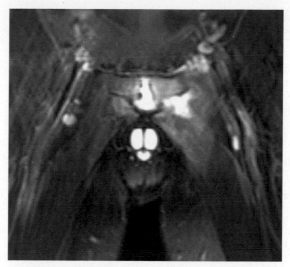

FIGURE 33.1 Enhancement (white areas) in and around the pubic symphysis represent infection and abscess.

DIAGNOSTIC CONSIDERATIONS

Testicular torsion
Epididymitis
Orchitis
Inguinal hernia
Abdominal wall hernia
Myositis, infectious (*Staphylococcus aureus*, eg)

Investigation

A repeat MRI was performed (Figure 33.1).

Results

- A 2.9 cm fluid collection is present within the pubic symphysis with adjacent edema of the superior pubic rami abutting the joint.
- A second fluid collection between the adductor brevis and pectineus muscles on the left that enhances with contrast.
- Edema of the adductor brevis, obturator externus, and pectineus muscles.

DIAGNOSIS

Septic arthritis, pubic symphysis joint, with adjacent abscess

Treatment/Follow-up

1. Surgical debridement. The abscess was drained, and the pus was cultured and grew *Fusobacterium necrophorum*.
2. Clindamycin 4 to 6 weeks.

TEACHING POINTS

Infection of the pubic symphysis is an unusual but not especially rare occurrence. Risk factors include recent vaginal delivery, recent urologic surgery, long-term indwelling Foley catheter, and participation in athletics in particular soccer and football.

The symptoms are often groin and/or scrotal pain, leg pain, hip pain, and a wide-based waddling gait. The usual organisms are *Staphylococcus aureus*, *Streptococcus pneumoniae*, *Pseudomonas aeruginosa*, *Mycobacterium tuberculosis*, and *Escherichia coli*. *Fusobacterium* sp. have been rarely reported.

Osteitis pubis is a sterile, inflammatory lesion of the pubic symphysis that occurs in athletes, *without fever and without infection*, and responds to rest and NSAIDs. It is an overuse irritation of the joint common in those who kick, such as punters.

Epilogue: The originally negative bone scan was reread as positive. The symmetry of uptake around the pubic symphysis and the nearby prominently enhancing bladder led to the initial misinterpretation.

Suggested Readings

Naredo Sanchez E, de Cal IW, Alegre Bernal N, et al. Fusobacterium osteomyelitis of the pubic symphysis in a healthy soccer player. *J Rheumatol*. 2000;27(8):2047-2048. PMID: 10955353.

Ross JJ, Hu LT. Septic arthritis of the pubic symphysis: review of 100 cases. *Medicine (Baltimore)*. 2003;82(5):340-345. PMID: 14530783.

Smith M, Martin RP, Matzkin E, Moyer ML. Osteomyelitis of the pubic symphysis. *Orthopedics*. 2003;26(12):1233-1235. PMID: 14690298.

34

Polycythemia NOT Vera

Andrew J. White

CHIEF COMPLAINT

Toddler who "cannot stand up anymore"

HISTORY OF PRESENT ILLNESS

A 17-month-old girl fell into her dresser drawer this morning while mother was getting her dressed, and afterward she could not stand up by herself. Mom did not think the child lost her balance; she did not trip, she was not pushed, and she did not hit her head. It was more like "a tall building slowly falling over." She did not lose consciousness and had no fever, but she was taken to the emergency department, where the physicians documented weakness on the right side and an Sao_2 of 70%.

There was no murmur and no rash.

PAST MEDICAL HISTORY

Hemoglobin was "high" on screen at 1 year. No cause was established despite an evaluation by a hematologist.

EXAMINATION

- Occasional blue fingertips/nail beds when she is cold.
- **Hgb 22, Hct 66**, and Plts 292. She underwent partial exchange transfusion to acutely lower the hematocrit.
- Head CT: Hyper- and hypodensities were present in L-frontal, temporal, and parietal areas; no intraventricular hemorrhage. Ventricles were normal size, there was no mass and no mass effect.

DIAGNOSTIC CONSIDERATIONS

- Polycythemia, idiopathic
- Stroke, due to polycythemia, with hemiparesis

At this stage, it was concluded that her idiopathic polycythemia, which had been worked up previously, was responsible for creating a prothrombotic state. The cause of the hypoxia, leading to the polycythemia, was pursued.

Investigation and Results

- Echocardiogram: Normal heart structure; bubble contrast showed **R→L shunt.**
- Chest CT: Large arteriovenous malformation (AVM) in the right middle lobe.
- Cardiac catheterization:
  - R-middle lobe AVM (occluded with a 10 mm plug).
  - Two aorticopulmonary collateral vessels (occluded with coils).

After the cardiac catheterization procedure, her Sao_2 was 100% on RA.

Mom recalled her aunt had an AVM in her lung, so she made a phone call and discovered that several family members had a disease they called Osler-Weber-Rendu disease.

DIAGNOSIS

1. **Hemorrhagic hereditary telangiectasia** (aka HHT or Osler-Weber-Rendu disease)
2. **Pulmonary AVM**, due to #1
3. **Polycythemia** from hypoxia, due to #2
4. **Embolic stroke**, due to #2 and 3

Follow-up/Treatment

• Genetic testing was performed which confirmed the diagnosis.
• Workup to identify the presence of AVMs in lungs, CNS, and liver.
• Prophylactic antibiotics for dental work, to prevent brain abscess via the R to L shunt.
• Nasal hygiene to minimize epistaxis.

TEACHING POINTS

HHT is a disease of abnormal vascular development that is underrecognized and underdiagnosed. It was once thought to be exceedingly rare but is now known to have a prevalence of about 1:5000 people. It is an autosomal dominant disorder that results from mutations in endoglin (called the HHT1 subtype), Alk1 (HHT2), SMAD4 (HHT3), or other molecules associated with the TGF-B signaling pathway. Highly penetrant, the phenotypic variance even within families is quite high, with some essentially asymptomatic and others severely affected. Complications include both hemorrhagic stroke from intracranial AVM bleeding but more often ischemic stroke from paradoxical embolism via pulmonary AVMs. Pulmonary AVMs may also bleed, leading to hemoptysis, which may be life-threatening. Shunting through these AVMs is right to left, leading to hypoxia and/or exercise intolerance, which may go unrecognized in children, or can be mistaken for asthma or deconditioning. About 5% of people with HHT develop pulmonary hypertension.

The diagnosis is made on either genetic testing (in about 90% of cases a mutation can be identified), or based on having three of four clinical criteria, which include the following:

1. Recurrent epistaxis. This may present in infancy or later in life or may never occur. Epistaxis typically becomes the most troublesome symptom for adult patients, who often have daily nosebleeds lasting hours each day. Compounded by GI blood loss, patients often need blood transfusions on a regular basis, and supplemental iron.
2. Cutaneous telangiectases. These are generally present on the hands, face, lips, and tongue, but they usually progress with age. Many children have no visible skin lesions whatsoever. If present, they can often be found on the backs of the hands, at the vermillion border, or tip of the tongue and are tiny in children.
3. Solid organ AVMs. Nearly 55% of patients with HHT have pulmonary vascular malformations, 15% have CNS AVMs and about 5% have liver AVMs. Small but numerous telangiectases may line the GI tract and cause blood loss.
4. Family history. A first-degree relative with HHT satisfies a diagnostic criterion.

Treatment is based on:

• Identification of AVMs with imaging. MRI of the brain detects vascular lesions reliably. Contrast echocardiography is used as a screening tool to infer the presence of pulmonary AVMs. CT or conventional angiography can confirm their presence and anatomy.
• Embolization. CNS and pulmonary AVMs may be embolized depending on size, location, and vessel anatomy. Surgical resection may also be utilized. The risk-benefit ratio of treatment should be weighed carefully, and based on size and location of AVM, with the age of the child, and risks of intervention versus nonintervention.

- Nasal hygiene. Moisture is usually sufficient in most children. Laser cautery is preferable to electrocautery in more difficult cases. Antiangiogenic therapy has been used.
- Genetic counseling is recommended.

In this child, the presence of a pulmonary AVM (PAVM) led to chronic hypoxia and resultant polycythemia. The polycythemia led to a small clot, which traveled through the PAVM and caused an ischemic stroke. The hematologist had not considered a shunt as a cause of the polycythemia and did not check the Sao_2.

Suggested Readings

Faughnan ME, Mager JJ, Hetts SW, et al. Second International Guidelines for the diagnosis and management of hereditary hemorrhagic telangiectasia. *Ann Intern Med.* 2020;173(12):989-1001. doi:10.7326/M20-1443

Gefen AM, White AJ. Asymptomatic pulmonary arteriovenous malformations in children with hereditary hemorrhagic telangiectasia. *Pediatr Pulmonol.* 2017;52(9):1194-1197.

Pahl KS, Choudhury A, Wusik K, et al. Applicability of the Curaçao criteria for the diagnosis of hereditary hemorrhagic telangiectasia in the pediatric population. *J Pediatr.* 2018;197:207-213.

35

Run Over

Jennifer Horst

CHIEF COMPLAINT

"I was run over by a car."

HISTORY OF PRESENT ILLNESS

A 14-year-old girl was sitting on the hood of a parked car smoking marijuana when she hopped off and was accidently hit and run over by another passing car going at low speed. She suffered an obvious injury to her right ankle, which was distorted and misshapen and bleeding, and she also complained of shoulder pain, abdominal pain, and other scattered musculoskeletal injuries. She did not lose consciousness and had no other apparent injuries. An ambulance was called and took her to an emergency room.

Family/Social History

- Diabetes, hypertension, and cancer in grandparents.
- Vaccinations up-to-date. Uses marijuana. Lives with parents.

EXAMINATION

- Vitals: T 36.9, HR 122, RR 15, BP 114/62, O_2 sats 88% on room air that improved to 100% on 2 L NC.
- Constitutional: Patient in severe distress due to ankle pain.
- HEENT: Normocephalic. PERRL. No scalp or facial hematoma. No facial swelling. No hemotympanum. No intraoral injuries. Airway intact. No septal hematoma.
- Neck: C-collar in place. No C-spine tenderness.
- Chest: Pain and tenderness over bilateral clavicle and shoulders. No bruising of chest wall.
- Heart: Tachycardic, no murmur.
- Lungs: Clear bilaterally.
- Abdomen: Soft but diffusely tender. Abrasions over left lower quadrant. Black tire marks diffusely over the abdomen.
- Pelvis: Diffuse tenderness.
- Extremities: Obvious deformity of right ankle with visible bone protruding through the skin; bilateral shoulder tenderness. +2 dorsalis pedis pulses intact bilaterally.
- Neurologic: GCS 14 to 15. Eyes closed at baseline, but with intermittent screaming in pain and open eyes. Answers questions appropriately but sparingly. Able to wiggle toes in both feet.
- Spine: No C-spine or L-spine tenderness. +T-spine tenderness.

DIAGNOSTIC CONSIDERATIONS

She was considered a "major trauma," and the trauma surgery team was called to evaluate her. In addition to the obvious ankle injury, being run over across the abdomen by a car may have caused any, or several, internal organ injuries, including splenic rupture, liver laceration, ruptured viscous, pelvic fracture, spine injuries, and aortic dissection, among other injuries.

Investigation and Results

- CXR normal—Clear lungs. No pneumothorax or clavicle fracture.
- C-spine x-ray—No fracture.
- Right tibia/fibula and ankle x-ray: Open dislocated intra-articular fracture obliquely oriented through the distal right tibia with protrusion of the fibula through the skin and gas within the joint.
- CT head without contrast: No intracranial abnormality.
- CT abdomen and pelvis with contrast: Soft tissue stranding in the left lower quadrant representing mild contusion without underlying osseous or hollow viscus injury.
- CT reconstruction thoracic: No fractures of thoracic or lumbar spine.

Diagnosis

1. **V03.10**, pedestrian on foot injured in collision with car
2. **Ankle fracture**, open, with dislocation, secondary to #1

Treatment/Follow-up

Fentanyl was given for pain. A normal saline bolus was administered, antibiotics were given for the open ankle fracture, and a booster TDaP was administered.

After exclusion of other serious injuries, she was taken to the operating room (OR) by orthopedic surgery for open reduction and internal fixation of the right open ankle fracture. The postoperative diagnosis was an open intra-articular fracture of distal tibia, right, type I or II. Left shoulder, right shoulder, and right clavicle x-rays were obtained the following day because of continued pain, and they were normal. Her shoulder pain improved, and she was discharged home a few days later.

However, she presented again 8 days later with persistent right thoracic back pain since discharge despite taking pain medication. She had intermittent shortness of breath as well as worsening pain when moving her right arm. On examination, she was particularly tender over the right clavicle. In addition, her right arm was "hanging in extension." A repeat clavicle x-ray revealed no fracture.

Computed tomography (CT) of chest was performed which revealed a posterior dislocation of the right clavicle at the sternoclavicular joint without evidence of vascular mediastinal injury. A CT angiogram revealed no vascular injury. She was again taken to OR by orthopedic surgery for open reduction and internal fixation of the sternoclavicular dislocation. She was discharged home the following day.

Final Diagnoses

1. **V03.10**, pedestrian on foot injured in collision with car
2. **Ankle fracture**, open, with dislocation, secondary to #1
3. **Clavicle dislocation**, posterior

Teaching Points

The clavicle is the first bone in the human body to ossify, but the physis of the clavicle is the last to fuse, usually between the ages of 20 and 25 years. In patients younger than 25 years, a sternoclavicular joint dislocation can be accompanied by a medial clavicular physis fracture.

Sternoclavicular joint (SCJ) dislocations due to trauma can dislocate anteriorly (most common) or posteriorly. Anterior dislocations often present with deformity with a palpable lump lateral to the sternum. Posterior dislocations can compress the mediastinal structures and may present with patients complaining of dyspnea, dysphagia, tachypnea, and stridor. Complications such as brachial plexus and vascular injuries, esophageal punctures, and tracheal compression are reported. Both anterior and posterior SCJ dislocations can present with palpable prominence that increases with arm abduction and elevation, decreased arm range of motion and instability, paresthesias in affected extremity, or venous congestion/diminished pulse compared to contralateral side.

Routine chest radiographs have a poor sensitivity for identifying SCJ dislocations. Most sources report CT imaging to be the best choice for imaging SCJ dislocations, which allow for three-dimensional (3D) reconstruction of the SCJ to determine its exact position and to identify any possible injury to mediastinal structures. Most adult EDs would obtain a dedicated CT to exclude dislocation in such a circumstance, rather than rely on radiographs.

Suggested Reading

Morell DJ, Thyagarajan DS. Sternoclavicular joint dislocation and its management: a review of the literature. *World J Orthop*. 2016;7(4):244-250.

36

It's Never Lupus

Andrew J. White

CHIEF COMPLAINT

"We just moved here and she needs a doctor."

HISTORY OF PRESENT ILLNESS

A 15-year-old girl with a history of systemic lupus erythematosus sought care with pediatric rheumatology after moving from Alaska.

At the **age of 11 years**, she presented with a hypertensive crisis and acute renal insufficiency. Left ventricular hypertrophy and retinopathy suggested long-standing hypertension. On physical examination, she had splenomegaly, ulnar deviation of several proximal interphalangeal joints of the fingers, and was short, but had no malar rash or other cutaneous signs of lupus. Laboratory test results included leukopenia (4k), anemia (Hb 10), and thrombocytopenia (80-120k), but her complement studies were normal and her ANA was negative, as were other tests for lupus (Smith, dsDNA). A kidney biopsy demonstrated "full-house" immunofluorescence, with sparse deposits in both subepithelial and subendothelial compartments on electron microscopy. Prominent glomerular sclerosis, interstitial fibrosis, and tubular atrophy were noted.

Diagnosis: Class 5 membranous "lupus-like" glomerulonephritis (since she did not meet other criteria for systemic lupus erythematosus).

Treatment: Intravenous methylprednisolone, mycophenolate mofetil, hydroxychloroquine, and antihypertensive medications.

At the **age of 12 years**, she developed elevated serum transaminases, thought to be due to the mycophenolate, which was discontinued and azathioprine was started.

She developed cytopenias, hypogammaglobulinemia (IgG 390), and low *Streptococcus pneumoniae* titers and was treated with intravenous immunoglobin (IVIG) and revaccinated.

Despite immunosuppressive therapy to treat cytopenia (presumably associated with lupus), the pancytopenia persisted and a bone marrow biopsy was performed. It showed myeloid hypoplasia, which improved with additional steroid treatment but seemed to worsen with azathioprine, which was therefore discontinued as it is known to cause bone marrow suppression. Due to worsening renal disease (HTN, proteinuria), a course of rituximab was given and then repeated when it had no effect.

At the **age of 13 years**, a repeat kidney biopsy showed less immunofluorescent deposits, but worsening interstitial fibrosis was present, as well as atrophy and features of focal segmental glomerulosclerosis.

At the **age of 14 years**, the transaminases remained elevated, leading to a liver biopsy showing prominent fibrosis and some cirrhosis. The pancytopenia persisted. Rituximab was given again, and dialysis was initiated due to progressive renal impairment, despite ongoing immunosuppressive therapy for lupus. Sirolimus was initiated. Repeat kidney biopsy demonstrated focal segmental glomerulosclerosis (FSGS) affecting 71% of the glomeruli, as well as interstitial fibrosis and tubular atrophy, but no immunofluorescence was detected this time. Repeat bone marrow aspiration: hypocellular, trilineage hematopoiesis; no malignancy. Additional immunosuppression had no apparent effect on her cytopenias, cirrhosis, or renal impairment.

At the **age of 15 years**, her family relocated to the Midwest where she continued to receive dialysis and immunosuppression. Repeat laboratory testing for systemic lupus erythematosus remained negative on several occasions.

No one in the family has lupus, or any renal problems.

EXAMINATION

- Vitals: 37.1, 131, 40, 103/83, 98%, height at 5%.
- Comfortable and in no distress.
- Skin warm and dry, no malar rash.
- Posterior pharynx clear, mucous membranes moist.
- No tonsillar hypertrophy.
- Neck supple, no lymphadenopathy.
- Lungs clear.
- No murmur.
- Soft, nondistended abdomen, nontender, no hepatosplenomegaly, no masses.
- No clubbing, cyanosis, but there was moderate pitting edema.
- CNS normal, moves all limbs, no arthritis, but there is clinodactyly.

DIAGNOSTIC CONSIDERATIONS

Her new physician did not understand how her classic lupus renal biopsy results could be present without evidence of systemic lupus. While the cytopenias could clearly be part of lupus, the lack of response to years of immunosuppression raised the possibility that they were medication side effects.

Investigation and Results

Whole exome sequencing was undertaken in an attempt to identify a syndrome (or a syndrome of predisposition to autoimmunity) that might explain her renal disease, liver disease, and apparent bone marrow failure (or medication side effects).

Two heterozygous mutations were discovered in WDR19, both pathogenic. Mutations in WDR19 are associated with several distinct clinical **ciliopathy syndromes**, including Jeune thoracic dystrophy, cranioectodermal dysplasia, Senior-Loken syndrome (renal disease and retinal degeneration), and the answer in this case.

DIAGNOSIS

Nephronophthisis

Final Diagnoses

1. Nephronophthisis 13, due to WDR19 mutations
2. Renal failure, due to #1
3. Hepatic fibrosis, due to #1
4. Portal hypertension, due to #1
5. Splenomegaly, due to #4
6. Thrombocytopenia, due to #5
7. Anemia, due to #2
8. Hypogammaglobulinemia, iatrogenic
9. Short stature, due to #1
10. Finger abnormalities, due to #1

It was, indeed, never lupus!

TEACHING POINTS

Nephronophthisis is a group of heterogeneous, autosomal recessive disorders that lead to kidney disease. It is the most common genetic cause of end-stage renal disease in children and adolescents. The first causative gene (NPHP1) was identified in 1997, but there are currently 19 associated genes, of which WDR19 is a minor contributor (0.5% of cases). Thirty-eight cases involving this gene have been reported in the literature, and this specific entity due to WDR19 is called **nephronophthisis 13**. Mutations in this gene are also associated with Caroli disease, which involves focal, saccular, or fusiform dilatation of the intrahepatic bile ducts, leading to hepatic fibrosis (and which also occurs in a form of autosomal recessive polycystic kidney disease due to PKHD1 gene).

The clinical symptoms of nephronophthisis are typically mild at first and include polyuria, polydipsia, secondary enuresis, growth retardation, and anemia. Hypertension typically presents later, once glomerulosclerosis has occurred. Extrarenal manifestations are uncommon (15% of all cases) and include skeletal abnormalities, retinal problems, and neurologic symptoms, as well as hepatic fibrosis and polydactyly. Immune complex deposition in the kidneys does occur, perhaps from anti-WDR19 antibodies.

Treatment is kidney transplantation.

Suggested Readings

Bredrup C, Saunier S, Oud MM, et al. Ciliopathies with skeletal anomalies and renal insufficiency due to mutations in the IFT-A gene WDR19. *Am J Hum Genet.* 2011;89:634-543.

Coussa RG, Otto EA, Gee HY, et al. WDR19: an ancient, retrograde, intraflagellar ciliary protein is mutated in autosomal recessive retinitis pigmentosa and in Senior-Loken syndrome. *Clin Genet.* 2013;84:150-159.

Gianviti A, Barsotti P, Barbera V, Faraggiana T, Rizzoni G. Delayed onset of systemic lupus erythematosus in patients with "full-house" nephropathy. *Pediatr Nephrol.* 1999;13:683-687.

Halbritter J, Porath JD, Diaz KA, et al. Identification of 99 novel mutations in a worldwide cohort of 1,056 patients with a nephronophthisis-related ciliopathy. *Hum Genet.* 2013;132:865-884.

Huerta A, Bomback AS, Liakopoulos V, et al. Renal-limited "lupus-like" nephritis. *Nephrol Dial Transplant.* 2012;27:2337-2342.

Lee JM, Ahn YH, Kang HG, et al. Nephronophthisis 13: implications of its association with Caroli disease and altered intracellular localization of WDR19 in the kidney. *Pediatr Nephrol.* 2015;30:1451-1458.

Park E, Lee JM, Ahn YH, et al. Hepatorenal fibrocystic disesaes in children. *Pediatr Nephrol.* 2016;31:113-119.

Pirkle J, Freedman B, Fogo A. Immune complex disease with a lupus-like pattern of deposition in an antinuclear antibody-negative patient. *Am J Kidney Dis.* 2013;62:159-164.

Stokman M, Lilien M, Knoers N. Nephronophthisis. In: Adam MP, Ardinger HH, Pagon RA, et al, eds. *GeneReviews.* University of Washington; 2016:1993-2021.

Wolf TF, Hildebrandt F. Nephronophthisis. *Pediatr Nephrol.* 2011;26:181-194.

37 Springtime Seizure

Kyle P. McNerney

CHIEF COMPLAINT

"Abnormal movements"

HISTORY OF PRESENT ILLNESS

A 7-month-old African-American male infant presented with abnormal movements. He had been healthy overall since his birth last fall, and he has never moved this way before. He attended an outdoor church picnic yesterday on a warm spring day, which was his first time outdoors for any substantial length of time. He was looked after by several family members during the picnic. He was not dropped, did not fall, nor was there any reported trauma. Today, he was lying on his back and suddenly had a 3-minute episode of full-body stiffness with rhythmic, jerking movements of his upper and lower extremities, and his eyes rolled up in his head. Mom called emergency medical services (EMS), but by the time of arrival, he had recovered. He was brought to the emergency department (ED) for evaluation.

PAST MEDICAL HISTORY

Healthy term infant born appropriate for gestational age (AGA) with birth weight 9 lb 9 oz. He was exclusively breastfed until 5 months of age when he started eating small quantities of fruits, vegetables, and meat. He sits independently, he does not crawl or pull to stand, and he babbles with consonants.

Medications

None

Family/Social History

No family members with seizures. He lives at home with his parents and three healthy older siblings. His mother took prenatal vitamins during pregnancy but discontinued them after he was born.

EXAMINATION

- Vitals: Temperature 37 °C. Heart rate 110 beats per minute. Respiratory rate 30 breaths per minute. Blood pressure 100/64 mm Hg. Spo$_2$ 97% on room air.
- General: Awake, alert, makes eye contact and cries.
- Skin: Warm and dry without rash or birthmarks. Palpable nodules on the anterior chest at costochondral junctions.
- HEENT: Normocephalic, conjunctivae clear, tympanic membranes pale-pink with intact light reflex, no rhinorrhea, mucous membranes moist, no lymphadenopathy. No teeth present.
- Pulmonary: Lungs clear to auscultation bilaterally.
- Cardiovascular: Regular rate and rhythm, no murmurs.
- Abdomen: Soft, nontender, nondistended, no hepatosplenomegaly or masses palpated.
- Extremities: Widened, flaring bone deformities at the wrists and knees. No leg bowing.

- Genitourinary: Tanner 1 male with testes descended bilaterally.
- Neurologic: Awake, alert, fussy but consolable. Extraocular movements intact. Sensation grossly intact. Moves all extremities well.

DIAGNOSTIC CONSIDERATIONS

Although not witnessed, the description of the movements was classic for a seizure. Trauma or nonaccidental trauma should always be considered in a new-onset seizure and may not be revealed on history. Infectious causes such as sepsis or meningitis would be likely to have fever and signs of infection on physical examination. Metabolic or electrolyte abnormalities can provoke a seizure, including hyponatremia, hypernatremia, hypoglycemia, or hypocalcemia, and the abnormal flaring noticed in this infant's distal extremities raise concern for a metabolic bone disease. Cardiovascular disease such as an arrhythmia or congenital heart disease can induce a seizure or mimic one with an unresponsive episode. Ingestion or exposure to medication could cause a seizure, and the risk of accidental ingestion increases as children become more mobile. Lastly, a central nervous system (CNS) malformation or an epilepsy syndrome such as West syndrome or Dravet syndrome can cause unprovoked seizures beginning in infancy.

Investigation

- Laboratory test: CBC, CMP, PTH, magnesium, phosphorus, 25-hydroxyvitamin D level
- Urinalysis and urine drug screen
- ECG
- Skeletal survey x-rays
- Consider head CT (deferred)

Results

Laboratory test was obtained, and the complete blood count demonstrated normal hemoglobin, white blood cell count, and platelet level. His complete metabolic panel showed normal sodium, potassium, chloride, bicarbonate, BUN, creatinine, and glucose. His ionized calcium was low at 2.6 mg/dL (reference interval 3.9-5.2 mg/dL), and his alkaline phosphatase was markedly elevated at 1015 U/L (110-320 U/L). Additional laboratory results showed decreased 25-hydroxyvitamin D level at 10 ng/mL (20-100 ng/mL), elevated PTH at 109 ng/mL (14-72 ng/mL), normal magnesium 1.7 mg/dL (1.6-2.6 mg/dL), and normal phosphorus 5.9 mg/dL (3.5-7 mg/dL). An x-ray skeletal survey demonstrated fraying and irregular widening of the metaphysis at the distal radius and ulna, distal femur, and proximal tibia bilaterally, with cupping of the distal ulna (Figures 37.1 and 37.2). There was no bowing of the femurs and no evidence of fractures. His ECG showed normal sinus rhythm. He had a normal urinalysis and negative urine drug screen.

DIAGNOSIS

1. **Seizure**, due to hypocalcemia
2. Vitamin D deficiency rickets
3. Hungry bone syndrome

Treatment/Follow-up

He was admitted to the intensive care unit (ICU) and given several boluses of intravenous (IV) calcium gluconate to treat persistent hypocalcemia and was then converted to oral calcium carbonate when the levels were stable. He was treated with vitamin D supplementation, 1000 IU/d, and he maintained normal calcium levels without any additional seizure episodes. Repeat x-rays demonstrated healing and resolution of his skeletal findings over the next 6 to 12 months.

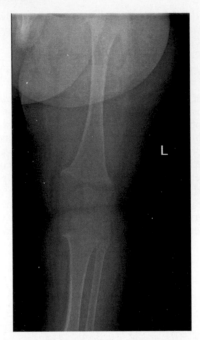

FIGURE 37.1 Fraying and irregular widening of the metaphysis at the distal femur and proximal tibia.

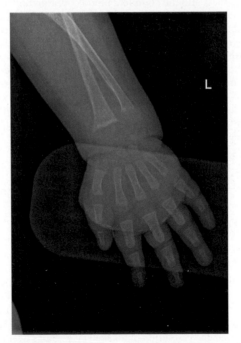

FIGURE 37.2 Fraying and irregular widening of the distal radius and ulna, with ulnar cupping.

TEACHING POINTS

A new-onset seizure in an infant can be provoked by events such as trauma, infection, metabolic or electrolyte derangement, intoxication or ingestion, or could represent the first presentation of neurologic disease or an epilepsy syndrome. Workup of an infant with a new-onset seizure will include screening laboratory tests (eg, CBC, electrolytes/glucose) and consideration of neurologic or nonneurologic causes. This infant's race, history of breastfeeding, lack of sun exposure, and physical examination findings consistent with rickets provided important clues for the diagnosis of hypocalcemic seizure secondary to vitamin D deficiency rickets.

Rickets is an impairment of bone mineralization with characteristic skeletal findings evident in the growth plates as a flaring of the distal long bones. Bone deformities occur more frequently in weight-bearing extremities due to increased bone remodeling. Crawling infants may have more prominent deformities in the wrists, whereas ambulatory children can develop more prominent lower extremity changes including leg bowing. Children can also present with generalized bone pain or irritability, delayed tooth eruption, frontal bossing and delayed closure of the fontanelle, softening of the cranial bones (craniotabes), bowed lower extremities, and enlargement of the costochondral junctions (rachitic rosary).

Vitamin D deficiency rickets is the most common cause of rickets and still occurs in both underdeveloped and developed nations. Vitamin D is a critical regulator of skeletal formation and is obtained through dietary intake/supplementation or exposure to ultraviolet (UV) light. Children considered at-risk for vitamin D deficiency include black or Hispanic children, children with obesity, children with malabsorption syndromes, or children on medications such as steroids, antiepileptic medicines, antifungal, or antiretroviral medicines. Vitamin D deficiency occurs more frequently in the winter due to decreased penetrance of UV-B light through the atmosphere. This effect is more prominent in northern latitudes, where vitamin D is unable to be synthesized even with direct sun exposure during the winter months. Infants with darker skin pigmentation have increased rates of vitamin D deficiency due to decreased vitamin D synthesis in the skin. Breastmilk alone does not provide an infant with adequate vitamin D intake, so vitamin D supplementation (400 IU/day) is recommended for all breastfeeding infants.

In vitamin D deficiency rickets, laboratory tests indicate decreased 25-hydroxyvitamin D level, elevated alkaline phosphatase level, elevated PTH levels, and low to normal calcium and phosphorous levels. 25-hydroxyvitamin D levels reflect the stored amount of vitamin D in the body and is the preferred test for vitamin D deficiency. This should not be confused with 1,25-dihydroxyvitamin D, which is the bioactive form of vitamin D but has a short serum half-life and does not reflect vitamin D status. Guidelines do not support the routine use of 1,25-dihydroxyvitamin D assessment in the evaluation of vitamin D deficiency. Vitamin D deficiency rickets can be provisionally diagnosed in children with a compatible history and physical examination, as well as characteristic laboratory test results, and the diagnosis is confirmed after appropriate skeletal healing in response to vitamin D therapy. Other considerations for the diagnosis of rickets include x-linked hypophosphatemia, impairments of vitamin D metabolism, severe renal or liver disease, or FGF23-mediated hypophosphatemia. Atypical rickets may require additional workup and referral to a pediatric bone specialist.

This infant's hypocalcemic seizure occurred the day after sunlight exposure at a Spring picnic. The acute hypocalcemia was precipitated by vitamin D generated from sun exposure. This phenomenon is described as "hungry bone syndrome," and it occurs when repletion of vitamin D leads to acute hypocalcemia due to rapid uptake of calcium into the bone. Consequently, calcium supplementation is recommended in the management of children with severe vitamin D deficiency, and some providers begin lower doses of vitamin D supplementation in severely vitamin D–deficient children. With adequate treatment of vitamin D deficiency, laboratory markers of rickets should show improvement within 1 month, and skeletal deformities begin to improve over a period of several months. If biochemical and radiologic improvement does not occur with vitamin D treatment, providers should confirm adherence to the regimen, adequate absorption of vitamin D, and consider alternative diagnoses.

Suggested Readings

Golden NH, Abrams SA, Nutrition CO. Optimizing bone health in children and adolescents. *Pediatrics*. 2014;134(4):e1229-e1243.

Holick MF. Resurrection of vitamin D deficiency and rickets. *J Clin Invest*. 2006;116(8):2062-2072.

Sahay M, Sahay R. Rickets–vitamin D deficiency and dependency. *Indian J Endocrinol Metab*. 2012;16(2):164-176.

Underland L, Markowitz M, Gensure R. Calcium and phosphate hormones: vitamin D, parathyroid hormone, and fibroblast growth factor 23. *Pediatr Rev*. 2020;41(1):3-11.

38

Kneed I Say More?
Andrew J. White

CHIEF COMPLAINT

He was born that way.

HISTORY OF PRESENT ILLNESS

A well-appearing, vigorous term baby boy was born to a healthy 29-year-old G1P1 mother. A leg abnormality was immediately noticed in the delivery room. There was no birth trauma and no trauma during pregnancy. Apgar scores were 9 and 9.

PAST MEDICAL HISTORY

Family/Social History

No one in the family has leg problems, although a grandfather did have a knee replacement for osteoarthritis.

EXAMINATION

The left leg was hyperextended at the knee to nearly 90° (Figure 38.1). It did not seem to be tender with palpation or range of motion, and there was no obvious fracture or instability. The foot was well perfused and pink. The rest of the examination was completely normal.

DIAGNOSIS

Genu recurvatum congenitum (ICD 10 Q68.2)

TEACHING POINTS

Genu recurvatum congenitum is a term used to describe a number of abnormal knee findings, from simple hyperextension to an irreducible, complete dislocation, which is usually called **congenital dislocation of the knee (CDK)**. It usually occurs in isolation but may occur together with other orthopedic anomalies such as club foot or dislocation of the hip. Occasionally, it is part of a syndrome such as arthrogryposis multiplex congenita, Marfan syndrome, Ehlers-Danlos syndrome, myelomeningocele, or Larsen syndrome (a disorder similar to Ehlers-Danlos that presents with multiple joint dislocations and cardiovascular anomalies and is due to mutations in filamin B [encoding a cytoskeleton component] or in collagen VII).

While rare, CDK occurs in about 1 birth per 100,000. Treatment is typically nonoperative and includes early reduction and serial casting, with therapy focused on gradual improvement in range of motion. The long-term outcome is surprisingly good.

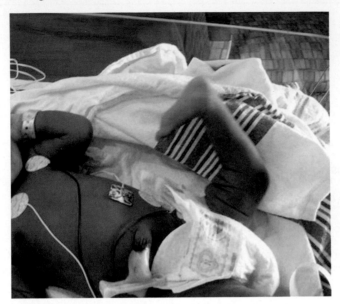

FIGURE 38.1 Markedly hyperextended left knee.

Suggested Readings

Cheng CC, Ko JY. Early reduction for congenital dislocation of the knee within twenty-four hours of birth. *Chang Gung Med J.* 2010;33(3):266-273.

Mehrafshan M, Wicart P, Ramanoudjame M, Seringe R, Glorion C, Rampal V. Congenital dislocation of the knee at birth—Part I: clinical signs and classification. *Orthop Traumatol Surg Res.* 2016;102(5):631-633.

39

Reflux Rebuff

Andrew J. White

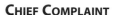

CHIEF COMPLAINT

Poor weight gain

HISTORY OF PRESENT ILLNESS

A 22-day-old girl was admitted for lack of weight gain and difficulty feeding since birth. She never latched on well and gets tired quickly during feeds. She was switched from breast milk to Nutramigen with no improvement of her symptoms. She had 8 to 10 bowel movements daily on breast milk, decreasing to 2 per day on Nutramigen. She had no episodes of vomiting or systemic signs such as fever, although she seems irritable during feeds.

PAST MEDICAL HISTORY

She was born at 39 weeks via C-section due to being large for gestational age. Her birth weight was **8 lb, 1 oz (75%)**. She stayed in the hospital for 5 days. She passed the newborn hearing screen. The mother was 30 years of age at delivery, and this was her first pregnancy, which was conceived naturally. The mother had no illnesses during pregnancy. She did receive ondansetron until the seventh month because of morning sickness and took prenatal vitamins for the entire pregnancy. She did not smoke or drink alcohol during pregnancy. Prenatal ultrasounds were normal.

A review of systems was negative except the child seems to have a pronounced startle reaction with noises, she has some wheezing, especially during feeding, and occasionally she will cough. She also has a rash.

Family/Social History

The patient lives with her parents. Father is 28 years of age, and he is healthy. The mother is 30 years of age and healthy. This is the only child for both parents. The father has a 24-year-old brother and a 21-year-old sister; both are healthy. The 44-year-old paternal grandmother was diagnosed at the age of 26 years with breast cancer. She underwent mastectomy but has not had genetic testing. The paternal grandfather (PGF) is 48 years of age, and he has hypercholesterolemia and hypertension. A niece of the PGF has arthrogryposis, and another niece has Goldenhar syndrome. PGF's sister is 35 years of age and has Down syndrome. He also has 11 additional siblings who are healthy. Both paternal grandparents are of German descent. The mother has 33-year-old and 37-year-old sisters who are both healthy. One daughter of the 37-year-old sister was evaluated for possible skeletal dysplasia because of short arms. The maternal grandparents are 60 years of age, and both are healthy.

EXAMINATION

The patient was alert, in no distress, and was interactive. Her blood pressure was 96/53, her heart rate was 124, her RR was 39, and temperature was 37.2. Oxygen saturation was 99%. Her weight was **3.67 kg (10%)**, and her length was **50 cm (10%)**; her OFC was **40 cm (99%)**. There were no dysmorphic features.

- HEENT: Normocephalic without skull deformities.
- Eyes: Normal extraocular movements.
- Mouth: Midline tongue, strong sucking; there was micrognathia.
- Neck: Supple without deformities or masses.
- Chest: Symmetric, normal breath sounds without wheezing or crackles.
- Heart: S1, S2 were normal without murmur.
- Abdomen: Soft and nontender without organomegaly.
- GU: Normal female Tanner stage 1.
- Musculoskeletal: There was no polydactyly, syndactyly, or clinodactyly. No bone deformities. Normal range of motion.
- Skin: There were no hyper- or hypopigmented lesions.
- Neurological: Normal tone and strength of muscles. Normal neonatal reflexes.

Diagnostic Considerations

The sole consideration on the admitting physician's note was

1. Reflux

Investigation

She underwent an upper GI with small bowel follow-through (Figure 39.1).

Results

The study was read as:
  "There are no abnormal vascular impressions upon the esophagus.
  There is no tracheoesophageal fistula.
  There is gastroesophageal reflux to the midupper esophagus without aspiration.

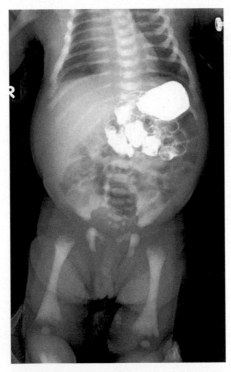

FIGURE 39.1 Upper gastrointestinal (GI) study.

There is no evidence of gastric outlet obstruction, and the duodenal-jejunal junction is in its normal, left upper quadrant location," **ie, a normal upper GI**.

However, a closer look at the films, particularly at the non-GI-related areas, led to a supplemental radiology report being filed, which read: "There are diffuse changes of osseous sclerosis with obliteration of medullary cavities with rachitic changes of the proximal/distal femurs, proximal tibias, and proximal humeri; most prominent at the distal femurs." These radiological findings are pathognomonic for infantile **osteopetrosis**.

Diagnosis

Osteopetrosis

Additional Investigation

1. CBC and diff
2. CMP, PTH, ionized calcium
3. Vitamin D level
4. Isoforms of CK (BB isoform is a good marker for osteoclast dysfunction)
5. Osteopetrosis genetic panel
6. Skeletal survey
7. Consultations with Hematology/Oncology and Ophthalmology

Results

Osteopetrosis testing: Compound heterozygote in TCIRG1. (1549G > A in exon 13 and 117 + 1G > A in the donor splice site.) Both are known disease-causing mutations.

Teaching Points

- **Osteopetrosis** is a rare disease (incidence of 1 in 250,000) characterized by impaired osteoclast function, which usually manifests in the first few months of life. Presenting symptoms are often macrocephaly and frontal bossing or respiratory and feeding problems due to choanal stenosis from impaired bone remodeling. In addition, the enlarging bone decreases the size of neural foramina, leading to blindness, deafness, and facial nerve palsy. Vision loss eventually occurs in all untreated patients, as does hearing loss. Cytopenias from impaired hematopoiesis (from the lack of bone marrow medullary space) may be severe and life-threatening (maximum life span in untreated patients is about 10 years). Calcium homeostasis is abnormal, and these children develop hypocalcemia, tetany, and secondary hyperparathyroidism. Severe dental caries are common. Stem **cell transplantation can be curative**, but cranial nerve dysfunction is usually irreversible, and therefore, transplant is sought early in life.
- Another clue to the diagnosis in this case was the growth chart. The OFC of 99% contrasts with the 10% of the other parameters, and macrocephaly is often the presenting manifestation of Osteopetrosis.
- **Look at your films!**

Suggested Readings

Palagano E, Menale C, Sobacchi C, Villa A. Genetics of osteopetrosis. *Curr Osteoporos Rep*. 2018;16(1):13-25.

Sobacchi C, Schulz A, Coxon FP, Villa A, Helfrich MH. Osteopetrosis: genetics, treatment and new insights into osteoclast function. *Nat Rev Endocrinol*. 2013;9(9):522-536.

Wu CC, Econs MJ, DiMeglio LA, et al. Diagnosis and management of osteopetrosis: consensus guidelines from the Osteopetrosis Working Group. *J Clin Endocrinol Metab*. 2017;102(9):3111-3123.

Down and Out

40

Nicole Benzoni, Brian T. Wessman

CHIEF COMPLAINT

"Found down"

HISTORY OF PRESENT ILLNESS

A 17-year-old man was brought by emergency medical services to the emergency department (ED). He was found unconscious lying in a public parking garage and was febrile and hypoxic to 79%. He had altered mental status but was intermittently able to answer some simple questions. He had some weakness on exertion, and he complained of feeling tired and short of breath, which he said he had been experiencing for about a week.

PAST MEDICAL HISTORY

Unknown

Medications

None

Family/Social History

He admits to intravenous (IV) drug abuse with heroin, frequent marijuana, and alcohol use, as well as occasional tobacco use.

EXAMINATION

His vital signs upon arrival to the ED were HR 112, RR 24, SpO$_2$ 99% (NC 2L), BP 93/48, T 36.9 °C. He was now more alert and oriented and admitted recent IV drug use. His physical examination was notable for some needle marks on his arms and a murmur near the cardiac apex, but he had good bilateral air movement, no nasal flaring, and his abdomen was soft and nonsurgical. Cranial nerves were grossly intact, and he was moving all extremities without apparent weakness or limitation.

Shortly after arrival, he had a transient drop in his blood pressure, and a decision was made to obtain central access.

DIAGNOSTIC CONSIDERATIONS

- Altered mental status, resolved
- Hypoxemia
- Fever
- Recent IV drug abuse
- Cavitary lung lesions
- Anemia
- Transaminase elevation
- Cardiomegaly
- Acidosis

Investigation

His initial laboratory test results included a Hg of 4.9 g/dL, a lactic acidosis, and a slight elevation in serum transaminase levels. Thought to be a laboratory error, the anemia was confirmed on repeat testing, and he was transfused 2 units of packed red blood cells.

Imaging studies included a chest radiograph (Figure 40.1), an abdominal computed tomography scan, and a transthoracic echocardiogram (Figure 40.2). He was started on empiric antibiotics and subsequently admitted to the intensive care unit.

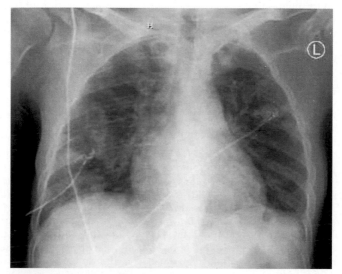

FIGURE 40.1   Chest radiograph showing multiple cavitary nodules throughout bilateral lung fields and an enlarged, globular-shaped cardiac silhouette.

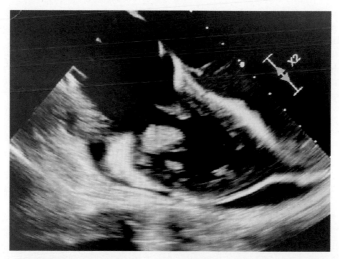

FIGURE 40.2   Representative image from the transthoracic echocardiogram focused on the right-sided cardiac structures. Note the globular vegetation on the tricuspid valve and the pericardial effusion along the free wall of the right ventricle.

Blood cultures grew methicillin-sensitive *Staphylococcal aureus* (MSSA) within 12 hours of being obtained.

DIAGNOSIS

Endocarditis, tricuspid, MSSA, secondary to IV drug use.

TEACHING POINTS

The differential for pulmonary cavitary lesions includes infectious disease (including septic emboli), autoimmune disease such as granulomatosis with polyangiitis, metastatic cancer, and perhaps unusual congenital causes. Acute or subacute time courses (<12 weeks) are more likely to be infectious (bacterial or fungal) in origin. Chronic (>12 weeks) disease processes favor a malignant, autoimmune, or more indolent infectious (fungal or mycobacterial) disease process.

Chronic infectious etiologies include *Mycobacterium tuberculosis*, which tends to involve the upper lobes in immunocompetent patients. Lower lobe involvement and pleural effusions are more apparent in immunocompromised patients. Fungal diseases such as aspergillosis can invade preexisting cavities within the lungs. Autoimmune diseases such as pulmonary sarcoidosis and granulomatosis with polyangiitis may also manifest as cavitary lesions.

Infective endocarditis (IE) can be right or left sided. In non-IV drug–using (IVDU) patients, left-sided (mitral valve) involvement is much more common. These patients are usually immunocompromised or have implanted devices or lines. Worldwide, *Staphylococcus aureus* is the most common etiology for all IE, although coagulase-negative *Staphylococcus epidermidis* is common in prosthetic valve endocarditis. The *HACEK* organisms which colonize the oropharynx and are classically associated with acute native valve endocarditis (*Haemophilus* spp., *Aggregatibacter* spp., *Cardiobacterium hominis*, *Eikenella corrodens*, and *Kingella* spp.) are uncommon but can be difficult to culture. Therefore, the American Heart Association recommends the collection of three blood cultures obtained within 1 hour of each other to improve the sensitivity and specificity of organism identification. Right-sided IE is almost always related to IVDU and is often caused by *S. aureus*.

This patient's fever, admitted IVDU, murmur, and acute presentation make bacteremia arising from the right side of the heart the most likely diagnostic etiology.

The standard for the diagnosis of endocarditis involves the modified Duke criteria (Table 40.1).

Note that the absence of fever is not enough to exclude endocarditis. Be particularly attuned in a patient with a new murmur and risk factors for valvular abnormalities Recall that endocarditis is not always infectious and may be caused by autoimmune or malignant processes. Systemic lupus erythematous has a particularly strong association with autoimmune endocarditis, known as Libman-Sacks endocarditis. In these patients, a complete transthoracic echocardiogram (TTE) may be diagnostic. If you still have a strong suspicion and TTE is unremarkable, a transesophageal echocardiogram (TEE) may be performed.

TABLE 40.1 Modified Duke Criteria

Diagnostic Requirements	Major Criteria	Minor Criteria
Two Major **or**	**Blood culture consistent with IE** • Typical organisms in two separate cultures **or** • One culture with *Coxiella burnetii*	**Vascular** phenomenon (eg, Janeway lesions, pulmonary emboli, conjunctival hemorrhage)
One Major + Three Minor **or**	**Sonographic evidence of endocarditis** • Echogenic vegetative mass **or** • Perivalvular abscess **or** • New dehiscence of prosthetic valve	**Immunologic** phenomenon (eg, Osler nodes, glomerulonephritis, Roth spots)
Five Minor		**Risk factors** (eg, Prosthetic valve or IVDU) **Fever** > 38 °C **Microbiologic:** (+) blood culture(s) that do not meet major criteria

IE, infective endocarditis; IVDU, intravenous drug using.

Suggested Readings

Baddour LM, Wilson WR, Bayer AS, et al. Infective endocarditis in adults: diagnosis, antimicrobial therapy, and management of complications. A scientific statement for healthcare professionals from the American Heart Association. *Circulation*. 2015;132:1435-1486. doi:10.1161/CIR.000000000000029

Li JS, Sexton DJ, Nathan M, et al. Proposed modifications to the Duke criteria for the diagnosis of infective endocarditis. *Clin Infect Dis*. 2000;30(4):633-638. doi:10.1086/313753

Liesman RM, Pritt BS, Maleszewski JJ, Patel R. Laboratory diagnosis of infective endocarditis. *J Clin Microbiol*. 2017;55(9):2599-2608. doi:10.1128/JCM.00635-17

Parkar AP, Kandiah P. Differential diagnosis of cavitary lung lesions. *J Belg Radiol*. 2016;100(1):100. doi:10.5334/jbr-btr.1202

Toom S, Xu Y. Hemolytic anemia due to native valve subacute endocarditis with Actinomyces israelii infection. *Clin Case Rep*. 2018;6(2):376-379. doi:10.1002/ccr3.1333

41

Hark, the Herald Angels Sing
Hannah C. B. White

CHIEF COMPLAINT

Painless rash

HISTORY OF PRESENT ILLNESS

A 16-year-old man presents with a rash on his abdomen which has been spreading. He noticed it several weeks ago as an oval area which was reddish on the edges but not in the center. The newer areas are much smaller. It does not itch; it does not bleed. He has had no fevers and no vomiting or diarrhea. He takes no medications. He thinks it might be ringworm because his girlfriend told him so.

PAST MEDICAL HISTORY

Healthy, but with a restricted, vegetarian diet

Family/Social History

No cats or dogs in the house. No recent travel. He has a girlfriend but denies sex.

EXAMINATION

Thin teenage boy with a rash (see Figure 41.1)

DIAGNOSIS

Pityriasis rosea

TEACHING POINTS

Pityriasis rosea is a benign idiopathic rash that resolves on its own in 6 to 8 weeks. The first lesion to appear is often called a "herald patch" as it precedes the disseminated rash by 1 to 2 weeks. Newer lesions occur mainly on the torso and may develop along the rib lines, giving the appearance of a Christmas tree shape on the back (*Hark, the herald angels sing…*).

In many cases, there is a preceding upper respiratory infection. Some patients find the rash pruritic. Rarely, fever, headache, nausea, and fatigue occur. The cause is unknown but may be due to a viral illness or reactivation of a previous virus.

HHV 6 and 7 have been implicated in some case reports but not universally.

The classic presentation and recognition of the herald patch in this case will allow the diagnosing physician (and the girlfriend!) to avoid unnecessary tests and/or treatment for ringworm, psoriasis, eczema, or even syphilis.

Treatment is unnecessary, although corticosteroids do provide relief if it is itchy.

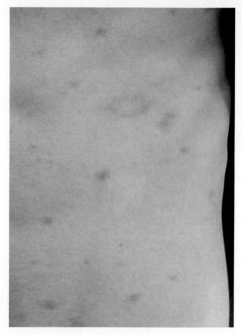

FIGURE 41.1   Erythematous papules and plaques, one larger than the others, with central clearing.

Suggested Readings

Drago F, Ciccarese G, Rebora A, Broccolo F, Parodi A. Pityriasis rosea: a comprehensive classification. *Dermatology*. 2016;232(4):431-437.
Eisman S, Sinclair R. Pityriasis rosea. *Br Med J*. 2015;351·h5233.

42

Slobber

Andrew J. White

CHIEF COMPLAINT

Rash

HISTORY OF PRESENT ILLNESS

A 3-month-old boy presented with 2 weeks of worsening rash. It started around his mouth, and mom thought it was irritation from the "slobber" from his pacifier. It started to spread, and a new "raspiness" to his cry prompted a visit to an urgent care center where he was diagnosed with impetigo and started on an oral antibiotic and topical mupirocin. He had been afebrile, maintaining good PO, had no upper respiratory infection (URI) symptoms, no respiratory distress, no vomiting or diarrhea, and no hair loss. The rash did not improve on the combination of antibiotics, so he came to the emergency department (ED).

PAST MEDICAL HISTORY

He has been breastfeeding well since birth, although he is small, at the 25% for weight.
No similar rashes in siblings.

EXAMINATION

General: Alert, active, healthy-appearing African-American male infant.
T-37.2, RR 38, HR 110 normal head shape. Anterior fontanelle was soft and flat.
Hair distribution was normal. Areas of skin breakdown and scaling in the scalp over the occipital region.
The pupils were equal and round. Extraocular muscle movements intact.
Nose and mouth were normal.
He had no dentition. Palate was intact and normally shaped. Ears were normally formed.
The skin of the face showed a rash around the mouth (Figure 42.1) with a denuded area surrounded by crusty dark black scaling. He also had rash on his ears and around his eyes, as well as on his chin and upper neck.
Chest shape was normal.
Lungs were clear.
Cardiac examination included a regular rate and rhythm with no murmur.
His abdomen was rounded and soft with no organomegaly.
GU: Circumcised male with testes descended bilaterally. He had a rash in the diaper area.
He also had a rash involving the elbows of both arms and a couple of patches of involvement on the skin of his fingers. The lower extremities were spared from rash.
Neurological examination was unremarkable.

DIAGNOSTIC CONSIDERATIONS

- Zinc deficiency
  - Congenital *aka* acrodermatitis enteropathica *aka* Danbolt-Closs syndrome *aka* Brandt syndrome
  - Acquired (eg, malabsorption from perhaps CF or celiac disease) or inadequate intake

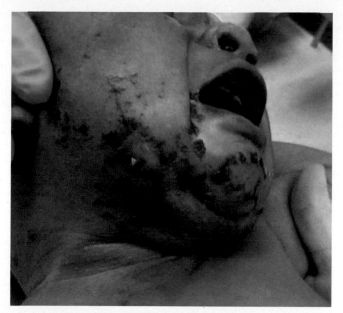

FIGURE 42.1   Denuded epithelium with dark crusty scale on the neck and chin.

- Biotin deficiency, which also has a classic perioral rash
- SSSS *aka* staphylococcal scalded skin syndrome, but the lack of a more disseminated rash makes staph toxin–mediated disease less likely

Investigation

1. Alkaline phosphatase level (this zinc-dependent enzyme is typically low in zinc deficiency and returns quickly from the laboratory test)
2. Zinc level
3. Biotin level
4. Sweat chloride
5. Sequencing of the SLC39A4 gene

Results

1. **Alk Phos was low** (Alk Phos was 56 U/mL—normal range is 110-320 U/mL).
2. **Zinc level was low (Zn 0.16 µg/mL—normal range is 0.6-1.2 µg/mL).**
3. SLCH39A4 is pending.

Diagnosis

Acrodermatitis enteropathica

Treatment/Follow-up

Zinc sulfate (or gluconate which is often better tolerated), at a dose of 3 mg/kg/d

Teaching Points

Acrodermatitis enteropathica is the clinical syndrome of zinc deficiency (rash, diarrhea, alopecia, and poor weight gain) caused by defects in the SLC39A4 gene, which is autosomal recessive, although the term is often applied to dietary zinc deficiency as well. The skin findings are typically present around the mouth, in the perianal area, and in an acral distribution (hence the term) and can be confused with diaper rash or eczema. Dietary causes are typically due to malabsorption syndromes such as cystic fibrosis and have even been reported in several cases of celiac disease. Treatment is supplementation with zinc, which makes sense for the acquired forms, but also works (for unclear reasons) in the congenital form. Recall that the SLC39A4 gene encodes a transmembrane protein that functions as a zinc transporter and allows the absorption of zinc from the gastrointestinal (GI) tract. Clearly, however, oral zinc supplementation is able to overcome the defective transporter and correct the deficiency. Zinc is better absorbed from breast milk than from formula, affecting the age of presentation (bottle-fed infants present earlier in life than breastfed infants). Zinc is present in meat and shellfish but not in most plant products, leading some to estimate that nearly 2 billion people suffer from zinc deficiency worldwide.

Suggested Readings

Kambe T, Fukue K, Ishida R, Miyazaki S. Overview of inherited zinc deficiency in infants and children. *J Nutr Sci Vitaminol (Tokyo)*. 2015;61:S44-S46.

Kury, Dréno B, Bézieau S, et al. Identification of SLC39A4, a gene involved in acrodermatitis enteropathica. *Nat Genet*. 2002;31:239-240.

Prasad AS. Zinc deficiency has been known for 40 years but ignored by global health organizations. *BMJ*. 2003;326(7386):409-410.

43

Off the Wall

Andrew J. White

CHIEF COMPLAINT

Foot rash

HISTORY OF PRESENT ILLNESS

A 13-year-old girl presents with a rash on her feet (Figure 43.1) that seems to be triggered by physical activity. It first began 6 months ago and has occurred intermittently, one to two times per month lasting for 2 to 3 days. When it occurs, it is located on her feet, soles, palms, and sometimes over her knees. It is usually red, flat, and painful but not to touch. It responds well to ibuprofen and resolves without scarring. Sometimes a few of her toes get purple. She had a fever today.

During these episodes, she usually does not have fatigue, fever, oral ulcers, muscle pain, or changes in bowel or bladder functions. She has had some recent pain in her hip and calf which she thinks are muscle strains from her competitive soccer playing. She is tired today but did not sleep well last night. She denies headaches or visual changes. She takes no medications and has had no other changes in health recently, no travel.

PAST MEDICAL HISTORY

No prior hospitalizations or surgeries

Medications

No medications

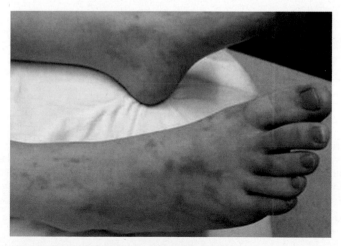

FIGURE 43.1   Red macular rash which mostly blanches.

Family/Social History

FH: No autoimmune diseases such as LE, RA, IBD, psoriasis
SH: No drug use, alcohol, or sex.

EXAMINATION

- **Vital signs:** T-37, HR 90, RR 20, BP 114/62, O_2 97%.
- **General:** Looks tired.
- **Skin:** Over the dorsum of her feet, there is an erythematous, macular, and mostly blanching rash with smaller macules over soles, extending proximally over shins. It is also present in smaller amounts on knees and palms. Not painful to touch.
- **HEENT:** Eyes are anicteric and noninjected. Pupils are equally round and reactive to light with intact extraocular movements. There is no active nasal drainage. Oral mucosa is moist with no oral ulcers, no tonsillar hypertrophy, erythema, or exudates.
- **Neck:** Supple with no lymphadenopathy.
- **Pulmonary:** Unlabored breathing, lungs are clear.
- **Cardiovascular:** Regular rate and rhythm, normal S1 and S2, and no murmurs, rubs, or gallops. Peripheral pulses are 2+ and symmetric.
- **Abdomen:** Soft, nondistended, nontender to palpation. No hepatosplenomegaly.
- **Back:** Straight spine with no lesions.
- **Extremities:** All joints have full range of motion without effusion or warmth. Strength is equal and symmetric.
- **Neurologic:** Alert and oriented with normal speech, symmetric cranial nerves. Equal and appropriate muscle strength.

DIAGNOSTIC CONSIDERATIONS

The admitting team wrote the following: "This is most likely cutaneous polyarteritis nodosa or other small vessel vasculitis such as leukocytoclastic vasculitis. Antiphospholipid antibody syndrome is also a possibility. Other causes could be lupus, inflammatory bowel disease, or cryoglobulinemia, the latter possibly triggered by infection, but this is less likely given the duration of nearly 6 months."

Investigation

1. Evaluate for SLE: ANA, C3, C4, UA, urine protein/creatinine
2. Exclude or confirm other vasculitides: ANCA, cryoglobulinemia
3. Acute hepatitis panel, antiphospholipid antibodies
4. Skin biopsy

Results

Laboratory test results:

- 9.7 > 11.6 < 250,
- PT/PTT normal
- AST 164, ALT 89
- ESR 28 mm/hr
- CRP 147 mg/L
- ANA negative
- **Skin biopsy result**: "Vascular congestion with purpura and focal eccrine gland necrosis. These findings are suggestive of **ischemia,** likely secondary to an underlying vasculopathic process. However, there is no definitive evidence of thrombus or other occlusion in these sections."

Course

She developed fever while in the hospital. The fever, coupled with the findings of ischemia on skin biopsy, suggested thromboembolic disease and led to an echocardiogram, which revealed

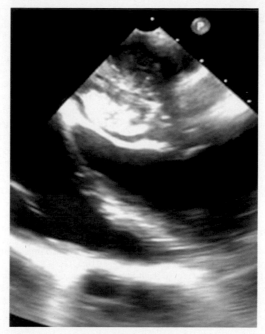

FIGURE 43.2   Echocardiogram with mass filling left atrium.

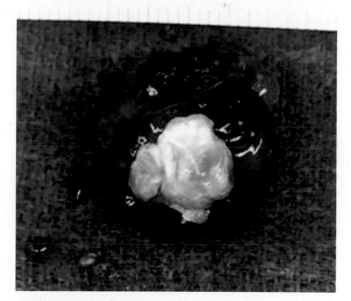

FIGURE 43.3   3 × 3 cm excised mass.

a large heterogeneous mass nearly filling the entire left atrium (see the bright object in Figure 43.2), suggestive of an atrial myxoma.

She went to surgery, and the 3 × 3 cm mass (Figure 43.3) was sent to pathology.

DIAGNOSIS

Atrial myxoma

TEACHING POINTS

Atrial myxomas are the most common type of cardiac tumor and are benign (nonmalignant) but can have serious consequences, such as embolic stroke. They are derived from mesenchymal cells and arise from the wall of the septum but are friable and may break free.

Most (75%) occur in the left atrium. They are more common in women. Ten percent of atrial myxomas are familial and occur as part of the Carney complex, an autosomal dominant disorder(s) characterized by cutaneous myxomas, schwannomas, hyperpigmentation, multiple lentigines, and endocrine hyperactivity. Most cases of Carney complex are due to mutations in PRKAR1A, a tumor-suppressor gene on chromosome 17, which encodes the type 1A regulatory subunit of protein kinase A. Treatment is surgical resection but there is a 3% recurrence rate.

Atrial myxomas should be on your differential diagnosis for **fever of unknown origin**, as they often secrete inflammatory cytokines such as IL-6. It is unclear if her symptoms were due solely to embolic phenomenon or to a vasculopathy secondary to the cytokine secreting mass, or to both.

Suggested Readings

Bernatchez J, Gaudreault V, Vincent G, Rheaume P. Left atrial myxoma presenting as an embolic shower: a case report and review of literature. *Ann Vasc Surg.* 2018;53:266.

Schiele S, Maurer SJ, Pujol Salvador C, et al. Left atrial myxoma. *Circ Cardiovasc Imaging.* 2019;12(3).

Yi SY, Han MJ, Kong YH, Joo CU, Kim SJ. Acute blindness as a presenting sign of left atrial myxoma in a pediatric patient: a case report and literature review. *Medicine (Baltimore).* 2019;98(38):e17250.

44

Rats!

Andrew J. White

CHIEF COMPLAINT

Vomiting, diarrhea, and now a rash

HISTORY OF PRESENT ILLNESS

An 8-year-old girl was transferred from another hospital after 5 days of vomiting and diarrhea. She was treated with ibuprofen for a 101 °F fever on day 2 of illness and then with 2 days of promethazine for continued vomiting. She developed a rash and had difficulty walking. Her appetite improved somewhat, but the day before transfer, her rash worsened and became painful, and she developed arthralgias and swollen metacarpophalangeal (MCP) and proximal interphalangeal (PIP) joints. She became jaundiced, and her urine output decreased.

Laboratory test results: BUN 115, Cr 2.4, platelets 22k, AST 188, ALT 65, and total bili of 9.2.

She was given a normal saline (NS) bolus and was started on maintenance intravenous fluid (IVF) prior to transfer.

PAST MEDICAL HISTORY

Hospitalization at the age of 6 years for pneumonia. No surgeries.

Family/Social History

Father has hypertension and hyperlipidemia.

She has dogs, cats, ferrets, rats, rabbits, and hamsters but has not had any bites or scratches. No recent travel, no known tick bites, no freshwater swimming.

EXAMINATION

T 38.4 HR 124 RR 32 BP 80/40 SpO$_2$ 92% on RA.

Weight 23.7 kg (30th percentile); height 133 cm (80th percentile).

Uncomfortable, does not like to be moved or touched.

Jaundice, petechiae on feet (Figure 44.1) and hands, purpura on heels, as well as a faint erythematous macular rash over the lower extremities.

Normocephalic, atraumatic, conjunctiva clear, no drainage. Scleral icterus, conjunctival injection. TM without erythema, bulging or perforation. No effusion. No nasal drainage or flaring. Lips cracked and bleeding, otherwise moist mucous membranes. Posterior pharynx clear, no oral lesions, no tonsillar hypertrophy.

Neck supple, no lymphadenopathy.

Lungs are clear, and there is no use of accessory muscles or retractions.

RRR, no murmurs, rubs, or gallops, normal S1, S2. 2+ distal pulses.

Abdomen soft, NTND, no HSM, no masses, NABS.

Spine straight with no deformities.

No clubbing or cyanosis. Edema of hand, fingers (MCP and PIP joints), and toes is present. Arthritis of finger joints.

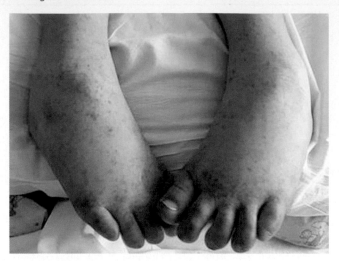

FIGURE 44.1 Petechiae on feet.

Awake, alert, answering questions appropriately. Cranial nerves intact, no motor or sensory deficits.

DIAGNOSTIC CONSIDERATIONS

* Purpura fulminans, secondary to meningococcus
* Rocky Mountain spotted fever (RMSF)
* Leptospirosis
* Ehrlichiosis
* Henoch-Schonlein purpura
* Rat-bite fever

Investigation

* CBC 8.1 > 11.9/34 < 22, 63s, 22b, 5L, 10M.
* CMP Na 128, K 3.1, Cl 93, CO_2 20, Gl 174, BUN 115, Cr 2.4, Ca 8.2, tot protein 6.4, Alb 2.6, tot bili 9.2, ALP 244, AST 188, ALT 65.
* Tot bili 9.6, direct bili 8.2, indirect 1.4.
* PT 9.3, INR 0.89, PTT 32.
* D-dimer 3.05, fibrinogen 625.
* ESR, 46, LD 403, CRP 18.1.
* Haptoglobin 104.
* Lipase 669, tot bili 7.0, direct bili 5.9, GGT 84, C3 70.2, Plt 26, BUN 84, Cr 1.4
* Abdominal sonography: Normal-appearing liver, kidneys, bladder, visualized pancreas. Splenomegaly.

Course

Lumbar puncture on day of admission showed no evidence of viral or bacterial meningitis. She was empirically started on IV antibiotics (vancomycin HD 1-3, ceftriaxone HD 1-6) and then switched to oral doxycycline for a 14-day course. Blood cultures were negative. Laboratory test results for ehrlichiosis, leptospirosis, and RMSF were negative. Babesiosis was considered, but infectious disease consultation deemed **rat-bite fever** the most likely diagnosis. She was treated with a 2-week course of doxycycline.

Discharge Diagnosis: Rat-bite fever.

At the follow-up appointment 1 month later, repeat RMSF testing demonstrated a positive antibody titer.

DIAGNOSIS

Final diagnosis: Rocky Mountain Spotted Fever

TEACHING POINTS

In the United States, rat-bite fever is most commonly caused by *Streptobacillus moniliformis*, part of the normal oral flora of rats and excreted in their urine but also transmitted by contact or ingestion of contaminated milk or food from squirrels, mice, gerbils, cats, and weasels. Contact is not necessarily a bite, *per se*, and can result from cage changing or animals licking breaks in the handler's skin (a habit the patient admitted her rat did frequently). Most animals are colonized, so increased precautions when changing cages with gloves and good hygiene are warranted, particularly in a child who scratches her skin frequently.

The disease involves abrupt onset of fever, chills, predominantly extremity-based (including palms, soles) rash, myalgias, vomiting, headache, and adenopathy. Course can be followed by migratory polyarthritis or arthralgia, and complications include relapsing disease, pneumonia, abscess formation, septic arthritis, myocarditis, endocarditis, or meningitis.

The causal agent can be isolated from blood, bite lesions, abscess aspirates, or joint fluid. Giemsa or Wright stain should also be performed on blood specimens. Cultures should be held up to 3 weeks as the organism may be slow to grow. A microbiologic diagnosis is difficult, particularly given overlapping symptomology with other animal- and tick-borne illnesses and their inherent nature of being hard to culture, so it comes as no surprise that the diagnosis was later changed in this case to RMSF.

Penicillin G for 7 to 10 days is the drug of choice for rat-bite fever, but ampicillin, cefuroxime, cefotaxime, or doxycycline can be used. The use of doxycycline may be especially helpful as proven in this case, if any suspicion of tick-borne illness remains. Untreated, the infection usually resolves on its own, though it may take a year to do so. Prognosis is generally positive, though arthralgias can persist for several months.

RMSF is a wide-spread disease caused by *Rickettsia rickettsii*, transmitted by *Dermacentor* ticks. It has been reported in almost all of the 50 states (except Hawaii, Alaska, and Maine), but five states (North Carolina, Oklahoma, Arkansas, Tennessee, and Missouri) account for over 60% of cases. Consequently, the term "Rocky Mountain" may impair the diagnostician's thinking. In the last several years, the incidence has been between two and eight cases per million (about 2000 cases per year in the United States). Initial symptoms include fever, headache, and myalgia. Later symptoms are the rash, which may be petechial and sometimes painful, joint pain, and conjunctivitis. In some cases, the rash never develops, further confounding the diagnosis. Prior to routine antibiotic usage, nearly 30% of cases were fatal. Early treatment is essential, and recognition of the nonspecific symptoms is difficult, particularly without a known tick bite.

Suggested Readings

Giorgiutti S, Lefebvre N. Rat bite fever. *N Engl J Med*. 2019;381(18):1762.
Woods CR. Rocky Mountain spotted fever in children. *Pediatr Clin North Am*. 2013;60(2):455-470.

45

Flip Flop

Andrew J. White

CHIEF COMPLAINT

"Discolored, painful toes"

HISTORY OF PRESENT ILLNESS

A 12-year-old girl presented with painful toes that started 1 to 2 months ago. She thought it might be a fungal infection. No treatment was started, but she saw a podiatrist who started her on an unknown topical cream; however, there was no improvement. Initially, her first and second toes were involved, but then all 10 toes became affected, with the most painful being the fifth toe on the left foot. The pain is 5/10 at its worst, usually precipitated by putting on tight-fitting shoes. Indeed, she wore "flip-flops" to her clinic visit on this cold, snowy winter day. Her fingers, toes, and ears are not involved. She does not remember any trauma or animal exposures prior to onset. She has had no fevers, joint pain, mouth sores, hair loss, weight loss, or swelling.

PAST MEDICAL HISTORY

- Congenital cataracts
- Seasonal allergies
- Pneumonia, at the age of 6 years

Medications

- Loratadine

Family/Social History

She lives with her parents and sister. She is in the seventh grade. She enjoys chess club and playing music.

No one in the family has rheumatoid arthritis (RA), lupus, or Raynaud phenomenon.

EXAMINATION

- Gen: Thin, well-appearing preteen.
- No oral ulcers. No tight skin around mouth.
- RRR, no murmur, 2+ radial pulses.
- Lungs clear.
- Abd: soft, NT/ND, +BS, no HSM.
- Ext: Left fifth toe erythematous, slightly enlarged, and tender to palpation (Figure 45.1). Blanches, cap refill 2 to 3 seconds. Toes are cool to the touch. Left first and second toe erythematous at distal segment. Right first and second toes erythematous and tender. Skin on toes dry and cracked in places.
- Neuro: Reflexes 2+ and symmetric.

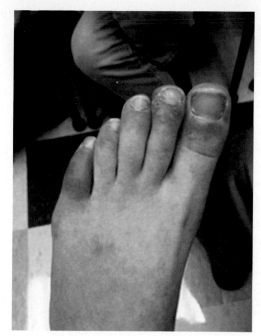

FIGURE 45.1 Patient's left foot.

Diagnostic Considerations

- Raynaud phenomenon
- Acrocyanosis
- Frostbite

Diagnosis

Chilblains

Teaching Points

Chilblains *aka* pernio is a milder form of frostbite that presents with inflammatory lesions from acute or repeated exposure to damp cold, above the freezing point. Frostbite, on the other hand, typically results from exposure to temperatures below freezing. The lesions are edematous, reddish, or purple and are often very painful or pruritic or burning. It is most common in young women, but both sexes and all age ranges may be affected. It is distinct from other nonfreezing cold injury, such as frostnip (cold-induced paresthesias that improve upon rewarming) and trench foot (prolonged exposure to cold and dampness leading to bullae and other tissue damage which is worse with tight boots and was seen often during World War I [WWI]), and is distinct from Raynaud phenomenon and acrocyanosis. Treatment involves dressing warmly. Lesions typically resolve in 2 to 4 weeks, without permanent damage.

Suggested Readings

Guly HR. Frostbite and other cold injuries in the heroic age of Antarctic exploration. *Wilderness Environ Med*. 2012;23(4):365-370. doi:10.1016/j.wem.2012.05.006

Larkins N, Murray KJ. Major cluster of chilblain cases in a cold dry Western Australian winter. *J Paediatr Child Health*. 2013;49(2):144-147.

Padeh S, Gerstein M, Greenberger S, Berkun Y. Chronic chilblains: the clinical presentation and disease course in a large paediatric series. *Clin Exp Rheumatol*. 2013;31:463-468.

Simon TD, Soep JB, Hollister JR. Pernio in pediatrics. *Pediatrics*. 2005;116(3):e472.

Sugiura K, Takeichi T, Kono M, et al. Severe chilblain lupus is associated with heterozygous missense mutations of catalytic amino acids or their adjacent mutations in the exonuclease domains of 3'-repair exonuclease 1. *J Invest Dermatol*. 2012;132(12):2855-2857. doi: 10.1038/jid.2012.210

46

I Told You It Hurt

Andrew J. White

CHIEF COMPLAINT

Headache

HISTORY OF PRESENT ILLNESS

A 7-year-old girl started complaining of headache 2 days ago. The pain was in the frontal area, and she had taken some acetaminophen without much relief. She went to school on the day of presentation, and her teacher noticed a large lump on her scalp. Her mother had not noticed the swelling until that day. There was no known trauma, although she did play tag 3 days ago but sustained no head injuries. Her mother was with her the next 2 days, and they watched movies and were fairly inactive. Her hair was newly braided about a week prior to presentation. She had no constitutional symptoms, was not an easy bruiser, had no gum or nose bleeds, and had no rash.

EXAMINATION

There was a 10×10 cm^2 wide boggy, protruding area on her right frontoparietal scalp. She had a few bruises on her shins but no petechiae or bruising elsewhere. Her neurologic examination was normal.

DIAGNOSTIC CONSIDERATIONS

- Cellulitis
- Kerion, a fungal scalp infection
- Unrecognized trauma
- Tumor (primary or metastatic)

Investigation

- Laboratory tests: Hg 10, platelets 281, normal PT, PTT, and INR.
- A CT scan of the head was obtained (see Figure 46.1) and read as follows: "Noncontrast images from a head CT show a large right subgaleal hematoma (white arrow). There is no underlying skull fracture."

DIAGNOSIS

Subgaleal hemorrhage, secondary to hair braiding

TEACHING POINTS

The scalp is composed of five layers: skin, connective tissue, galea aponeurotica, loose areolar tissue, and periosteum. Fluid between the various layers represent different diagnoses. Caput succedaneum is transient edema and serosanguinous fluid collection above the galea aponeurotica. Cephalohematoma is bleeding beneath the periosteum. Subgaleal hemorrhage

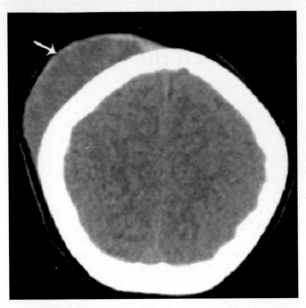

FIGURE 46.1 In this single view of the computer tomography (CT) scan, the arrow indicates the subgaleal hematoma.

is bleeding in the loose areolar tissue. Unlike cephalohematoma, subgaleal hemorrhage can cross suture lines.

Subgaleal hemorrhage that occurs after the neonatal period is usually associated with tangential or radial force applied to the scalp in which veins crossing the subgaleal space rupture. One review of subgaleal hemorrhage suggested that children have a more vascular subgaleal space with a thinner scalp that could potentially predispose them to hemorrhage. They described subgaleal hemorrhage in a variety of patients aged 2 months to 52 years. Of these hemorrhages, 80% were located in the frontal or parietal scalp, and 93% of cases were in children younger than 10 years. Fifty-one percent had associated skull fracture, and there was concern for a possible bleeding diathesis in 0.05%.

Case reports of subgaleal hemorrhage from minor trauma exist. The hemorrhage can occur immediately or may be delayed as long as 14 days after the event. The onset is usually insidious, occurring over several days, and frequently accompanied by headache.

Treatment is watchful waiting. Complications may include calcification or extension into the orbit which may be treated with surgical drainage. Consideration of laboratory evaluation for coagulation defects or serial measurement of hemoglobin depends on the specific clinical scenario. Radiographic imaging may also be considered to exclude skull fracture.

Suggested Readings

Adeloye A, Odeku EL. Subgaleal hematoma in head injuries. *Int Surg.* 1975;60(5):263-265.
Vu T, Guerrera M, Hamburger EK, Klein BL. Subgaleal hematoma from hair braiding: case report and literature review. *Pediatr Emerg Care.* 2004;20(12):821-823.

47

A Little Mottling

William B. Orr, Susan J. Bayliss, Jennifer A. Wambach

CHIEF COMPLAINT

Poor perfusion

HISTORY OF PRESENT ILLNESS

A late preterm infant female was born at 35 weeks estimated gestation to a healthy 26-year-old G3P2 mother with normal antenatal testing for rubella, syphilis, hepatitis B, and human immunodeficiency virus (HIV). Pregnancy was complicated by intrauterine growth restriction and preterm labor 3 weeks prior to delivery, for which mother was given betamethasone and nifedipine.

The infant was delivered via C-section due to nonreassuring antenatal surveillance. She cried at birth, was vigorous, and received routine neonatal care. Apgar scores were 8 and 9. At birth, she had a diffuse, deep purple, nonblanchable, reticulated rash with violaceous patches on her extremities, abdomen, and back that were most prominent on her left arm and leg, without areas of ulceration (Figure 47.1).

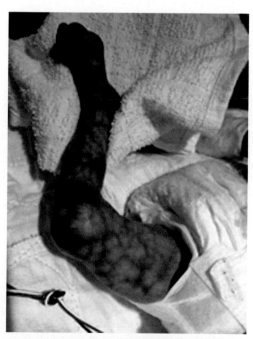

FIGURE 47.1 Left lower extremity demonstrates diffuse, dark purple, nonblanchable, reticulated rash.

PAST MEDICAL HISTORY

None

Family/Social History

Family history was positive for congenital cataracts.

EXAMINATION

No other abnormalities were identified on physical examination. She was admitted to the neonatal intensive care unit.

DIAGNOSTIC CONSIDERATIONS

The physicians in the delivery room were puzzled and had no plausible explanation.

Results

Her laboratory studies were within normal limits including white blood cell count, hemoglobin, prothrombin time, partial thromboplastin time, and international normalized ratio. Blood culture was negative. Biopsy was not performed. The infant was not given antibiotics as there were minimal septic risk factors. Echocardiogram, abdominal ultrasound, and ophthalmologic examinations were normal.

DIAGNOSIS

Pediatric Dermatology was consulted and immediately recognized and diagnosed:
Cutis marmorata telangiectatica congenita (CMTC).

Treatment/Follow-up

The infant was treated with diffuse application of petrolatum to areas of dry skin to help reduce the risk for ulceration.

TEACHING POINTS

CMTC was first described by Cato van Lohuizen in 1922 in a child with skin findings including livedo reticularis, telangiectases, and superficial ulceration. CMTC is a rare, sporadic, congenital cutaneous disorder with persistent cutis marmorata, telangiectasia, and phlebectasia, often with skin atrophy and rarely with ulceration. Most commonly present at birth, CMTC has also been diagnosed during infancy from 3 months to 2 years of age. There is a slight female predominance, and CMTC has been identified among individuals of diverse ethnic backgrounds. The lower extremities are most commonly affected followed by the trunk, upper extremities, and rarely the face. Although the majority of cases are unilateral (67%), there are reports of bilateral and even generalized lesions. CMTC is most frequently associated with hypotrophy of the affected limb (rarely hypertrophy). Other associated anomalies include congenital glaucoma (up to 10% of patients with facial involvement), retinal detachment, macrocephaly, syndactyly, hip dysplasia, clubfoot, high-arched palate, tendinitis stenosans, aplasia cutis congenita, hypospadias, lipoma, multicystic renal disease, and Kartagener syndrome. Neurologic deficits, seizures, and developmental delays have also been reported in ~10% of affected individuals. CMTC can be seen in Adams-Oliver syndrome (AOS) which includes aplasia cutis congenita and malformations of the limbs. Screening patients with CMTC for associated anomalies is recommended including ophthalmologic, cardiac, and orthopedic assessments.

Histology of the affected tissue in CMTC demonstrates swollen endothelial cells, abnormal dilation and congestion of the capillaries in the papillary dermis, proliferation of the vascular channels in the reticular dermis, dilated veins, and venous lakes. Diagnosis can be made from clinical examination alone and does not require a skin biopsy. The prognosis is generally favorable with reduction of the erythema during the first 2 years of life with supportive dermatologic care including petrolatum and monitoring for skin ulceration or infection. However, there is usually a persistent net-like pattern on the skin. Laser therapy has been performed with variable outcomes.

The etiology and pathogenesis of CMTC remain unknown. Proposed etiologies include failure of development of the mesodermic vessels in early embryogenesis, peripheral neural dysfunction, or somatic mosaicism for a lethal gene mutation. Localized atrophy and ulceration may result from vascular occlusion. Most cases are sporadic, but familial cases have been reported. Recently, a child with CMTC (diffuse livedo reticularis of trunk and extremities, dark red mottled patches and telangiectasia of the face), bilateral glaucoma, dysmorphic facial features, generalized cerebral atrophy, pial angiomatosis, seizures, motor and speech developmental delays, hepatomegaly, and hypospadias was identified with whole-exome sequencing to be homozygous for a nonsense variant in *ARL6IP6*.

Suggested Readings

Abumansour IS, Hijazi H, Alazmi A, et al. ARL6IP6, a susceptibility locus for ischemic stroke, is mutated in a patient with syndromic cutis marmorata telangiectatica congenita. *Hum Genet.* 2015;134(8):815-822.

Amitai DB, Fichman S, Merlob P, Morad Y, Lapidoth M, Metzker A. Cutis marmorata telangiectatica congenita: clinical findings in 85 patients. *Pediatr Dermatol.* 2000;17(2):100-104.

Bui T, Corap A, Bygum A. Cutis marmorata telangiectatica congenita: a literature review. *Orphanet J Rare Dis.* 2019;14(1):283.

De Maio C, Pomero G, Delogu A, Briatore E, Bertero M, Gancia P. Cutis marmorata telangiectatica congenita in a preterm female newborn: case report and review of the literature. *Pediatr Med Chir.* 2014;36(4):90.

del Boz Gonzalez J, Serrano Martin MM, Vera Casano A. Cutis marmorata telangiectatica congenita. Review of 33 cases. *An Pediatr (Barc).* 2008;69(6):557-564.

Fayol L, Garcia P, Denis D, Philip N, Simeoni U. Adams-Oliver syndrome associated with cutis marmorata telangiectatica congenita and congenital cataract: a case report. *Am J Perinatol.* 2006;23(3):197-200.

Happle R. Mosaicism in human skin. Understanding the patterns and mechanisms. *Arch Dermatol.* 1993;129(11):1460-1470.

Kienast AK, Hoeger PH. Cutis marmorata telangiectatica congenita: a prospective study of 27 cases and review of the literature with proposal of diagnostic criteria. *Clin Exp Dermatol.* 2009;34(3):319-323.

Picascia DD, Esterly NB. Cutis marmorata telangiectatica congenita: report of 22 cases. *J Am Acad Dermatol.* 1989;20(6):1098-1104.

Van Lohuizen C. Uber eine seltene angeborene Hautanomalie (cutis marmorata telangiectatica congenita). *Acta Derm Venereol.* 1922;3:202-211.

48

Tic Toc, Doc

Alexa Altman Doss

CHIEF COMPLAINT

"My legs gave out"

HISTORY OF PRESENT ILLNESS

An 11-year-old boy presented to his primary care doctor after two episodes of his legs giving out in the past week. He feels like he cannot control his legs during these episodes. He was awake and recalls the entire event.

Mother noted he has been more irritable over the last few weeks and has started napping again after school. She also says his mouth kept opening with his jaw dropping down yesterday while he was watching TV. The patient said he did not have much control over his jaw at the time but this resolved after taking a nap.

Two months ago, he had a febrile upper respiratory infection that spread easily through the whole family.

PAST MEDICAL HISTORY

- Mild persistent asthma controlled on Flovent 44, 2 puffs BID
- Obesity, BMI >95th percentile

Family/Social History

Father with obstructive sleep apnea. Sister with moderate persistent asthma. He lives with mother, father, and one younger sister. Attends school and is in sixth grade.

EXAMINATION

- Vitals: T 37.1, HR 82, RR 14, BP 112/74, weight 59 kg
- General: Alert, no acute distress
- HEENT: Head normocephalic, atraumatic, pupils equal reactive and responsive to light, conjunctiva normal, EOMI, TM normal bilaterally, no nasal congestion, moist mucus membranes, no pharyngeal erythema, tonsils 1+ bilaterally, neck supple, no cervical lymphadenopathy
- Pulmonary: Lungs clear to auscultation bilaterally, no wheezing, rales or rhonchi, no retractions
- Cardiovascular: Heart regular rate and rhythm, no murmurs, rubs, or gallops, normal S1 and S2, radial pulses 2+ bilaterally
- Abdomen: Soft, normal bowel sounds, nondistended, nontender, no hepatosplenomegaly.
- Extremities: No clubbing, cyanosis, or edema
- Skin: Warm, dry, no rashes, capillary refill <2 seconds
- Neurologic: Awake, alert, oriented ×3, answers questions appropriately for age, cranial nerves II-XII intact, patellar and Achilles reflexes 2+, muscle strength 5/5 in bilateral upper and lower extremities, normal tone, normal gait, negative Romberg, normal heel-to-toe walk, and normal finger-to-nose test

DIAGNOSTIC CONSIDERATIONS

- Epilepsy
- Obstructive sleep apnea
- Tic disorder
- Sydenham chorea
- Poor sleep hygiene
- Narcolepsy with cataplexy
- Syncope
- Drug exposure
- Hypothyroidism
- Rapid-onset obesity, hypoventilation, hypothalamic and autonomic dysfunction (ROHHAD)

Investigation

- Initial laboratory tests BMP, magnesium, phosphate, CBC, TSH, T4, ferritin, and urine drug screen are all unremarkable.
- Video EEG: captured one fall, but no seizure activity was present on EEG.
- Brain MRI: normal.

Results

Impression: Tic disorder, although these typically present earlier at about 6 years of age.

Over the next 3 months, he began taking naps daily, sometimes taking a nap twice daily despite sleeping 7.5 to 8.5 hours each night. The episodes of his legs giving out and falling became more frequent, now up to three times per week. Occasionally, there has been an association with falling when he was laughing. He developed more episodes of jaw dropping or tongue movements when riding in the car or watching TV. He also had intermittent ptosis.

He was admitted for further workup, and he had a video EEG that captured the above episodes but did not show seizure activity. A sleep study and a multiple sleep latency tests excluded obstructive sleep apnea and periodic limb movement disorder. His mean sleep latency was 5.5 minutes. He also had three episodes of sleep-onset REM periods. These findings are suggestive of narcolepsy. Laboratory tests included HLA typing that was positive for HLA DQB1*0602.

DIAGNOSIS

Narcolepsy, with cataplexy

Treatment/Follow-up

- Sleepiness was treated with armodafinil. Cataplexy treated with sodium oxybate and atomoxetine. Good sleep hygiene was enforced. Weight loss was highly encouraged.
- Over the next 2 months, his excessive daytime sleepiness and cataplexy significantly improved. He lost 5 lb by decreasing snacking and plans to start basketball for exercise.

TEACHING POINTS

Narcolepsy is a life-long neurologic disorder that can often be initially misdiagnosed due to lack of symptom recognition. Symptoms include excessive daytime sleepiness, cataplexy, sleep paralysis, and hypnagogic or hypnopompic hallucinations. These symptoms can gradually appear over time, typically starting with excessive daytime sleepiness, leading to a delay in diagnosis. Narcolepsy is divided into two forms, type 1 and type 2. Type 1 patients, previously called narcolepsy with cataplexy, are characterized by cataplexy and low orexin (hypocretin 1) levels in CSF. Orexin is a neuropeptide needed to maintain wakefulness. The majority of patients with narcolepsy type 1 are also positive for HLA DQB1*0602. Childhood narcolepsy type 1 can also be associated with obesity at the time of symptom onset. Type 2 patients, previously called narcolepsy without cataplexy, do not have cataplexy and have normal orexin.

Cataplexy: Approximately, 70% to 80% of patients experience cataplexy. Cataplexy is an abrupt loss of muscle tone that can be triggered by strong emotions. Patients are awake during these episodes that last seconds to minutes. Cataplexy episodes in children typically involve the face and include ptosis, tongue protrusions, jaw dropping, and head drop.

Treatment focuses on managing symptoms, as there is no cure for narcolepsy. Education is provided on good sleep hygiene; patients may benefit from a short, scheduled nap. Daytime exercise is encouraged to increase alertness. School modifications may be required. Patients who are overweight should also aim for a healthy weight. Daytime sleepiness can be treated with stimulant medications. Cataplexy can be treated with sodium oxybate, amitriptyline, venlafaxine, imipramine, or atomoxetine.

Suggested Readings

Babiker MO, Prasad M. Narcolepsy in children: a diagnostic and management approach. *Pediatr Neurol*. 2015;52(6):557-565. doi:10.1016/j.pediatrneurol.2015.02.020

Kotagal S, Hartse KM, Walsh JK. Characteristics of narcolepsy in preteenaged children. *Pediatrics*. 1990;85(2):205-209.

Kotagal S, Krahn LE, Slocumb N. A putative link between childhood narcolepsy and obesity. *Sleep Med*. 2004;5(2):147-150. doi:10.1016/j.sleep.2003.10.006

Koziorynska EI, Rodriguez AJ. Narcolepsy: clinical approach to etiology, diagnosis, and treatment. *Rev Neurol Dis*. 2011;8(3-4):e97-e106.

Nevsimalova S. Narcolepsy in childhood. *Sleep Med Rev*. 2009;13(2):169-180. doi:10.1016/j.smrv.2008.04.007

Nishino S, Ripley B, Overeem S, Lammers GJ, Mignot E. Hypocretin (orexin) deficiency in human narcolepsy. *Lancet*. 2000;355(9197):39-40. doi:10.1016/S0140-6736(99)05582-8

49

Epulis

Luke T. Viehl

CHIEF COMPLAINT

"White spots on her gums"

HISTORY OF PRESENT ILLNESS

A 5-week-old girl presented to her pediatrician's office due to "white spots" on her lower gums. Parents noticed the white spots approximately 1 week ago, and they have increased slightly in size and are now somewhat red. She has been fussy since birth, and her pediatrician had started her on famotidine and switched formulas several times. She has had no other symptoms.

PAST MEDICAL HISTORY

Born at 40 and 2/7 weeks via spontaneous vaginal delivery (SVD). Uncomplicated pregnancy with reassuring serologies. Meconium-stained fluids at delivery but did not receive respiratory support. Currently on Nutramigen.

Medications

None

Family/Social History

Family history: No history of gastrointestinal (GI) disorders or milk protein intolerance.
Social history: Lives at home with parents who are both nurse practitioners. No recent travel or exposures.

EXAMINATION

- VS: T 37.5 °C; HR 130; RR 32; SpO$_2$ 100%.
- General: She is active and irritable; difficult to console but will briefly calm with swaddling and rocking.
- HEENT: An approximately 0.5-cm diameter erythematous swelling is present along the labial surface of the right mandibular gingiva, but the mouth and oropharynx are otherwise clear. Fontanelle is soft and flat, TMs normal, no nasal drainage.
- CV: Regular rate and rhythm, no murmurs.
- Pulm: Normal breath sounds bilaterally without any distress.
- Abdomen: soft, nontender/nondistended, no HSM.
- GU: Normal Tanner 1 female external genitalia.

DIAGNOSTIC CONSIDERATIONS

- Hemangioma
- Nonaccidental trauma
- Congenital **epulis**
- Thrush

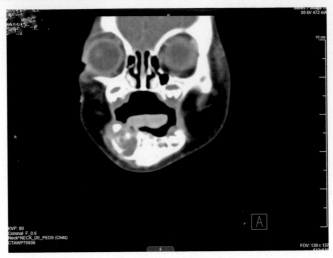

FIGURE 49.1 Coronal image shows large tumor centered at the right mandible resulting in multiple missing teeth and floating teeth within the tumor.

Investigation

She was referred to an ENT clinic for further evaluation. The lesion had doubled in size in the interim. Propranolol was started for the possibility of a hemangioma. In addition, she had become increasingly inconsolable with near-constant crying despite q4 acetaminophen with only brief 1- to 2-hour periods of rest.

She was seen 1 week later, and the lesion had again doubled in size despite propranolol therapy. A CT was obtained with a representative image shown in Figure 49.1.

The decision was made to biopsy the lesion, which revealed the ultimate diagnosis.

DIAGNOSIS

Melanotic neuroectodermal tumor of infancy

Treatment/Follow-up

After the biopsy results returned, she underwent segmental mandibulectomy of approximately 3 cm with placement of external distractor. A gastrostomy tube was placed to enable feeding. Her distractor has since been removed, but the gastrostomy remains due to continued issues with swallowing coordination. Her mouth and chin have cosmetic defects, but she continues to be followed by ENT and Plastic Surgery and will undergo reconstruction in the near future.

TEACHING POINTS

This class of tumor is benign but grows rapidly and aggressively. It is often located in the maxilla and can destroy the underlying bone. It is typically grayish blue in color with a firm surface and spherical shape. Surgical removal is often curative with rare recurrence. Adjuvant therapy with chemotherapeutic agents or radiation is not routinely utilized.

These neoplasms were first described in 1918. There was significant confusion regarding the origin of this tumor. As such, these tumors have gone by several different names including congenital melanocarcinoma, retinal anlage tumor, pigmented congenital epulis, or melanotic progonoma. These tumors can present in several different locations but predominantly arise from the craniofacial region, especially the maxilla (~62%), skull (~16%), and mandible (~8%). Other sites are more rare, but these tumors have been reported arising from the brain, epididymis, mediastinal structures, ovary, uterus, and appendicular long bones. Interestingly, 10% to 15% of these tumors have been associated with elevation of urinary vanillylmandelic acid, further confirming their neural crest cell origin.

An epulis is a congenital, rare and benign hamartomatous growth found on the alveolar ridge seen in newborn infants. Occasionally they may lead to respiratory or feeding difficulties, due to mass effect. The pathogenesis is unknown and they are thought synonymous with a gingival granular cell tumor of the newborn. Treatment is surgical resection.

Suggested Readings

Andrade NN, Mathai PC, Sahu V, Aggarwal N, Andrade T. Melanotic neuroectodermal tumour of infancy—a rare entity. *J Oral Biol Craniofac Res*. 2016;6(3):237-240. doi:10.1016/j.jobcr.2016.06.005

Olson JL, Marcus JR, Zuker RM. Congenital epulis. *J Craniofac Surg*. 2005;16(1):161-164. doi:10.1097/00001665-200501000-00033

50

Big Boy Colic

Andrew J. White

CHIEF COMPLAINT

Seven-year-old boy with vomiting

HISTORY OF PRESENT ILLNESS

He vomited twice the night before and five times on the morning he went to the emergency room. There were streaks of small amounts of blood on the most recent episode. He has not vomited before, and he has had no diarrhea, constipation, fevers, or upper respiratory infection (URI) symptoms. He has been more tired lately, but he dressed himself that morning, walked to the bus stop, and was awake and alert, before calling his mom after vomiting again, this time with some crampy belly pain. Mom was worried about the blood in the vomit, and the new symptom of what she called "colicky" pain, and so she took him to the emergency department (ED).

PAST MEDICAL HISTORY

- Asthma, mild intermittent
- ADHD, not treated
- Anemia, newly diagnosed 3 weeks ago, treated with iron

EXAMINATION

He was sleepy and difficult to arouse. Tachycardic with a 3/6 SEM and cap refill was >5 seconds. Abdomen was soft. No rash, 2+ reflexes at the knees.

A stat CBC was sent: Hemoglobin of **4.1 mg/dL; MCV was 68;** and **RDW was 26**. Electrolytes were normal, as were serum transaminases, lipase, and amylase.

DIFFERENTIAL

Early diagnostic thoughts were not recorded, but **acute GI blood loss** must have been on the short list, with resultant poor perfusion of the CNS.

A blood transfusion was initiated, and admission to the general pediatrics ward was planned; however, his mental status did not improve and seemed to worsen.

He then developed new-onset respiratory distress, which rapidly progressed to respiratory failure within an hour.

He was intubated, and a stat CXR revealed pulmonary edema. The blood transfusion was paused because of the possibility of a transfusion-related acute lung injury (TRALI), and he was sent for a head CT to exclude intracranial hemorrhage as an etiology for his declining mental status.

The CT showed no acute bleed, and he was admitted to the PICU, where he remained intubated, ventilated, and obtunded.

A flat plate of the abdomen, ordered as part of the investigation for GI bleeding, revealed the diagnosis and is shown in Figure 50.1.

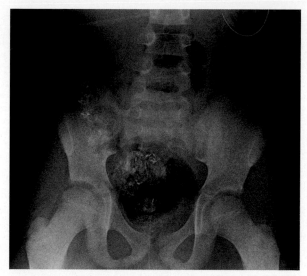

FIGURE 50.1   A flat plate of the abdomen, ordered as part of the investigation for gastrointestinal (GI) bleeding, showing radiodensities within the lumen of the gut.

DIAGNOSIS

1. **Lead poisoning**, due to ingestion of paint chips
2. Encephalopathy due to #1
3. Anemia, iron deficient, due to and/or exacerbated by #1
4. Pica, due to #3, and contributing to #1
5. **Lead colic** (the cause of the chief complaint)
6. Respiratory failure, unknown etiology, possibly TRALI

Treatment/Follow-up

1. Evacuation of GI tract
2. Chelation. Dimercaprol injectable 91 mg q 4 hours **and** edetate calcium disodium injectable 450 mg q 12 hours
3. Slow resumption of transfusion
4. Supportive respiratory care in ICU

TEACHING POINTS

Lead is among the first metals to be mined and used by humans because of its low melting point, malleability, and corrosion resistance. The toxic effects of lead were discovered as early as the second century BD by the Greek physician Nikander, who observed colic and paralysis with lead toxicity. A century later, the Greek physician Dioscorides wrote that with lead, "the mind gives way." In the Roman empire, the Middle Ages, and the Industrial Revolution, lead exposure was mostly occupational. However, the introduction of lead-based residential paint in the 19th century brought lead within reach of children. The addition of tetraethyllead to gasoline from the 1920s to the 1980s to prevent engine knocking further contributed to lead exposure through contamination of air, dust, and soil. Australian physicians made the connection between lead-based paint and increased toxicity in children in the early 1900s. Lead-based paint was banned in most of the developed world by the mid-1930s, but aggressive lobbying by the US Lead Industries Association prevented a US ban until the late 1970s. The lead industry led a campaign to discredit the studies and began featuring children prominently in their advertising. The Dutch Boy brand and logo was one manifestation of this marketing.

The manifestations of lead toxicity in children are primarily a result of ingestion or inhalation of lead dust from lead-based paint residue in the home as well as lead dust in soil. Ingestion of paint chips is less common but is of concern in cases of concurrent iron-deficiency anemia that can cause pica. The multisystem toxicity is largely due to lead's ability to bind to sulfhydryl groups on enzymes and mimic other divalent cations, such as iron, calcium, and zinc. Lead is excreted very slowly in small amounts in urine and even smaller amounts in feces, hair, nails, and sweat. Children younger than 2 years retain about one-third of absorbed lead whereas adults retain less than 1%. There is no known safe level of lead and no apparent threshold for physiologic effects. Because most biochemical reactions in the body involve divalent cations that can be displaced by lead, the effects of lead toxicity are widespread:

1. **Neurologic:** Effects range from developmental delay, cognitive deficits, and behavioral problems to encephalopathy (at blood lead levels of about 100 µg/dL) to coma and death. Although lumbar puncture is a standard diagnostic modality for encephalopathy, lumbar puncture should be avoided in cases of severe lead toxicity as lead can cause increased intracranial pressure.

2. **Hematologic:** Decreased hemoglobin synthesis can occur with blood lead levels greater than about 40 µg/dL. In addition, iron-deficiency anemia is a common comorbidity with lead poisoning, both because of poor nutrition in at-risk populations as well as increased gastrointestinal (GI) absorption of lead due to iron deficiency. Basophilic stippling of red blood cells (RBCs) may be seen but is not specific for lead toxicity.

3. **Renal:** Acute, high-level lead poisoning can cause a Fanconi-type syndrome, with glucosuria, aminoaciduria, and renal phosphate wasting. Rarely, more prolonged (decades-long), high-level exposure can cause lead nephropathy, a chronic tubulointerstitial nephritis that can progress to end-stage renal disease.

4. **GI:** Lead colic, resulting in vomiting, abdominal pain, and constipation, occurs rarely.

5. **Endocrine:** Lead inhibits vitamin D metabolism, possibly contributing to decreased growth and delayed puberty.

Treatment for any elevated blood lead level begins with removal of the lead source as well as correction of coexisting iron, calcium, and zinc deficiency. The Centers for Disease Control and Prevention (CDC) recommends abdominal radiograph and subsequent bowel decontamination for children with blood lead level over 20 µg/dL. Chelation is not indicated for blood lead levels between 20 and 44 µg/dL as it may reduce the lead level but has not been shown to improve clinical outcomes. Oral chelation therapy is recommended for children with blood lead levels over 45 µg/dL. Hospitalization, while not essential, provides the opportunity to monitor adverse effects of chelation and removes the child from the lead source. Oral meso-2,3-dimercaptosuccinic acid (DMSA, or Succimer) is the first-line therapy, with IV edetate calcium disodium (CaNa$_2$EDTA) as a backup for children who cannot adhere to treatment. For severe lead toxicity (blood lead level over 70 µg/dL), hospitalization in an intensive care unit and combined chelation therapy with IM dimercaprol (British anti-Lewisite, or BAL) and IV CaNa$_2$EDTA are indicated. CaNa$_2$EDTA should not be confused with Na$_2$EDTA, as the latter will cause hypocalcemia. Two-agent chelation reduces mortality in severe lead toxicity from 66% to 1% to 2%, although it does not affect the chronic neurocognitive effects of lead toxicity.

Suggested Readings

Bellinger DC. Lead. *Pediatrics*. 2004;113:1016.

Centers for Disease Control and Prevention. *Managing Elevated Blood Lead Levels among Young Children: Recommendations from the Advisory Committee on Childhood Lead Poisoning Prevention*; 2002.

Major RH. Some landmarks in the history of lead poisoning. *Ann Med*. 1931;3:218.

Markowitz G, Rosner D. "Cater to the children": the role of the lead industry in a public health tragedy, 1900-1955. *Am J Public Health*. 2000;90:36.

Selevan SG, Rice DC, Hogan KA, Euling SY, Pfahles-Hutchens A, Bethel J. Blood lead concentration and delayed puberty in girls. *N Engl J Med*. 2003;348:1527.

51

A Definite Eating Disorder

Laura A. Duckworth

CHIEF COMPLAINT

Generalized swelling, fatigue

HISTORY OF PRESENT ILLNESS

A 9-year-old girl was brought to the emergency department (ED) by her mother because of loose stools, fatigue, and swelling in her legs and face. For over a week, she has been having at least six watery, nonbloody stools a day, which was up from her normal 1 to 2 stools per day. She has intermittent nonspecific abdominal pain prior to defecation. She has had extreme fatigue, sometimes sleeping all day. Two days ago, she developed facial swelling, which then progressed to leg swelling the next day. No fevers, vomiting, hematochezia, cough, or congestion.

PAST MEDICAL HISTORY

- A 27-week premature infant, complicated by necrotizing enterocolitis (NEC). Did not go home on oxygen.
- Short gut syndrome due to NEC. G-tube was removed 5 years ago. She has 36 cm of remaining small bowel with an ileocolonic anastomosis at the hepatic flexure and has no ileocecal valve.
- Micronutrient deficiencies (vitamin D, E, B12) that were supplemented in the past, but she is no longer receiving them.
- Developmental delay.
- Latent nystagmus and exotropia, followed by ophthalmology.

Medications

She is not currently taking any medications on a daily basis.

Family/Social History

Lives at home with mom, and they follow a vegan diet with limited red meat consumption. Mother cooks with noniodized sea salt.

EXAMINATION

- Vitals: HR 145 beats/min; RR 16 breaths/min; T 38.1 F; BP 119/74 mm Hg; SpO$_2$ 100% on room air.
- General appearance: Comfortable, cooperative, no acute distress.
- HEENT:
  - Head: Normocephalic, atraumatic.
  - Ears: TMs normal bilaterally.
  - Eyes: Disconjugate gaze (at her baseline). Conjunctival pallor. No scleral icterus.
  - Nose: No nasal discharge.
  - Mouth/throat: Mucus membranes moist. Posterior pharynx clear.
  - Neck: No cervical lymphadenopathy.
- Cardiovascular: Tachycardia. Regular rhythm. 2/6 systolic murmur. 2+ distal pulses.

- Pulmonary: Lungs clear to auscultation bilaterally. Respiratory effort is normal. No wheezes, rales, or rhonchi.
- Abdominal: Flat, nontender, nondistended. Large horizontal well-healed surgical scar. No hepatosplenomegaly.
- Skin: Pale. Warm, dry. Capillary refill 2 to 3 seconds.
- Extremities: No clubbing or cyanosis. Nonpitting edema to bilateral feet.
- Neurologic:
  - Mental status: Awake, alert, answers questions appropriately but sometimes slow to respond.
  - Cranial nerves: Face symmetric, tongue midline. PERRL, right > left exotropia.
  - Motor: Normal tone. Full strength in upper and lower extremities bilaterally.
  - Reflexes: 2+ biceps and patellar reflexes. 2 beats of ankle clonus bilaterally.
  - Cerebellar: No ataxia, tremor, or nystagmus.

DIAGNOSTIC CONSIDERATIONS

Edema complicating the nonspecific problems of diarrhea and fatigue suggest either a protein-losing enteropathy or perhaps HUS.

Investigation

The workup started with screening laboratory tests of CBC, CMP, and UA (to evaluate for proteinuria) but then was quickly expanded once the CBC returned.

Laboratory Results

- CBC: **Hemoglobin 3.0 g/dL** (MCV 98.8), **platelets 26,000 K/mm³**, WBC 5.8 K/mm
- CMP: Na 141 mmol/L, K 2.6 mmol/L, Cl 106 mmol/L, CO_2 25 mmol/L, BUN 8 mg/dL, Cr 0.63 mg/dL, glucose 126 mg/dL, Ca 8.2 mg/dL, total bilirubin 1.5 mg/dL, total protein 5.8 g/dL, albumin 3.6 g/dL, alkaline phosphatase 102 U/L, ALT 36 U/L, AST 226 U/L
- UA 1+ protein, 1+ bilirubin, 1+ leukocyte esterase
- Vitamins/minerals: Vitamin B12 < 150 pg/mL (undetectably low), vitamin D < 8 ng/mL (low), vitamin E 3.8 mg/L (low end of normal), zinc 0.7 mcg/mL (normal), selenium 93 ng/mL (normal), folate 17.0 ng/mL, thiamine 129 nmol/L (normal)

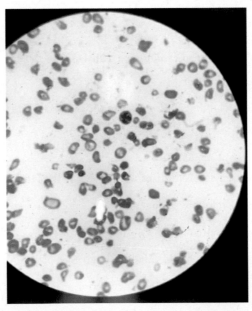

FIGURE 51.1 Peripheral blood smear.

- Hemolysis laboratory results: LDH > 2500 U/L, haptoglobin < 10 mg/dL, direct antiglobulin test negative
- Iron profile: Iron 169 mcg/dL (high), TIBC 355 mcg/dL (normal), transferrin saturation 48% (high), ferritin 137 ng/mL (normal)
- Reticulocytes 5.8% (inappropriately normal)
- Thyroid studies: TSH 13.75 mcIU/mL (high), free T4 1.40 ng/dL (normal), thyroperoxidase antibody < 20 U/mL
- Methylmalonic acid 7.46 nmol/mL (high)
- Peripheral smear (Figure 51.1): Normal WBC quantity with immature granulocytes and hypersegmented neutrophils, no blasts; RBCs low in number with anisocytosis, polychromasia, some ovalocytes, and some RBC fragments; thrombocytopenia

DIAGNOSIS

Anemia due to vitamin B12 deficiency.
   Coexisting **vitamin A and E deficiency**, also contributing to anemia.

Treatment/Follow-up

1. Mother is a Jehovah's witness and refused blood transfusion for her daughter on religious grounds. Since the child was relatively stable other than tachycardia (her blood pressure and saturations were normal), she was not given any blood products during admission.
2. Vitamin supplementation: Vitamin B12 IM, ferric gluconate IV, fat-soluble vitamins (DEKAs) PO. Hemoglobin reached nadir of 2.4 but slowly improved to reached 6.5 g/dL at discharge.
3. 2 L of oxygen via nasal cannula to optimize oxygen-carrying capacity.
4. Negative infectious studies (respiratory pathogen panel, urine, blood, and stool cultures).

TEACHING POINTS

In children, vitamin B12 deficiency can present with nonspecific symptoms including developmental delay, irritability, fatigue, poor feeding, and failure to thrive. Other symptoms may include the nervous system, such as paresthesias, ataxia, hypotonia, and mood changes or poor school performance.

   The etiology is generally due to either decreased intake, abnormal absorption, or inborn errors of B12 transport or metabolism. Most dietary B12 is obtained from animal source foods; thus, people with a primarily vegetarian or vegan diet, or infants breastfed by mothers with this diet, are at risk for vitamin B12 deficiency. Absorption of vitamin B12 is a complex process that starts with release of B12 from dietary proteins by gastric acid and binding to R-binder proteins in the stomach. After release from R-binder proteins by pancreatic enzymes, it combines with intrinsic factor in the small intestine (produced by gastric parietal cells) and is absorbed in the terminal ileum. Thus, any deficiencies in these steps can lead to malabsorption of vitamin B12 (ie, lack of intrinsic factor, medications that decrease gastric acid such as proton-pump inhibitors [PPIs], pancreatic insufficiency, parasitic infections or small intestinal bacterial overgrowth [SIBO], or disruptions of the ileal surface such as in Crohn disease, celiac disease, short gut syndrome, etc.). The dual features in this case of a vegan diet and short gut syndrome created a virtual "eating disorder" that led to the presentation.

   Laboratory findings in B12 deficiency not only show a low B12 level but, prior to treatment, will also show high levels of methylmalonic acid and total homocysteine, two precursors of metabolic reactions in which B12 is an essential cofactor.

   Treatment dosage in children has not been well established. Intramuscular injections are usually the mainstay of treatment; however, some recent studies in children have shown that oral dosing can also be effective. However, for this particular patient, intramuscular administration was an appropriate given her short gut syndrome and questionable ability to absorb. For severe anemia, potassium supplementation is frequently needed during initial treatment.

   Vitamin B12 deficiency can present with concurrent thrombocytopenia and signs of hemolysis such as elevated lactate dehydrogenase (LDH) and schistocytes, similar to microangiopathic hemolytic anemia. However, in contrast to some other forms of hemolytic anemia, reticulocytopenia is usually seen due to ineffective erythropoiesis and intramedullary destruction. LDH elevations are seen due to destruction of immature nucleated red blood cells in the bone marrow.

Suggested Readings

Rasmussen SA, Fernhoff PM, Scanlon KS. Vitamin B12 deficiency in children and adolescents. *J Pediatr.* 2001;138:10-17.

Sezer RG, Akoğlu HA, Bozaykut A, Özdemir GN. Comparison of the efficacy of parenteral and oral treatment for nutritional vitamin B12 deficiency in children. *Hematology.* 2018;23(9):653-657.

Stabler S. Vitamin B12 deficiency. *N Engl J Med.* 2013;368:149-160.

Tran PN, Tran MH. Cobalamin deficiency presenting with thrombotic microangiopathy (TMA) features: a systematic review. *Transfus Apher Sci.* 2018;57(1):102-106.

52

Incomplete and Atypical

Andrew J. White

CHIEF COMPLAINT

Peeling skin

HISTORY OF PRESENT ILLNESS

A 10-year-old boy presented with 2 weeks of hand and foot swelling and skin peeling. He had several days of rhinorrhea and cough, and then after a week or so, he complained of his palms and soles being red, hot, and painful. These symptoms progressed to include swelling of his hands and feet, with a leathery texture of the skin, and, more recently, peeling of the skin on his hands that started at his fingertips. Also, in the last few days, he has had the onset of a symmetric, scaly red rash on the dorsal region of his feet and at the sides of his waist. He has had no fever, no enlarged lymph nodes, no arthralgias, no oral mucosal changes, and no red eyes.

He was initially seen at an urgent care center and started on methylprednisone. He was then seen at another hospital, but no diagnosis was made. WBC 12.4 (on steroids at the time), Cr 0.8, and total protein 6.1. CRP < 0.1 and ESR 5 mm/h.

He again sought medical care because his fingertips became red again, and mom noticed the peeling and was concerned about an atypical presentation of Kawasaki disease, which she had read about on the internet. With one of the five criteria, and 0 days of fever, this was felt to be unlikely, as it would be incomplete and atypical.

PAST MEDICAL HISTORY

Healthy

Family/Social History

- **Family history**: Sudden cardiac death in sister. Hodgkin disease in mom.
- **Social history:**
  - He traveled to the Smoky Mountains 3 weeks ago but had no ticks.
  - Pets: Three cats and two fish.
  - Sports: He plays soccer competitively.

EXAMINATION

- Comfortable and in no distress
- T 37.5, HR 100, RR 32, blood pressure 104/70
- No murmur
- Clear lungs
- Peeling skin on hands (see Figure 52.1)

DIAGNOSTIC CONSIDERATIONS

1. Incomplete, atypical, nonfebrile Kawasaki disease (ie, **not** Kawasaki disease)
2. Parechovirus

165

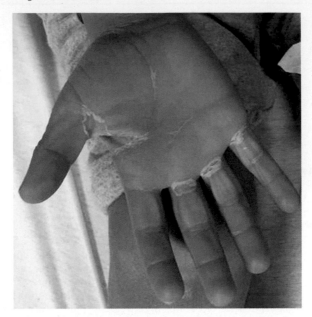

FIGURE 52.1   Peeling skin on hands.

3. Toxin-mediated disease (SSS)
4. Erythromelalgia

Investigation

- Laboratory tests: CBC normal (WBC 8.9), mono negative, enterovirus PCR negative, multiplex negative. Echo normal (no dilated coronaries).
- Dermatology was consulted, and upon examining the child, made the diagnosis.

DIAGNOSIS

Pityriasis rubra pilaris (PRP), ICD10 L 44.0

TEACHING POINTS

PRP is a rare skin condition characterized by keratotic papules and erythematous plaques with scale and palmoplantar keratoderma. Most cases are sporadic, although just over 5% of cases have a family history and are inherited in an AD manner.

There are several types recognized:

1. Classic adult PRP
2. Atypical adult PRP
3. Classic juvenile PRP
4. Circumscribed juvenile PRP
5. Atypical juvenile PRP (which is often the familial type)

The familial form is caused by a mutation in CARD14, on 17q25.3. As this is in the caspase pathway, the molecular mechanism may involve impaired apoptosis of epithelium (*pure speculation by the editor*). The etiologies in the nonfamilial forms have not yet been identified, but disease onset has been associated with infection, hypothyroidism, myositis, and malignancy, as well as skin trauma and ultraviolet (UV) exposure.

The differential diagnosis includes seborrheic dermatitis, psoriasis, drug eruption, and atopic dermatitis.

Treatment includes topical corticosteroids, as well as mild systemic immunomodulators such as methotrexate or cyclosporine. Anti-TNF therapy may be useful. Treatment in general is challenging, and the response to treatment of the familial form has been described as poor. In up to 80% of the adult cases, spontaneous remission occurs after 3 to 5 years.

Suggested Readings

Beamer JE, Newman SB, Reed WB, Cram D. Pityriasis rubra pilaris. *Cutis.* 1972;10:419-421.

Fuchs-Telem D, Sarig O, van Steensel MAM, et al. Familial pityriasis rubra pilaris is caused by mutations in CARD14. *Am J Hum Genet.* 2012;91:163-170.

Sehgal VN, Srivastava G. (Juvenile) pityriasis rubra pilaris. *Int J Dermatol.* 2006;45:438-446.

Zeisler EP. Pityriasis rubra pilaris—Familial type. *Arch Derm Syphilol.* 1923;7:195-208.

53

Follow the Leader

Andrew J. White

CHIEF COMPLAINT

Fever and fast breathing

HISTORY OF PRESENT ILLNESS

A 19-month-old boy with asthma presents with **fever** and **rapid breathing**. He felt warm the past 6 days (did not take temperature) and for the past 3 days has had rapid breathing, wheezing, and grunting. Mom gave nebulized albuterol at home which helped at first but no longer helps. He also has clear rhinorrhea and vomited once. He has had no cough and no diarrhea. Decreased PO intake of food but good PO intake of liquid and good urine output. In the emergency department (ED), he was febrile and had an RR in the 70s. He was given acetaminophen, and once the temperature decreased, he improved.

Chest x-ray (CXR) showed pneumonia with effusion (Figure 53.1), and he was started on ampicillin, intravenous (IV) fluids, and admitted.

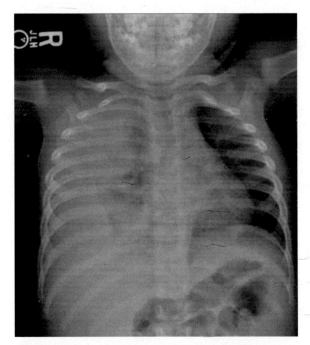

FIGURE 53.1   Chest x-ray.

Past Medical History

- Behind on immunizations. Up-to-date as of 9 months.
- Asthma. Home nebulizer.

Family/Social History

None

Examination

- Vital signs: 37.1, 131, 40, 103/83, 98%.
- Comfortable and in no distress.
- Skin warm and dry, no rash.
- Posterior pharynx clear, mucous membranes moist.
- No tonsillar hypertrophy.
- Neck supple, no lymphadenopathy.
- Crackles and diminished breath sounds on right side, normal breath sounds on left side. No wheeze, no stridor.
- Soft, nondistended abdomen, nontender, no hepatosplenomegaly, no masses.
- Spine straight with no deformities visualized.
- No clubbing, cyanosis, or edema.
- CNs normal, moves all limbs.

Diagnostic Considerations

The admitting team's diagnostic thoughts: "19-month-old with 6 days fever and 3 days respiratory symptoms—wheeze, grunting, shortness of breath, no cough. Symptoms initially responsive to albuterol, but now with little response. Most likely diagnosis is **community-acquired pneumonia**. Differential also includes aspiration pneumonia and foreign body aspiration. He currently appears well when afebrile, worse appearing when temperature rises. No supplemental O_2 currently. The pleural effusion should be drained and cultured."

Plan:

1. Ampicillin IV
2. Surgery consult for drainage of effusion and chest tube placement

Diagnostic clue: Later that day, when the teaching attending was observing the medical student perform an H & P on this child, a clue was uncovered. Mom mentioned they had moved here 7 months ago. The student did not pursue this line of questioning, but the attending was curious and asked:

"You moved from where?" he asked

"A small town in rural Texas." Mom replied.

Again, the student let this response sit.

The attending, once again, followed up with: "Why did you move away from Texas—most folks love it there?"

"Well, Dad has been in and out of prison too many times and we needed to get away," she replied.

An additional diagnostic consideration was now more likely **tuberculosis**.

Investigation

As the patient was about to head to the operating room shortly, the team moved quickly to notify infectious diseases and the operating room staff and the surgeons, who were able to successfully perform the procedure (chest tube placement) in negative pressure isolation and with appropriate protective gear (N95 masks), preventing what would have been exposure of many individuals to tuberculosis.

Results

PPD was positive at 18 × 20 mm. Antituberculous therapy was initiated, chest tube was removed after 3 days, and the patient improved and was discharged home after a week.

DIAGNOSIS

Tuberculosis

Treatment/Follow-up

1. Isoniazid, ethambutol, rifampin, pyrazinamide, and vitamin B6 for 2 months, followed by two drug therapy for 4 months.
2. Notification of Department of Health.

TEACHING POINTS

- Think TB. While relatively common in the United States, it is rarely considered in children.
- A retelling of the story, as is done in teaching hospitals, sometimes leads to new clues and should not be viewed as onerous to family/patient/physician—instead it can be **useful**.

Suggested Readings

Carvalho I, Goletti D, Manga S, Silva DR, Manissero D, Migliori G. Managing latent tuberculosis infection and tuberculosis in children. *Pulmonology*. 2018;24(2):106-114. doi:10.1016/j.rppnen.2017.10.007. PMID: 29502937.
Chiappini E, Lo Vecchio A, Garazzino S, et al. Recommendations for the diagnosis of pediatric tuberculosis. *Eur J Clin Microbiol Infect Dis*. 2016;35(1):1-18. doi:10.1007/s10096-015-2507-6. PMID: 26476550.
Khurana AK, Dhingra B. What is new in management of pediatric tuberculosis? *Indian Pediatr*. 2019;56(3):213-220. PMID: 30954994.
Nahid P, Dorman SE, Alipanah N, et al. Official American Thoracic Society/Centers for Disease Control and Prevention/Infectious Diseases Society of America clinical practice guidelines: treatment of drug-susceptible tuberculosis. *Clin Infect Dis*. 2016;63(7):e147-e195. doi:10.1093/cid/ciw376. PMID: 27516382; PMCID: PMC6590850.

54

Vampire Bites

Andrew J. White

CHIEF COMPLAINT

"We think vampires are attacking her."

HISTORY OF PRESENT ILLNESS

An 11-year-old girl was seen for anemia. Three years ago, she had an upper respiratory tract infection with influenza B, and routine laboratory tests found a dramatically low hemoglobin of **3 g/dL**, which was unexpected and unexplained, and workup revealed only iron deficiency. She was treated with monthly iron infusions, without improvement, but which have continued intermittently to date. She now also receives blood transfusions, two units every 2 weeks, and does become symptomatic when anemic in between transfusions. She has no gross blood in her stool and never has. A recent stool guaiac was positive; however, it was not felt to be the etiology of her blood loss as it had been negative on over 30 occasions previously. Parents suggest a **vampire** must be attacking her while she sleeps, as this is the only logical source of her blood loss, and since she has seen dozens of doctors and had countless tests, all without an answer.

She has had none of the following symptoms: vision problems, fever, emesis, difficulty swallowing, chest pain, difficulty breathing, hematemesis, abdominal pain when she is not anemic, melena, blood in her stool, scleral icterus, or jaundice. She has not started her menses yet. The parents have not seen any bite marks on her neck or other areas.

PAST MEDICAL HISTORY

A lumbar paraspinal mass has been present since birth and is growing smaller, documented by serial imaging. On biopsy, it was shown to be a hemangioma.

- A condensed summary of her workup has included (*in addition to the normal things you would expect but are not listed here*):

TMPRSS6 (the test for IRIDA—iron refractory iron deficiency anemia), paroxysmal nocturnal hemoglobinuria, erythropoietin levels, lead, hemoglobin analysis, chromosomal microarray, MRI of the pelvis and abdomen, chest x-ray, MRI enterography, bone marrow biopsy (×2), colonoscopy and upper GI endoscopy ×2, video capsule endoscopy, spinal angiogram of paraspinal mass, and biopsy of the paraspinal mass.

All of the above were normal and unremarkable and failed to explain her refractory iron deficiency anemia.

Medications

- MiraLAX
- Blood transfusions
- Iron infusions

Family/Social History

Social history: She lives with mom, dad, and a 12-year-old brother. She is in the sixth grade and is on the B honor roll. She enjoys art and music but sits out PE because she tires easily.

Family history: Maternal grandmother with breast and ovarian cancer and hyperglycemia; paternal grandfather with low blood pressure.

EXAMINATION

Height 144.6 cm (35%), weight 41.8 kg (65%), and BMI of 19.9 (75%). Blood pressure 108/60, temperature 36.4, heart rate 92, and respirations 18. She is alert and cooperative. Normocephalic, atraumatic. Pupils are equally round and reactive to light. Extraocular movements intact. She does not have any scleral icterus. Her oropharynx is moist and clear. No tonsillar hypertrophy. TMs are normal bilaterally. No thyromegaly, no cervical adenopathy. Heart: Regular rate and rhythm. There is a 3/6 systolic murmur. Lungs are clear with no wheezes, crackles, or rhonchi. Abdomen is soft, nontender, nondistended; no splenomegaly. She is Tanner II. Extremities are warm, well perfused. There is no evidence of venipuncture marks nor scars on the arms or neck. No clubbing present. Good capillary refill. No pitting of her nails. Her skin is normal without signs of telangiectases or hemangiomata. She has a scar over her left paraspinal muscles at L1, which is the site of her biopsy, and a scar where her port was placed in her left anterior chest. The port is palpable. She has 5/5 strength in bilateral hands, deltoids, triceps, hamstrings, quadriceps, and plantar flexion and dorsiflexion. She has symmetric +2 patellar reflexes. She has normal sharp sensation, negative Romberg, and normal gait.

DIAGNOSTIC CONSIDERATIONS

Established diagnoses:

1. Hemangioma, lumbar, paraspinal
2. Anemia, iron deficient, refractory, idiopathic, severe

Thought process: With normal **production** (BM biopsies had no evidence of marrow failure) and no evidence of red cell **destruction** (CBC smears without schistocytes and negative coombs), the etiology of anemia must be due to blood **loss**. The prior endoscopy studies may have missed the specific area of blood loss, and the video capsule, while able to visual more territory, does not see all. Another distinct diagnostic option was that someone was indeed removing her blood via syringe (**Munchausen by proxy),** and the vampire story may have been a reflection of that blood loss mechanism. The child was reexamined with particular attention paid to her vasculature and was asked privately about the vampire story. The repeat examination and her answers were not concerning, and so a potentially diagnostic study was performed.

Investigation

A tagged red cell scan was performed with 11 mCi Tc-99m.

Result

"There is an area of radiotracer activity in the right lower quadrant of the abdomen in the initial images. On delayed images, this radiotracer activity appears to be **in the distal small bowel**. This is an abnormal finding that indicates a GI source of bleeding."

She was taken to the operating room, with GI in attendance for possible intraoperative endoscopy. An excerpt from the operative note: "...Visualized portions of the stomach and spleen appeared normal. Visualized portions of the colon appeared normal. Upon initial inspection of the small bowel, **there were abnormal purple, bulky vascular lesions present within the bowel wall**. Nine of the larger vascular lesions were identified and resected..."

On histology, "variably sized, irregular, thick and thin walled, anastomosing venous channels are present, primarily located in the muscularis propria and submucosa, extending to the serosal and mucosal surfaces. Multiple thrombi are present. Staining was negative for the juvenile hemangioma marker Glut-1. Endothelial cells were positive for CD31 and negative for the lymphatic marker D2-40, confirming **venous** origin."

DIAGNOSIS

Blue rubber bleb nevus syndrome (BRBNS)

TEACHING POINTS

BRBNS is a rare disorder characterized by multifocal venous malformations of the skin, soft tissue, and GI tract. First reported in 1860, it was more fully characterized by William Bean in 1958. Approximately 200 cases have been reported in the literature. Patients suffer from chronic anemia from GI bleeding that usually begins in childhood; only rarely do they suffer from massive hemorrhage. A nearly ubiquitous hallmark of the syndrome is the presence of several to hundreds of purplish, cutaneous lesions. While the mechanism is unknown, two families with affected persons in three and five successive generations (supporting an autosomal dominant inheritance) were reported by Walshe in 1966. Most cases, however, are not familial.

After the diagnosis was made, a repeat histologic examination of the paraspinal mass biopsy was repeated and did not show evidence of venous origin. At the 1-month follow-up visit, the hemoglobin had risen to 9.8 mg/dL, without any intervening transfusion.

Questions remaining:

- Why were most of her guaiac studies negative?
  - Likely answer: The bleeding was intermittent, or perhaps the guaiac technique was poor.
- Why did the prior endoscopies not visual the vascular malformations?
  - Likely answer: They do not visual all the mucosa.
- Why did she have no cutaneous blue rubber blebs?
  - Answer: They are not always present.

Suggested Readings

Bean WB. *Vascular Spiders and Related Lesions of the Skin*. Charles C Thomas; 1958:178-185.
Ertem D, Acar Y, Kotiloglu E, Yucelten D, Pehlivanoglu E. Blue rubber bleb nevus syndrome. *Pediatrics*. 2001;107:418-421.
Walshe MM, Evans CD, Warin RP. Blue rubber bleb naevus. *Br Med J*. 1966;2:931-932.

55

Chips Ahoy, Matey

Andrew J. White

CHIEF COMPLAINT

Leg pain

HISTORY OF PRESENT ILLNESS

A 7-year-old boy with autism began having trouble walking and would hold onto things like chairs or a railing to support himself. This progressed over 2 weeks to the point where he refused to walk at all. He complained of pain in his legs (all over), left wrist, ankle, and toes and would also occasionally point to his lower abdomen. Acetaminophen helps somewhat with the pain. There has been no trauma or injury. He has been receiving physical therapy without improvement. He has also had poor p.o. intake and for the last 2 weeks has had increasingly loose stools. His stools are loose at baseline and occur every other day. He now is carried to the toilet, and when there, he appears flushed and has tremors and screams during attempts at defecation. He has also started picking at his gums, which is new for him; he often picks at his earlobes and fingers repetitively, as part of his autistic spectrum disorder, causing areas of excoriation and bleeding. He has not had fevers, cough, or rhinorrhea; no nausea or vomiting; and no dysuria.

He was seen by orthopedics 3 weeks before admission, who performed x-rays, which were negative. When the refusal to walk continued, a magnetic resonance image (MRI) of his lumbosacral spine and brain were obtained and were both normal. Physical therapy was initiated but without improvement. He was also evaluated by a neurologist, who prescribed baclofen and tizanidine, which have not improved his symptoms. He was seen by second neurologist on the day of admission, who referred him for inpatient evaluation.

PAST MEDICAL HISTORY

Autism, diagnosed at 2.5 years of age. No chromosome microarray analysis (CMA) or fragile X testing has been sent. He is able to say a few phrases. Prior to the events leading to this admission, he had been running and walking independently and able to ride a scooter with ease.

Family/Social History

Limited diet. He eats only **Chips Ahoy** cookies, M&M's, crackers with peanut butter, and eclairs. He does not eat meat, fruits, or vegetables.

EXAMINATION

- Vitals: Temperature 37.6, heart rate 130, respiratory rate 20, blood pressure 121/80, SpO$_2$ 98%.
- General: Distressed and repeating phrases but lying in bed comfortably.
- Skin: Warm and dry. Capillary refill less than 2 seconds. Rash on cheeks and bilateral shins. Excoriated patches on the right ear and several fingers.
- HEENT: Normocephalic, atraumatic. Conjunctivae clear without injection or scleral icterus.
- Mouth: Gums with beefy red, hypertrophied excoriations, without purulent drainage (Figure 55.1).

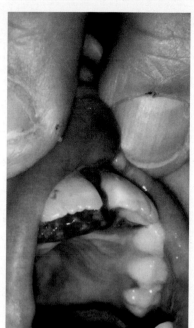

FIGURE 55.1   Gums with beefy red, hypertrophied excoriations, without purulent drainage.

- Neck: Supple without lymphadenopathy.
- Lungs: Clear to auscultation bilaterally.
- Cardiovascular: Regular rate and rhythm.
- Abdomen: Soft, nontender, nondistended, normoactive bowel sounds.
- Neurologic: Awake, alert, anxious.

    Extraocular movements intact. Face symmetric. Normal sensation and strength on face. Normal strength of shoulder shrug. Moves all extremities against resistance. Keeps left upper extremity held against body with minimal movement. Increased tone in lower extremities. Achilles contractures. Keeps knees flexed. Resists extension. Full sensation to light touch in all four extremities. Reflexes 2+.

DIAGNOSTIC CONSIDERATIONS

- Septic arthritis
- Osteomyelitis
- Fracture
- Muscular dystrophy
- Juvenile dermatomyositis
- Rickets

Investigation and Results

- Vitamin D was 38 mg/mL
- CK was 131 U/L
- CRP was 39 mg/dL
- ESR was 68 mm/hr
- CMP was within normal limits
- CBC with hemoglobin of 7.7 g/dL, microcytic

Rheumatology was consulted due to the high ESR and the leg pain, and they suspected vitamin C deficiency based on previous experience and because of the restrictive diet. Vitamin C level was drawn and sent and returned a week later with an undetectable level.

MRI of the lower extremities demonstrated abnormal signal enhancement in the lower extremity metaphyses and subperiosteal fluid in distal femurs; classic findings for **scurvy**.

In retrospect, a white metaphyseal band was visible on the plain film obtained by orthopedics and is classic for scurvy.

He was treated with IV vitamin C and had brisk and dramatic improvement in his pain. Resolution of the gum hypertrophy and hemorrhage was rapid. The leg pain resolved, and he had improved range of motion and use of his wrist. He had continued difficulty walking due to the flexion contractures of his knees.

Nutrition, speech, and psychology were involved to help with his food aversion.

DIAGNOSIS

1. **Scurvy** (vitamin C aka ascorbic acid deficiency) ICD-10 = E54
2. Autism spectrum disorder
3. Flexion contractures, knees, ankles, secondary to disuse
4. Anemia, iron deficiency

Treatment/Follow-up

1. Ascorbic acid 150 mg p.o. two times daily
2. Multivitamin with iron, one chewable tablet p.o. once daily
3. Melatonin 6 mg p.o. once daily at bedtime
4. MiraLAX 8.5 g p.o. once daily in the morning

TEACHING POINTS

Scurvy has been recognized for centuries as a potentially fatal disease but has fallen off the radar screen of many clinicians in recent decades with the improvement in dietary intake of fresh fruits and vegetables. Current estimates of its prevalence in the United States is less than 1%, although, in practice, it has been detected much less frequently. The clinical manifestations of gum hypertrophy and perifollicular hemorrhage are well known, but the complaints of leg pain, myalgia, and arthralgia are less well recognized. Children who develop scurvy, by definition, have a restricted diet, and these children may carry a diagnosis of autism spectrum disorder, or ARFID (avoidant/restrictive food intake disorder). Supplementation with vitamin C results in rapid improvement.

Suggested Readings

Duggan PC, Westra SJ, Roseberg AE. Case records of the Massachusetts General Hospital. Case 23-2007: a 9-year-old boy with bone pain, rash, and gingival hypertrophy. *N Engl J Med.* 2007;357(4):392-400.

Fain O. Musculoskeletal manifestations of scurvy. *Joint Bone Spine.* 2005;72:124-128.

Ratanachu-Ek S, Sukswai P, Jeerathanyasakun Y, Wongtapradit L. Scurvy in pediatric patients: a review of 28 cases. *J Med Assoc Thai.* 2003;86(suppl 3):S734-S740.

Schleicher RL, Carroll MD, Ford ES, Lacher D. Serum vitamin C and the prevalence of vitamin C deficiency in the United States: 2003-2004 National Health and Nutrition Examination Survey (NHANES). *Am J Clin Nutr.* 2009;90(5):1252-1263.

56

A Shower an Hour

Nicholas R. Zessis

CHIEF COMPLAINT

"I've been throwing up for the last year."

HISTORY OF PRESENT ILLNESS

A 17-year-old boy came alone to the emergency department because he had nausea and vomiting for 1 year. It is episodic and sometimes lasts for 1 to 2 days and often as long as 1 week. He will have emesis anywhere from one to two times per day up to one to two times per hour during these spells. He may go weeks to months without an attack. The attacks are sometimes associated with diffuse abdominal pain. He has not been able to identify a trigger. It is not more or less prevalent at any time of day. It sometimes occurs at night.

He has not lost any weight and has no odynophagia or dysphagia. No headaches, vision changes, diarrhea, fever, back pain, or urinary symptoms. He has had no melena, hematochezia, or skin changes.

He has been evaluated by his pediatrician, as well as an urgent care center, and other emergency departments with an unremarkable workup (he can only recall blood tests and imaging). He thinks he was supposed to see a gastrointestinal (GI) physician but did not follow-up because his symptoms had resolved.

He presents today because this current episode has been the most unrelenting exacerbation he has experienced, having lasted about 10 days with nausea and emesis, missing almost 7 days of school.

PAST MEDICAL HISTORY

Healthy, no prior admissions, no prior surgeries, fully vaccinated

Medications

He does not take daily medications, although he has previously taken ondansetron with minimal relief.

Family/Social History

There is no one in the family with inflammatory bowel disease, celiac disease, or peptic ulcer disease.

He is an only child and lives with his mom and dad. He is a senior in high school, a B to C student. He started smoking marijuana because his friends started doing it and now smokes several times a week. He uses no additional drugs and denies additional ingestion. He has never been sexually active. He denies suicidal or homicidal ideation. No recent travel.

EXAMINATION

- Vitals: T 36.8 °C, HR 110 bpm, RR 16 bpm, BP 114/76 mm Hg, SpO$_2$ 99% on room air, BMI 21.1 kg/m^2.
- Mild bilateral conjunctival injection, otherwise an unremarkable examination.

DIAGNOSTIC CONSIDERATIONS

Recurrent etiologies such as cyclic vomiting syndrome, intermittent bowel obstruction, gallbladder disease, porphyria, metabolic disorders, cannabis hyperemesis syndrome, adrenal hyperplasia, SMA syndrome, Munchausen syndrome, and pseudotumor cerebri or other causes of increased ICP are plausible. Also, *chronic etiologies* (GERD, PUD, EoE/esophagitis, achalasia, food allergy, lead toxicity, motility disorders, secretory tumors, rumination, psychogenic, eating disorders, and vestibular disorders) were considered.

Investigation and Results

- CBC, hepatic function panel, GGT, lipase, ESR/CRP, two-view abdominal plain films, guaiac stool were normal
- BMP: Na 135 mEq/L, K 2.7 mEq/L, Cl 89 mmol/L, HCO_3 32 mmol/L, BUN 22 mg/dL, creatinine 0.89 mg/dL, glucose 71 mg/dL, and Ca 9.8 mg/dL
- Urinalysis with 2+ ketones, specific gravity 1.024
- Urine drug screen: Positive for marijuana

Initial Impression

On admission, the team thought the most likely diagnosis was cyclic vomiting syndrome, complicated by dehydration and hypokalemic hypochloremic metabolic alkalosis. In the emergency department, he was given

- A 1 L normal saline bolus
- Oral ondansetron
- Oral KCl supplement
- And plans were made to admit to General Pediatrics

Inpatient Course

The mother arrived at the bedside when the patient presented to the floor. The intern was taking more history from the mom, when the patient, in an agitated and restless manner, interrupted with:

Patient: *"Bro, do you have, like, a shower here?"*
Intern: "…Er, I think so. One more question about the vomiting, do you…"
Patient: *"But bro, the water though, it's, like, hot, right? I need it hot, bro."*
Intern: (scratches head and looks at mom) "How often does he take hot showers at home?"
Mom: *"At least 20 to 25 times a day,"* she says with a straight face.
Intern: "So…like, every hour?"
Mom: *"Pretty much. What about his skin color, he doesn't usually look like that?"*

Examination on Presentation to General Medicine

- Vitals: T 39.8 °C; HR 125 bpm; RR 22 bpm; BP 142/94 mm Hg; SpO_2 99% on room air.
- Diffusely flushed skin, diaphoretic, mildly agitated.
- Dilated pupils, dry mucous membranes.
- Tachycardic rate, regular rhythm, strong distal pulses, cap refill 3 seconds.
- Tachypneic, clear throughout without retractions.
- Soft abdomen, nondistended, nontender, without hepatosplenomegaly; bowel sounds are hyperactive.
- Mild intermittent tremor present in upper extremities.
- 4+ patellar reflexes with sustained ankle clonus. The reflexes of his upper extremities are 2+.

Additional History

He had been getting frequent prescriptions for ondansetron around town, many of them within the last week. Mom is unsure how many doses he has taken but denies additional medication use.

Revised Diagnostic Considerations

Serotonin syndrome, neuroleptic malignant syndrome, anticholinergic toxicity, malignant hyperthermia, sympathomimetic toxicity, and meningitis/encephalitis.

DIAGNOSIS

1. **Cannabis hyperemesis syndrome**
2. **Serotonin syndrome**

Treatment/Follow-up

- Serotonin syndrome
  - Discontinue ondansetron already ordered in his chart; ie, no serotonergic agents.
  - CR monitor, maintenance IV fluids, NPO.
  - Short-acting benzodiazepine: Shortly afterward, his vitals and neuromuscular findings greatly improved; he escaped transfer to the PICU as a result.
  - ECG obtained: QTc of 480 ms.
  - Electrolyte panel obtained with repletion if needed.
  - Toxicology consult
    - Standard hyperthermia measures, avoid antipyretics.
    - Serial ECGs and electrolytes.
    - CK level: Normal.
    - Start cyproheptadine.
- Cannabis hyperemesis syndrome
  - Marijuana cessation counseling.
  - Rehydration.
  - Toxicology consult
    - Topical capsaicin cream applied to abdomen, which was poorly tolerated.
    - Benzodiazepines prn for nausea, haloperidol prn to abort severe hyperemesis, though the latter was not needed.
- Discharge: He improved and was discharged home with topical capsaicin.

TEACHING POINTS

- Cyclic vomiting syndrome, diagnosis
  - At least five attacks in any interval or minimum of three attacks during 6-month period
  - Episodic attacks of intense nausea/vomiting lasting 1 hour to 10 days, occurring at least 1 week apart
  - Stereotypical pattern and symptoms
  - Vomiting during attacks occurs at least four times per hour for at least 1 hour
  - Return to baseline between episodes
  - A diagnosis of exclusion
- Cannabis hyperemesis syndrome (CHS)
  - Classically thought to occur only with prolonged marijuana use (>2 years) and at a high dose (about daily), although case reports more recently describe instances of less significant ingestion leading to CHS.
    - In this patient, the emergency department initially discounted the possibility of cannabis hyperemesis syndrome, as they felt he was not smoking enough marijuana.
    - The finding of relief from hot water is pathognomonic for CHS.
  - The literature is unclear regarding the time to resolution of symptoms after cessation of marijuana use due to a lack of follow-up data.
  - Many patients relapse, as marijuana use can temporarily improve nausea.
- Serotonin syndrome (SS)
  - A clinical diagnosis; it manifests from mild tremors to life-threatening hyperthermia and shock.

- In its most severe form, it can require aggressive treatment of hyperthermia (will not respond to acetaminophen, as hyperthermia is due to increased muscular metabolism), sedation, intubation, and paralysis.
  - Investigate for rhabdomyolysis as a result.
- Diagnosis: Hunter criteria fulfilled if patient has taken a serotonergic agent, plus:
  - Spontaneous clonus.
  - Inducible clonus and agitation or diaphoresis.
  - Ocular clonus and agitation or diaphoresis.
  - Tremor and hyperreflexia.
  - Hypertonia.
  - Temperature >38 °C and ocular clonus or inducible clonus.
- Neuromuscular findings are typically more prominent in the lower extremities.
- Management principles.
  - Discontinuation of all serotonergic agents.
  - Supportive care aimed at normalization of vitals.
  - Sedation with benzodiazepines.
  - Administration of serotonin antagonists.
  - Reassessment for resuming use of causative serotonergic agents.
- Although there are case reports describing the role of ondansetron in precipitating SS, it is generally believed that ondansetron alone cannot cause SS.

Suggested Readings

Dunkley EJ, Isbister GK, Sibbritt D, et al. The Hunter Serotonin Toxicity Criteria: simple and accurate diagnostic decision rules for serotonin toxicity. *QJM.* 2003;96(9):635-642.

Gollapudy S, Kumar V, Dhamee MS. A case of serotonin syndrome precipitated by fentanyl and ondansetron in a patient receiving paroxetine, duloxetine, and bupropion. *J Clin Anesth.* 2012;24(3):251-252.

Li BU, Lefevre F, Chelimsky GG, et al. North American Society for Pediatric Gastroenterology, Hepatology, and Nutrition consensus statement on the diagnosis and management of cyclic vomiting syndrome. *J Pediatr Gastroenterol Nutr.* 2008;47(3):379-393.

Simonetto DA, Oxentenko AS, Herman ML, et al. Cannabinoid hyperemesis: a case series of 98 patients. *Mayo Clin Proc.* 2012;87(2):114-119.

Sorensen CJ, DeSanto K, Borgelt L, et al. Cannabinoid hyperemesis syndrome: diagnosis, pathophysiology, and treatment—a systematic review. *J Med Toxicol.* 2017;13(1):71-87.

Venkatesan T, Levinthal DJ, Li BUK, et al. Role of chronic cannabis use: cyclic vomiting syndrome vs cannabinoid hyperemesis syndrome. *Neurogastroenterol Motil.* 2019;31(suppl 2):e13606.

57

Phone a Friend
Kevin Baszis

CHIEF COMPLAINT

Abdominal pain and rash

HISTORY OF PRESENT ILLNESS

A 17-year-old male with familial Mediterranean fever (FMF) has had a rash on his right lower leg for 3 weeks and intermittent abdominal pain for 2 weeks, as well as a rash on his trunk and extremities for 1 day.

It started when he noticed a lump on his ankle. It began to spread, turn red, and cause swelling of the ankle. He was diagnosed with cellulitis and treated with oral clindamycin. The colchicine he was on to treat the FMF was held due to possible drug interaction.

Two weeks later, he developed intermittent right upper quadrant (RUQ) pain that was sharp and radiating to his left shoulder. He distinguished this from his typical FMF abdominal pain, which is usually in the left lower quadrant (LLQ). He had chills and nausea but no obvious fever or vomiting over the past 2 weeks. There was no worsening or improvement of the pain with eating, nor any change in his bowel movements.

He then developed a raised, red, nonitchy rash on his chest that spread to his back and upper and lower extremities, prompting presentation to the emergency department (ED).

PAST MEDICAL HISTORY

- Familial Mediterranean fever

Medications

- Colchicine 0.6 mg daily but recently being held

Family/Social History

- Younger sister with FMF

EXAMINATION

- General appearance: Comfortable.
- Skin
  - Papular blanching rash extending from chest to back, neck, and abdomen.
  - On the right medial ankle extending to the posterior calf, there is a confluent, erythematous, indurated, warm plaque that is tender to palpation.
- Musculoskeletal
  - No effusion in right ankle.
  - R ankle soft tissue is mildly swollen relative to the L.
- Eyes: Conjunctiva clear, no drainage or injection. No scleral icterus.
- Nose: No drainage.
- Pulmonary: Lung sounds clear.
- Cardiovascular: No murmur.

- Abdomen: Nondistended. Tender over the RUQ as well as pain in the RUQ when palpating the LLQ. He has guarding but no rebound.
- Back: No CVA tenderness.
- Neurologic: Alert and chatty, 2+ reflexes, 5/5 strength.

DIAGNOSTIC CONSIDERATIONS

1. Cellulitis, resistant to clindamycin, right leg.
2. Drug rash, secondary to clindamycin.
3. Abdominal pain, secondary to clindamycin.

Investigation

- CBC, CMP, amylase, lipase, GGT, CRP
- CXR

Results

- WBC 10 k
- CMP, amylase, lipase, GGT normal
- CRP 68.3 mg/L
- CXR: perihilar atelectasis

DIAGNOSIS

He was in the process of being admitted for IV vancomycin to treat resistant cellulitis when the ED hospitalist phoned a rheumatologist friend and shared a picture from the patient's phone (Figure 57.1).

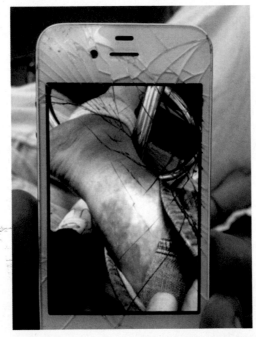

FIGURE 57.1 Picture of a phone with a picture of the leg rash, visible despite the cracked glass.

The friend suggested an alternative diagnosis:

1. **FMF flare,** with erysipeloid rash on the leg (due to poorly compliant teen, now off colchicine entirely)
2. **Drug rash on trunk,** secondary to clindamycin
3. **Abdominal pain,** secondary to FMF

Treatment/Follow-up

1. Stop antibiotics
2. Restart colchicine
3. Start corticosteroids

TEACHING POINTS

FMF is an autosomal recessive autoinflammatory disease due to mutation in the MEFV gene, which encodes for a protein quaintly named pyrin. It has a high prevalence in the Middle East, with a carrier frequency as high as one in seven in some populations. Short-lived (2-3 days) episodes of fever often accompanied by severe abdominal pain/peritonitis are typical and often lead to unnecessary exploratory laparotomy. Arthritis, pleuritis, pericarditis, and myositis are also common, as is the erysipeloid rash, which may be misdiagnosed as cellulitis. Scrotal inflammation, mimicking torsion, may also occur. Colchicine is effective at preventing most attacks and preventing the long-term complication of amyloidosis.

Suggested Readings

Barzilai A, Langevitz P, Goldberg I, et al. Erysipelas-like erythema of familial Mediterranean fever: clinicopathologic correlation. *J Am Acad Dermatol.* 2000;42(5 pt 1):791-795.
Berkun Y, Eisenstein E, Ben-Chetrit E. Fmf—clinical features, new treatments and the role of genetic modifiers: a critical digest of the 2010-2012 literature. *Clin Exp Rheumatol.* 2012;30(3 suppl 72):S90-S95.
Kolivras A, Provost P, Thompson CT. Erysipelas-like erythema of familial Mediterranean fever syndrome: a case report with emphasis on histopathologic diagnostic clues. *J Cutan Pathol.* 2013;40(6):585-590. doi:10.1111/cup.12132
Sag E, Bilginer Y, Ozen S. Autoinflammatory diseases with periodic fevers. *Curr Rheumatol Rep.* 2017;19(7):41.

58

Fish Eggs or Coffee Beans
Alex S. Plattner

CHIEF COMPLAINT

Vomiting

HISTORY OF PRESENT ILLNESS

A 17-year-old girl has had a burning sensation in her throat, chest, and abdomen for 2 to 3 weeks, and it hurts to swallow both liquids and solids. She has lost 20 lb over that time. The day prior to presentation, she felt a burning sensation in her chest while getting out of the shower and vomited the remnants of an apple. She then vomited material she described as "fish eggs or coffee beans." Subsequently, she has only been able to tolerate liquids. She has had no fevers but has had chills, occasional night sweats, and frequent headaches. She did not present immediately due to lack of transportation. She went to her pediatrician who sent her to the emergency department.

She has also had "spells" intermittently for the last 8 months, where she feels dizzy and hot, followed by weakness in her lower extremities. She sometimes asks to be carried or to sit in a wheelchair. She was seen at a different hospital 5 months ago with a normal laboratory workup. She was expelled from school a few months prior for too many days missed. Recent exposures include dogs, cats, snakes, pigs, ticks, and travel to Boston.

PAST MEDICAL HISTORY

She recently regained insurance and had not seen her pediatrician for over a year prior to this visit. Vaccines are up-to-date.

Medications

She does not take any medications.

Family/Social History

She does not know a family history.

EXAMINATION

- General: Thin-appearing teenage girl sitting in bed. Looks tired but in no distress.
- HEENT: Pupils equal and reactive, extraocular movements intact, normal conjunctivae, moist mucous membranes, oropharynx clear, neck supple without palpable cervical adenopathy.
- CV: Normal rate and rhythm, normal heart sounds without murmur.
- Pulm: Clear bilaterally, good air movement, normal effort.
- Abd: Soft, nontender, nondistended, no masses or organomegaly.
- MSK: No edema, tenderness, or deformity.
- Skin: Warm and dry without rash or bruising.
- Neuro: Alert and oriented to person, place, and time. Strabismus but otherwise normal CNs II-XII. Normal tone and g normal strength in all extremities. Gait examination not performed/deferred due to patient request.

DIAGNOSTIC CONSIDERATIONS

Initial differential diagnosis was concerning for a primary gastrointestinal (GI) bleed causing her coffee ground emesis; however, infections, malignancies, and neurologic etiologies could also cause bloody emesis due to frequent retching forming Mallory-Weiss tears. Her history of chills, night sweats, and significant weight loss is concerning for malignancies. Additionally, frequent headaches with vomiting raised concern for increased intracranial pressure (ICP). Her report of "spells" could be behavioral symptoms, seizures, intoxication, or an additional sequela of increased ICP.

Investigation and Results

- CBC: WBC 12.3 (72% N, 21% L, 6% M), Hgb 13.9, Plt 182
- CMP: Na 137, K 3.1, Cl 109, CO_2 19, BUN 9, Cr 0.67, glucose 92, Ca 9.2, Bili 0.4, protein 6.9, albumin 4.2, Alk Phos 64, ALT 13, AST 15
- TSH: 2.14
- Lipase: 15
- ESR/CRP: 7/1.4
- PT/INR/PTT: 14.2/1.0/25.8
- Urine hCG: Negative
- HIV: Negative

Overnight, the bedside nurse was called to the room by the patient's father and found the patient on her back, moving her arms back and forth, and kicking her legs in a nonrhythmic motion. These movements were suppressible. She was able to communicate with nurse and answer questions appropriately during this episode. Afterward, she was able to walk to the bathroom with assistance. She had 10+ similar episodes that evening. Neurology was consulted and concluded that the movements did not represent seizure activity. It was unclear if these movements were truly behavioral or related to an underlying condition. However, due to these symptoms, a head computed tomography (CT) was obtained the following morning (Figure 58.1).

A mass and hydrocephalus were visualized, and a magnetic resonance image (MRI) localized the tumor to the suprasellar region (Figures 58.2 and 58.3).

Laboratory workup, including LH, prolactin, GH, IGF-1, FSH, and ACTH, were within normal limits and helped to exclude pituitary adenoma. Ophthalmology was consulted and detected right-sided temporal pallor, decreased visual acuity, CN VI palsy, and bilateral papilledema.

DIAGNOSIS

Pilocytic astrocytoma

Treatment/Follow-up

She underwent partial resection of the tumor, which was identified as a pilocytic astrocytoma.

TEACHING POINTS

Pilocytic astrocytomas are a relatively rare form of pediatric brain tumors characterized by their well-circumscribed nature and generally good prognosis. In a study of 51 patients with a pilocytic astrocytoma, the overall survival was 82% at 10 and 20 years, with 89% of those surviving patients experiencing no persisting morbidity. Surgical removal is the mainstay of treatment; adjunctive chemotherapy and/or radiation may also be used. In a single-center, retrospective review of 31 patients with pilocytic astrocytomas, 10-year disease-specific survival was unaffected by the extent of tumor removal. However, there was a significantly greater risk of subsequent tumor growth or appearance of new lesions in patients who did not undergo total resection of the original mass.

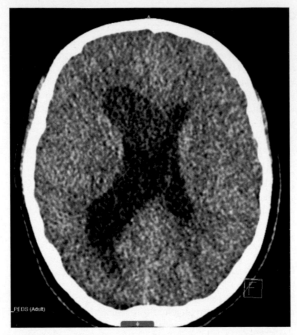

FIGURE 58.1 Axial view computed tomography (CT) shows a mass in the anterior portion of the right lateral ventricle.

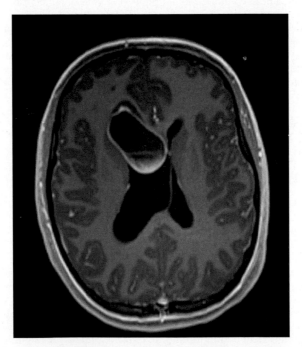

FIGURE 58.2 Axial view magnetic resonance image (MRI) shows a rim-enhancing lesion located at the anterior portion of the right lateral ventricle.

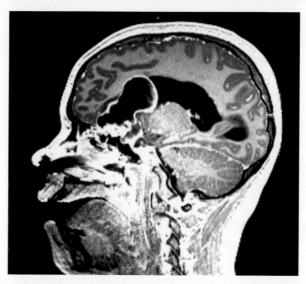

FIGURE 58.3 Sagittal view magnetic resonance image (MRI) shows a rim-enhancing lesion located at the anterior portion of the lateral ventricles.

Suprasellar masses most often present with visual impairment due to their proximity to the optic chiasm. Other symptoms may include headache, weakness, and/or vomiting due to increased ICPs, as seen in this patient.

Suggested Readings

Forsyth PA, Shaw EG, Scheithauer BW, O'Fallon JR, Layton DD Jr, Katzmann JA. Supratentorial pilocytic astrocytomas. A clinicopathologic, prognostic, and flow cytometric study of 51 patients. *Cancer*. 1993;72(4):1335-1342.

Park JH, Jung N, Kang SJ, et al. Survival and prognosis of patients with pilocytic astrocytoma: a single-center study. *Brain Tumor Res Treat*. 2019;7(2):92-97.

Synder PJ. Gonadotroph adenomas. In: Melmed S, ed. *The Pituitary*. 2nd ed. Blackwell Science Inc.; 2002:575.

59

One Foot in the Graves

Jennifer D. May

CHIEF COMPLAINT

Heavy breathing

HISTORY OF PRESENT ILLNESS

A 5-day-old 36-week boy was transferred from another hospital for worsening heavy breathing, respiratory distress, and tachycardia. He was born to a mother with Graves disease and was doing well and was asymptomatic for the first 3 days of life (DOLs).

The mother is a 28-year-old woman with Graves disease which was diagnosed during pregnancy after she presented with proptosis. She was treated with propylthiouracil (PTU) and then methimazole; however, she remained hyperthyroid throughout pregnancy. Mother's thyroid-stimulating immunoglobulins were elevated at 5.7 (normal is <1.3 on the thyroid stiffness index [TSI]), thyroid-stimulating hormone (TSH) <0.01 µIU/mL, and free T4 1.4 ng/dL.

The infant's thyroid studies were obtained on DOL 3 and included TSH < 0.01, free T4 > 7.7, and thyrotropin receptor antibodies >40. He was started on methimazole at 0.2 mg/kg divided BID; however, over the next 2 days, his tachycardia worsened, he began to need supplemental oxygen, and he became more jittery and irritable. Chest x-ray on DOL 5 demonstrated cardiomegaly.

EXAMINATION

- Vitals: Temp: 36.5 °C; pulse: 190; resp: 48; BP: 75/35; Spo_2: 90%; Fio_2: 40%
- Head: Small anterior fontanelle soft, open, flat, no molding
- Eyes: Normally spaced, open spontaneously, exophthalmos is present
- Red reflex: Present
- Ears/nose/throat/palate: No ear pits or tags, nares patent, palate high-arched
- Respiratory: Clear to auscultation, no retractions, good air exchange
- Cardiovascular: Regular rate and rhythm, no murmurs, lower extremity pulses equal bilaterally, normal capillary refill
- Abdomen: Round, soft, nontender, nondistended, no organomegaly, three vessel cord
- Genitalia: Normal phallus, bilateral descended testes, normal genitalia for gestational age, and uncircumcised
- Anus: Appears patent
- Spine: Straight and intact, no sacral dimple or tuft
- Extremities: No clavicular crepitus, hips stable with no clicks or clunks
- Neurologic: Awake; increased tone, irritable, good suck and grasp; tremulous

DIAGNOSTIC CONSIDERATIONS

- Neonatal Graves disease (NGD) secondary to maternal hyperthyroidism
- NGD secondary to TSH-activating mutation
- NGD secondary to McCune-Albright syndrome

Investigation and Results

- Infant's laboratory test results:
  - Thyrotropin receptor Ab > 40 (normal < 1.75 IU/L)
  - TSH < 0.01 μIU/mL (low)
  - Free T4 > 7.7 ng/dL (normal 1-3)
  - Free T3 25.9 pg/mL (normal range 2.3-4.1)
- Echocardiogram: Severely depressed biventricular systolic function (LV EF 21%), hypertrophy of the right ventricle with estimated RVp > 90 mm Hg, and moderate TR and MR

DIAGNOSIS

1. **Neonatal Graves disease**
2. **Cardiomyopathy** secondary to thyrotoxicosis

Treatment/Follow-up

He was treated with inhaled nitric oxide for pulmonary hypertension, milrinone and nipride for afterload reduction, and propranolol for beta-blockade. He was intubated (with extracorporeal membrane oxygenation [ECMO] team on standby) for worsening cardiorespiratory function on DOL 7.

The dose of methimazole was increased to better inhibit the synthesis of thyroid hormone. Potassium iodide was added to reduce thyroid hormone synthesis and acutely block thyroid hormone release, along with stress dose steroids to reduce peripheral T4 to T3 conversion, and cholestyramine to facilitate elimination of intestinal unconjugated thyroid hormone. On this medical management, he stabilized and gradually improved and was extubated on DOL 19. His cardiac function improved, and a repeat echocardiogram on DOL 22 showed normal systolic function but still with left ventricular hypertrophy (LVH) and right ventricular hypertrophy (RVH).

Discharge medications included sildenafil, methimazole, clonidine, prednisone, and propranolol, the last three of which were prescribed in weaning doses with a goal of cessation in 1 month.

TEACHING POINTS

NGD is caused by the activity of maternal TSH receptor–stimulating antibodies (TRAbs), transported across the placenta during pregnancy, leading to overproduction of thyroid hormone. The clinical manifestations of NGD can range from irritability, diarrhea, and poor weight gain to hemodynamic instability, pulmonary hypertension, heart failure, and death.

While the prevalence of Graves disease in pregnant women is 0.1% to 0.4%, only about 1% to 5% of neonates born to mothers with Graves disease will go on to develop NGD.

Recommendations for neonates born to mother with Graves disease include obtaining TRAb levels shortly after birth, and TSH and T4 at DOL 3 to 5 and again at DOL 10 to 14, or sooner, if the infant becomes clinically symptomatic. A TRAb level three times the upper limit of normal places the neonate at high risk of NGD.

Treatment may include the following: methimazole, to block the synthesis of T4 and T3 by inhibiting the enzyme thyroid peroxidase; propranolol, to counter the downstream effects of T3; Lugol solution aka potassium iodide (acutely inhibits T4 and T3 secretion and inhibits iodine organification in the thyroid gland); glucocorticoids, which also inhibit T4 to T3 conversion; cholestyramine, to bind excreted thyroid hormone metabolites and prevent their reabsorption by enterohepatic recirculation; lithium, to block thyroid hormone secretion; and plasmapheresis, to directly removal the TRAbs.

Therapy is continued until the maternal TRAbs are cleared. The half-life of TRAbs in the infant may be anywhere from 3 to 12 weeks.

Suggested Readings

Alexander EK, Pearce EN, Brent GA, et al. 2017 guidelines of the American Thyroid Association for the diagnosis and management of thyroid disease during pregnancy and the postpartum. *Thyroid.* 2017;3:315-389.

Samuels ST, Namoc SM, Bauer AJ. Neonatal thyrotoxicosis. *Clin Perinatol.* 2018;45:31-40.

Van Der Kaay DC, Wasserman JD, Palmert MR. Management of neonates born to mothers with Graves disease. *Pediatrics.* 2016;137(4):2015.

60

Mixed

Tarin M. Bigley

CHIEF COMPLAINT

"My fingers are blue and they hurt."

HISTORY OF PRESENT ILLNESS

A 15-year-old boy presented for several days of left fifth digit color change and pain. Initially, the fingertip would become pale and numb, followed by periods of his finger being blue or purple. His left second finger then started to demonstrate similar color changes. He saw his doctor who sent an antinuclear antibody (ANA) that was positive at 1:640. Several days before the onset of symptoms, he developed nausea and dysphagia and had several episodes of vomiting, so he was started on omeprazole. He had decreased appetite and lost 6 lb. He also had transient, diffuse myalgias and arthralgias, as well as fatigue and weakness that were improving upon presentation to rheumatology clinic. He did not have any other recent illnesses, medication, or drug exposure.

PAST MEDICAL HISTORY

* Sleep apnea due to enlarged tonsils and adenoids, now resolved
* Tonsillectomy and adenoidectomy in 2017 to treat sleep apnea

Family/Social History

* Adopted.
* Lives with family.
* Plays several sports, currently in football.
* He traveled to England and Italy several months ago.
* No known sick exposures.
* He denies drug use.
* He takes Juice Plus, but no other supplemental or alternative medication.

EXAMINATION

* Vitals: HR 78, RR 16, BP 118/64, Temp 36.7 °C, Ht 171.4 cm, Wt 65.3 kg, BMI 22.22 kg/m².
* Constitutional: He appears well-developed and well-nourished.
* HEENT: Normocephalic and atraumatic. Oropharynx is clear and moist with mild pharyngeal erythema. Pupils are equal, round, and reactive to light. Conjunctivae and EOM are normal.
* Neck: Normal range of motion. Neck supple. No thyromegaly present.
* Cardiovascular: Normal rate, regular rhythm, no murmur, rub, or gallop.
* Pulmonary/chest: Effort normal. He exhibits no tenderness.
* Abdominal: Soft, nondistended. There is no tenderness.
* Musculoskeletal: Normal range of motion. Tenderness of MCPs, PIPs, DIPs, wrists, elbows, shoulders, knees, ankles, MTPs. Strength 5/5 throughout, normal muscle bulk.
* Lymph nodes: He has no cervical adenopathy.
* Neurological: He is alert and oriented to person, place, and time. A sensory deficit is present in cyanotic fingers.

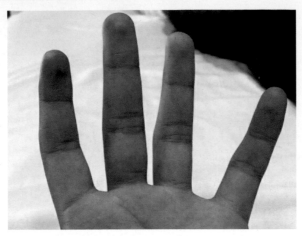

FIGURE 60.1   Fingers at time of presentation.

- Skin: Skin is warm and dry without rash. Capillary refill takes less than 2 seconds except there is pallor in bilateral fifth digit finger some pallor, cyanosis of bilateral index fingertips (Figure 60.1) and tips of bilateral fifth digits of hands, delayed cap refill. Good pulses axillary, brachial, dorsalis pedis.

DIAGNOSTIC CONSIDERATIONS

- Raynaud phenomenon: Primary versus secondary
- Acrocyanosis post viral infection
- Cryoglobulinemia post viral infection
- Cold agglutinin disease

Investigation and Results

- **ANA 1:1280, dsDNA 5 (low positive), anti-RNP > 8, anti-Smith 5.7, C4 11.9 (low), C3 82 (low), ANCA 1:2560** (pANCA, PR3, and MPO negative), RF negative, myositis and scleroderma antibody panel positive only for anti-RNP and anti-Smith.
- CBC, ESR, CRP, muscle enzymes normal.
- EBV IgG and IgM negative, hepatitis panel negative, and parvovirus IgG positive and IgM negative. *Mycoplasma pneumoniae* **IgM and IgG positive.**
- Cold agglutinin and cryoglobulin negative.
- Drug screen negative.
- Urinalysis and urine protein: Creatine normal.
- CXR normal, echocardiogram normal, CTA right upper extremity with normal vasculature.

DIAGNOSIS

Mixed connective tissue disease, with refractory Raynaud disease

Treatment/Follow-up

He was started on a baby aspirin, gabapentin, and amlodipine. The presence of autoantibodies and symptoms of mixed connective tissue disease (MCTD) led to the initiation of hydroxy-chloroquine. He also completed a course of azithromycin given his positive *Mycoplasma* IgG and IgM. However, the symptoms worsened and progressed to involve most fingers with severe features including persistence of ischemia and necrotic ulcerations (see Figure 60.2, note ulcerations of his second and fifth digit). He was admitted and treated with IV prostaglandin, rituximab, and a course of prednisone. He was also started on nitroglycerin paste, bosentan,

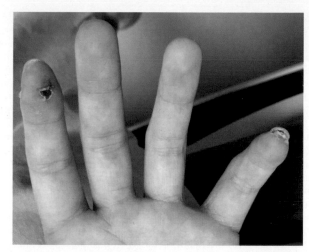

FIGURE 60.2   Digital ulceration with ischemia.

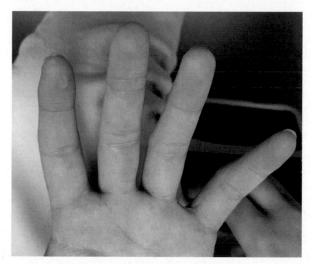

FIGURE 60.3   Resolution and healing of digital ulceration.

and sildenafil. The omeprazole was discontinued. He responded well, and the medications have gradually been decreased to hydroxychloroquine, sildenafil, and amlodipine. Although he continued to have occasional color changes with cold exposure, he otherwise fully recovered (Figure 60.3). His dsDNA antibody became normal, and anti-Smith antibody was low titer, while his anti-RNP antibody has remained high titer.

TEACHING POINTS

This patient had a complicated presentation and course. His episode of emesis and nausea with arthralgias and myalgias prior to the onset of finger color changes, the findings of *Mycoplasma pneumoniae* IgM indicating a recent infection, and the initiation of omeprazole were all considered as potential precipitating factors of his presentation. The presence of several autoantibodies was highly suggestive of an underlying autoimmune condition, in this case, MCTD.

The criteria for the diagnosis of MCTD have not been validated in the pediatric population. MCTD is generally considered an overlap syndrome in which patients have a high titer anti-U1 ribonucleoprotein (RNP) antibodies and features of systemic lupus erythematosus (SLE), systemic sclerosis, polymyositis, or dermatomyositis. It is characterized by clinical findings including Raynaud phenomenon, swollen hands, synovitis, myositis or myalgias, and skin rashes such as malar rash, scleroderma, and Gottron papules. ANA is typically high titer (>1:640). If anti-Smith or dsDNA antibodies are present, they are lower titer than anti-RNP, but their presence and persistence suggest that the patient is likely to develop SLE. While it is unclear if this patient will develop one of these diseases, his most impressive symptom was Raynaud phenomenon. It has been posited that when Raynaud phenomenon causes tissue damage, it should be referred to as Raynaud disease.

Raynaud phenomenon itself presents as a sudden onset of sharply demarcated color changes of the digits of the hands and sometimes the feet. It is caused by vasoconstriction of the digital arteries and arterioles, resulting in pallor, followed by cyanosis, and finally redness as vasoconstriction resolves and blood flow resumes. The thumbs are rarely involved. In Raynaud phenomenon, vasoconstriction usually occurs in response to cold exposure or, more accurately, exposure to a reduction in environmental temperate. Other stimuli such as stress can also induce vasoconstriction. The prevalence is estimated to be 3% to 20% of women and 3% to 14% of men and is higher in younger age groups (teenagers rather than toddlers) and those with a family history. Patients often describe numbness, tingling, pins and needles, aching, and, less commonly, ischemia resulting in ulcerations.

Diagnosis of Raynaud phenomenon involves a history of at least two color changes, usually pallor and cyanosis, after cold exposure. Primary Raynaud phenomenon describes patients who do not have a known underlying diagnosis. It is most common in young women, and there may be an association with migraine headaches or other vascular dysfunction. Secondary Raynaud occurs in the presence of an underlying disease. It is important to differentiate primary Raynaud from secondary Raynaud by history, examination, and sometimes laboratory studies. Rheumatologic conditions including SLE, MCTD, systemic sclerosis, dermatomyositis, Sjogren syndrome, and other autoimmune vasculitides should be given consideration and screened for in patients with Raynaud. Those patients with nail bed capillary changes such as telangiectasias or an ANA > 1:160 are more likely to have an underlying rheumatologic condition. Some studies suggest that there is an annual incidence of transition of primary to secondary Raynaud of about 1% and that development of an autoimmune disease is not uncommon. Other diagnostic considerations should include hypothyroidism, drug or toxin exposure such as polyvinyl chloride, ergotamines, nicotine, sympathomimetics, chemotherapeutics (especially cisplatin and bleomycin), cryoglobulinemia, cold agglutinin, paraneoplastic syndrome, vascular occlusion such as thrombus, and repetitive use of vibrational tools resulting in vascular injury.

The approach to management of Raynaud phenomenon depends on the severity of presentation and underlying diagnosis. Those with secondary diagnoses should undergo treatment of their underlying condition. Patients who do not have ischemic manifestations such as ulceration and whose symptoms do not cause decreased function in their daily life can be managed with supportive care and lifestyle modifications. These include avoiding exposure to decreases in temperature by wearing gloves, socks, and other warm clothing, as well as avoiding vasoconstrictive agents, such as caffeine and tobacco. If symptoms are severe or unresponsive to the maneuvers listed above, calcium channel blockers (CCBs) are first-line for pharmacologic management. When CCBs fail, topical nitrate, phosphodiesterase type 5 inhibitors (typically sildenafil), and sometimes angiotensin II receptor blockers (ARBs) and selective serotonin reuptake inhibitors (SSRIs) are considered. Patients with severe, progressive, or refractory ischemia are started on aspirin and IV prostaglandin. Digital or regional block and rarely sympathectomy are considerations for patients who do not respond to any pharmacologic treatment.

Suggested Readings

Berard RA, Laxer RM. Pediatric mixed connective tissue disease. *Curr Rheumatol Rep*. 2016;18(5):28.

Chikura B, Moore TL, Manning JB, et al. Sparing of the thumb in Raynaud's phenomenon. *Rheumatology*. 2008;47:219.

Freedman RR, Mayes MD. Familial aggregation of primary Raynaud's disease. *Arthritis Rheum*. 1996;39:1189.

Hirschl M, Hirschl K, Lenz M, et al. Transition from primary Raynaud's phenomenon to secondary Raynaud's phenomenon identified by diagnosis of an associated disease: results of ten years of prospective surveillance. *Arthritis Rheum*. 2006;54:1974.

Kallenberg CG, Wouda AA, Hoet MH, van Venrooij WJ. Development of connective tissue disease in patients presenting with Raynaud's phenomenon: a six year follow up with emphasis on the predictive value of antinuclear antibodies as detected by immunoblotting. *Ann Rheum Dis.* 1988;47:634.

Leppert J, Aberg H, Ringqvist I, Sörensson S. Raynaud's phenomenon in a female population: prevalence and association with other conditions. *Angiology.* 1987;38:871.

Spencer-Green G. Outcomes in primary Raynaud phenomenon: a meta-analysis of the frequency, rates, and predictors of transition to secondary diseases. *Arch Intern Med.* 1998;158:595.

Suter LG, Murabito JM, Felson DT, Fraenkel L. The incidence and natural history of Raynaud's phenomenon in the community. *Arthritis Rheum.* 2005;52:1259.

Zahavi I, Chagnac A, Hering R, et al. Prevalence of Raynaud's phenomenon in patients with migraine. *Arch Intern Med.* 1984;144:742.

61

Back to Basics

Lauren Gregory

CHIEF COMPLAINT

"He used to walk, but now he crawls."

HISTORY OF PRESENT ILLNESS

A 2-year-old boy presented with a worsening abnormal gait and low back pain. Four weeks ago, he refused to let his parents put him in his car seat and screamed that his back hurt. This was an atypical behavior for him. Two and a half weeks ago his parents noticed that his gait appeared abnormal. He now prefers to crawl rather than walk. To stand, he pushes off the ground with his hands and then pushes his hands onto his thighs. One week ago, he visited his grandparents in Kentucky where he vomited four times. He had no other symptoms and no further episodes of emesis. He has intermittently taken ibuprofen for his back pain, which provided some relief.

His pediatrician obtained a bilateral hip ultrasound, plain films of his hips and pelvis, CBC, and inflammatory markers. Both imaging studies were normal. CBC and CRP were normal, and the ESR was mildly elevated. He was then referred to a pediatric orthopedic surgeon who concluded that these symptoms could be due to inflammation or a soft-tissue strain. A repeat CBC was again normal, but the ESR remained elevated.

A sedated MRI of the pelvis and lumbar spine was ordered, but he presented to the ER prior to those studies being obtained, due to complete refusal to walk.

PAST MEDICAL HISTORY

- Term infant
- Milk allergy

Medications

- Ibuprofen PRN

Family/Social History

- Mother and brother—congenital hip dysplasia. Mother—carrier for Krabbe disease.
- Lives with his parents and younger brother in a house. Does not attend daycare. He is fully vaccinated.

EXAMINATION

- Vitals: T 37.2, HR 97, RR 24, BP 98/64, SpO$_2$ 99% RA.
- General: Comfortable and in no distress when in parent's lap, cries when made to stand.
- Head: Normocephalic, atraumatic.
- Eyes: Conjunctiva clear.
- Nose: No drainage.
- Mouth: No lip or oral mucosa lesions. Moist mucous membranes.
- Neck: Supple.
- Lungs: Breathing comfortably, clear to auscultation bilaterally.

- Cardiac: Regular rate and rhythm, no murmurs.
- Abdomen: Soft, distended, bowel sounds present, nontender to palpation, no organomegaly.
- Extremities: Well-perfused, no deformity.
- Back: Tender to palpation over sacrum.
- Skin: No rashes.
- MSK: Full active and passive range of motion of hips, knees, ankles, and feet bilaterally. Hips and knees are not tender to palpation.
- Neuro: Awake, alert. EOMI, face symmetric. Moves all extremities. Sensation grossly intact. No obvious muscle weakness. Decreased axial muscle tone. Reflexes 2+ bilaterally in upper and lower extremities. Coordination normal. Moved from sitting to standing by walking his hands forward on his legs. Walked with his pelvis tilted forward.

DIAGNOSTIC CONSIDERATIONS

Given the presence of Gower sign and decreased axial tone, neuromuscular disorders including Duchene muscular dystrophy and Becker muscular dystrophy were considered, as well as transverse myelitis. Given the presence of back pain, osteomyelitis, diskitis, trauma, malignancy, and spinal mass were considered.

Investigation

- CBC, CMP, magnesium, phosphorus, CK, ESR, CRP.
- Neurology was consulted and recommended an MRI brain and spine.

Results

- CBC: WBC 10.7, Hgb 12.1, Hct 36.6, Plt 407, 41% neutrophils, 0.2% immature granulocytes, 53% lymphocytes
- CMP, magnesium, phosphorus: Within normal limits
- ESR 30, CRP 1.3
- CK 60
- MRI: Intervertebral disk and adjacent vertebral body end plate enhancement with associated marrow signal abnormality, consistent with diskitis and osteomyelitis at the L5-S1 level

DIAGNOSIS

1. **Diskitis** of lumbosacral region.
2. **Osteomyelitis** of vertebra of lumbosacral region.
3. Bone biopsy was obtained by interventional radiology, and culture showed no growth, but PCR for **Kingella species** was positive.

Treatment/Follow-up

He was discharged home on cefazolin for *Kingella* osteomyelitis and diskitis. He was treated with 2.5 weeks of IV antibiotics and was then switched to cefalexin for an additional 4 weeks of treatment. ESR normalized and his physical examination returned to baseline during this time.

TEACHING POINTS

In the pediatric population, diskitis most commonly occurs in toddlers and young children. *Staphylococcus aureus* is the most common infectious cause of diskitis in children, although in half of the cases, no organisms are identified. Vertebral osteomyelitis is less common than diskitis, and it typically occurs in older children and adolescents. Osteomyelitis in children is usually due to hematogenous infection, though it can occur secondary to direct inoculation via trauma and surgery. The common bacterial causes of osteomyelitis vary by age group; *S. aureus* is the most common cause of acute hematogenous osteomyelitis in all age groups.

    Kingella kingae is a facultative anaerobic, beta-hemolytic gram-negative organism. Asymptomatic colonization of the oropharynx is common in young children (6 months), but incidence of colonization decreases to 10% to 12% by the second year of life and then declines to very low levels. *Kingella* is difficult to culture with routine cultures. PCR testing for *Kingella* is available.

Suggested Readings

Conrad D. Acute hematogenous osteomyelitis. *Pediatr Rev*. 2010;31(11):464-471. doi:10.1542/pir.31-11-464

Samara E, Spyropoulou V, Tabard A, et al. Kingella kingae and osteoarticular infections. *Pediatrics*. 2019;144(6):e20191509. doi:10.1542/peds.2019-1509

62

One Year

Nicholas W. DeKorver

CHIEF COMPLAINT

Neck pain and swelling

HISTORY OF PRESENT ILLNESS

A 9-year-old boy presented with right-sided neck pain and an enlarging mass. He noticed the mass 1 month prior to presentation, and at first, it caused no discomfort, but as it enlarged, he developed pain that was worse with swallowing. He had no fevers, no night sweats, and no abdominal symptoms.

PAST MEDICAL HISTORY

- Up-to-date on vaccinations
- Left elbow surgery, fracture

Medications

Loratadine

Family/Social History

He lives at home with his mother, father, and sister, with a cat but no other animal exposures. No travel outside the United States. No consumption of undercooked meats or unpasteurized dairy. No exposure to persons with chronic cough or tuberculosis. He sees a dentist regularly.

EXAMINATION

Vitals: T 36.5 °C, 97.7 °F, HR 104, RR 22, BP 120/74, SpO$_2$ 96%

He was alert, interactive, oriented, and in no distress. Head was normocephalic and atraumatic. Conjunctivae were clear; pupils were equal, round, and reactive. Extraocular movements were intact. External ear canals and TM normal bilaterally. No nasal drainage. Oropharynx was without erythema, and mucus membranes were moist. There was a 4 × 3 cm^2 midneck mass located to the right of the midline (see Figure 62.1), which was mobile, and tender to palpation, but without overlying erythema. The mass did not elevate with protrusion of the tongue or swallowing. Scattered shotty lymphadenopathy of the anterior cervical chain bilaterally. Lungs clear to auscultation; no increased work of breathing. Heart had regular rate and rhythm. No murmurs. Abdomen was soft, nontender to palpation, with normal bowel sounds. Extremities were well perfused and without effusions, erythema, or edema. No rashes. Normal neurologic examination.

DIAGNOSTIC CONSIDERATIONS

The differential for a neck mass is very broad and includes congenital, inflammatory, and neoplastic processes. Congenital etiologies include, but are not limited to, branchial cleft cysts, thyroglossal duct cysts, hemangiomas, dermoid cysts, laryngoceles, and teratomas.

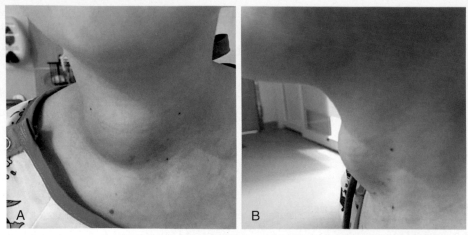

FIGURE 62.1   A 4 × 3 cm² neck mass located to the right of midline. **A**, Front view. **B**, Side view.

Inflammatory etiologies include both infectious lymphadenopathy (viral, bacterial, and parasitic) and noninfectious lymphadenopathy (sarcoidosis, Castleman disease, and Kawasaki disease). Neoplastic etiologies include lymphoma, neuroblastoma, rhabdomyosarcoma, thyroid masses, and lipomas, among others.

Investigation and Results

Laboratory testing included a CBC, CMP, and TSH, which were all unremarkable. Testing for specific infectious diseases (*Bartonella*, tuberculosis, *Histoplasma*, *Toxoplasma*, and *Blastomyces*) was negative. Ultrasound of the mass showed a lobulated lesion that lacked internal flow and was connected by a fistulous tract (Figure 62.2A). The mass compressed the right internal jugular vein and was thought to represent an infected brachial cleft cyst. CT of the neck and chest with contrast demonstrated a necrotic right-sided neck mass with calcified mediastinal and right hilar adenopathy, right upper lobe nodules, and small surrounding perilymphatic nodules (Figure 62.2B). He was taken to the OR for biopsy. Microscopic analysis of the fluid and tissue was performed. Flow cytometry for clonal B-cell populations was negative. Samples were sent for aerobic, anaerobic, acid-fast bacilli, and fungal cultures.

Imaging was most suggestive of actinomycosis, which pathology confirmed, and he was started on IV Augmentin.

DIAGNOSIS

Actinomycosis

Treatment/Follow-up

He was switched to oral Augmentin 2 days later and discharged home to complete 1 year of antibiotics. DHR flow for chronic granulomatous disease was negative. On follow-up, he was doing well on antibiotic therapy, and the mass was much smaller in size and no longer painful.

TEACHING POINTS

- Actinomycosis is a rare, chronic disease caused by members of the *Actinomyces* species of anaerobic, gram-positive, filamentous bacteria. Infection often leads to abscess formation, fistulas, sinus tracts, and tissue fibrosis.
- Diagnosing actinomycosis can prove challenging for several reasons: (1) infections often respond briefly to a short course of broad-spectrum antibiotics reducing the yield of cultures within 7 to 10 days of antibiotic therapy; (2) culturing *Actinomyces* requires strict anaerobic

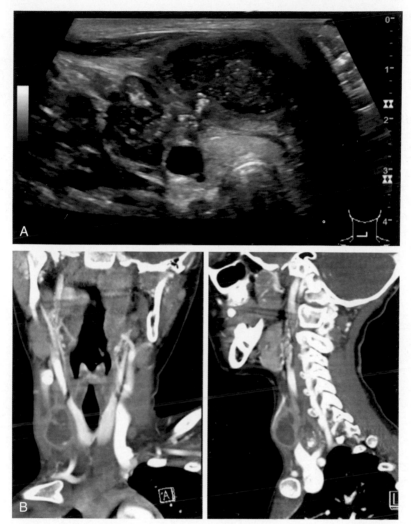

FIGURE 62.2   A, Ultrasound of neck mass and connecting fistula. **B,** Computed tomography (CT) imaging demonstrating neck mass and calcifications in anterior and lateral views.

processing and growth conditions and a long incubation time both of which increase failure rates; (3) histology can miss sulfur granules and characteristic bacteria shape due to extensive fibrosis and tissue damage. Cultures are negative in more than 50% of cases. Histopathology and staining detects sulfur granules and bacteria in roughly 75% of cases.

- Treatment for actinomycosis varies for severe or extensive and mild disease, but high-dose penicillin or amoxicillin is given, either IV or oral depending on severity. Surgical drainage of abscesses is often required. Duration of treatment often extends 1 to 2 months after resolution of infection to reduce the risk of recrudescence. In many cases, this may take months or even longer than a year of therapy.
- Branchial cleft cysts are the most common congenital neck lesions, accounting for 20% to 30% of all pediatric neck masses. They often present from late childhood to early adulthood with a localized acute infection of the lesion.
- Thyroglossal duct cysts often present with acute infection, as a midline anterior neck mass that may move with swallowing. A track or fistula that passes through the hyoid bone to the base of the tongue may be present. Compression of the mass may expel material through the fistula.

Suggested Readings

Chen A, Otto KJ. Differential diagnosis of neck masses. In: Flint PW, Haughey BH, Lund VJ, et al, eds. *Cummings Otolaryngology—Head and Neck Surgery*. Elsevier; 2010:1636-1642.

Ferry T, Valour F, Karsenty J, et al. Actinomycosis: etiology, clinical features, diagnosis, treatment, and management. *Infect Drug Resist*. 2014;7:183-197.

Geddes G, Butterly MM, Patel SM, Marra S. Pediatric neck masses. *Pediatr Rev*. 2013;34(3):115-125.

Rankow RM, Abraham DM. Actinomycosis: masquerader in the head and neck. *Ann Otol Rhinol Laryngol*. 1978;87(2):230-237.

Smego JRA, Foglia G. Actinomycosis. *Clin Infect Dis*. 1998;26(6):1255-1261.

63

Not Just Baby Fat

Katherine Velicki, Nicholas W. DeKorver

Chief Complaint

Leg swelling

History of Present Illness

A 4-month-old infant developed swelling in her feet and legs that appeared 3 weeks ago and gradually worsened. She was seen by her pediatrician for her well-child visit, and laboratory tests were sent because of the swelling. The albumin was 1.4 and a plasma protein of 3.0, and she was directly admitted to pediatric nephrology service for presumed nephrotic syndrome. She did have a runny nose 2 weeks prior to the swelling that has resolved completely. She has no fever, weight loss, fussiness, trouble breathing, dark stools, or blood in her urine. She has had soft, yellow stools with a consistency between cottage cheese and yogurt, occurring every 3 hours for the past 2 weeks.

Past Medical History

- Born full term at 40 weeks by uncomplicated vaginal delivery.
- She had an episode of jaundice at 2 weeks of age that resolved without treatment.
- Up-to-date on vaccinations.

Family/Social History

She is exclusively breastfed and lives with her mother, father, older sister, and two cats. She is "the favorite" at daycare, which she attends 5 days per week.

Examination

Vitals: T 36.9, HR 147, BP 100/82, RR 34, SpO$_2$ 100% on RA

Well-appearing baby with large body habitus, weighing in the 96th percentile. She was awake, alert, interactive, and did not cry until the end of her physical examination, after which she was easily consoled by her mother. There was edema and skin mottling of the bilateral lower extremities, extending from hips to feet. No organomegaly and no palpable abdominal mass. Mild diaper rash but no blood in diaper. Erythematous rash on her neck with satellite lesions.

Diagnostic Considerations

In addition to suspected infantile nephrotic syndrome, other possible etiologies include protein-losing enteropathy, protein malnutrition, liver pathology, and cardiac failure. Lower extremity edema alone should also raise the possibility of lymphatic abnormalities or impaired venous obstruction.

Investigation and Results

Repeat laboratory tests confirmed hypoalbuminemia and hypoproteinemia. Urinary protein/creatinine ratio was within normal limits, calling into question the diagnosis of nephrotic syndrome.

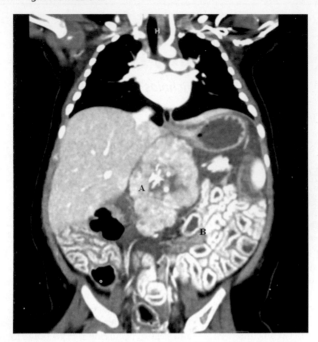

FIGURE 63.1 Contrasted computed tomography (CT) of chest-abdomen-pelvis. Imaging revealed a large (7.4 × 4.7 × 4.0 cm), midline, enhancing, centrally necrotic retroperitoneal mass with calcifications (**A**) and diffuse bowel wall edema (**B**).

Abdominal imaging by ultrasound was ordered to examine the kidneys and urinary system and showed a retroperitoneal mass. Additional imaging by CT with contrast demonstrated a large (7.4 × 4.7 × 4.0 cm) midline, enhancing, centrally necrotic retroperitoneal mass with calcifications, suggesting a diagnosis of extra-adrenal neuroblastoma (Figure 63.1). The mass encased the abdominal aorta, renal, celiac, splenic, common hepatic, and superior mesenteric arteries, but all remained patent. There were no signs of metastasis on imaging. Diffuse mucosal thickening and enhancement of the small bowel and rectum consistent with diffuse enteritis and proctitis was noted. Biopsies obtained via exploratory laparotomy revealed a poorly differentiated small round blue cell tumor with immunohistochemistry positive for synaptophysin, chromogranin, and vimentin. Two markers of catecholamine-secreting tumors, vanillylmandelic acid (VMA) and homovanillic acid (HVA), were elevated at 205.0 and 94.7, respectively.

DIAGNOSIS

Neuroblastoma, retroperitoneal, extra-adrenal

Treatment/Follow-up

Pathology confirmed neuroblastoma, classified as International Neuroblastoma Staging System (INSS) Stage 4 due to bilateral lymph node involvement. A metaiodobenzylguanidine (MIBG) scan confirmed that there were no distant metastases, and bone marrow biopsies of the bilateral iliac crests showed no evidence of malignancy. The patient received carboplatin and etoposide treatments through a right internal jugular port-a-catheter. Edema was treated with fluid restriction and infusions of albumin and furosemide. She was discharged with oncology follow-up and on a chemotherapy protocol.

TEACHING POINTS

Mechanisms for edema include increased capillary hydrostatic pressure, decreased capillary oncotic pressure, and increased capillary permeability. The initial consideration for this patient was infantile nephrotic syndrome leading to hypoproteinemia and reduced capillary oncotic pressure.

• Congenital nephrotic syndrome presents from birth to 3 months of age and infantile nephrotic syndrome from 3 months to 1 year of life. Mutations in NPHS1, NPHS2, and WT1 are responsible for the majority of cases. WT1 mutations are also responsible for Denys-Drash syndrome comprised of pseudohermaphroditism, Wilms tumor, hypertension, and degenerative renal disease.

• Neuroblastoma accounts for 7% to 10% of childhood cancers and is the most common cancer in infants younger than 12 months. Neuroblastoma often presents as an abdominal mass. Lower extremity edema can be present if the tumor is large and compresses venous or lymphatic drainage. These tumors are derived from neural crest cells and frequently express genes for norepinephrine transport and catecholamine metabolism. Testing for catecholamine pathway end products VMA and HVA can aid in diagnosis, as 70% to 90% of patients with neuroblastoma will have elevated levels. There are a small number of case reports of nephrotic syndrome in patients with neuroblastoma. Development of nephrotic syndrome in these cases was believed to be due to deposition of neuroblastoma-associated immune complexes on the glomerular basement membrane or secondary to increased intraglomerular pressure due involvement of the renal vessels.

• While this patient did not have nephrotic range proteinuria, the more likely etiology for the low protein and edema was protein-losing enteropathy. Protein-losing enteropathy has been described in neuroblastoma and may be due to lymphatic obstruction and lymphangiectasia.

Suggested Readings

Citak C, Karadeniz C, Dalgic B, et al. Intestinal lymphangiectasia as a first manifestation of neuroblastoma. *Pediatr Blood Cancer.* 2005;46(1):105-107. doi:10.1002/pbc.20530

Gerdes JS, Katz AJ. Neuroblastoma appearing as protein-losing enteropathy. *Am J Dis Child.* 1982;136(11):1024. doi:10.1001/archpedi.1982.03970470068017

Gurney JG, Ross JA, Wall DA, et al. Infant cancer in the U.S. *J Pediatr Hematol Oncol.* 1997;19(5):428-432. doi:10.1097/00043426-199709000-00004

Hinkes BG, Mucha B, Vlangos CN, et al. Nephrotic syndrome in the first year of life: two thirds of cases are caused by mutations in 4 genes (NPHS1, NPHS2, WT1, and LAMB2). *Pediatrics.* 2007;119(4):e907-e919. doi:10.1542/peds.2006-2164

Kim SH, Park HM, Lee JH, et al. A case of infantile nephrotic syndrome associated with neuroblastoma. *Child Kidney Dis.* 2018;22(2):91-96. doi:10.3339/jkspn.2018.22.2.91

Kontras SB. Urinary excretion of 3-methoxy-4-hydroxymandelic acid in children with neuroblastoma. *Cancer.* 1962;15(5):978-986. doi:10.1002/1097-0142(196209/10)15:5<978::aid-cncr2820150514>3.0.co;2-j

Poggi GM, Fognani G, Cuzzubbo D, et al. Neuroblastoma presenting with acute kidney injury, hyponatremic-hypertensive-like syndrome and nephrotic proteinuria in a 10-month-old child. *Case Rep Oncol.* 2011;4(2):400-405. doi:10.1159/000331211

Reifen R, Sherman P. Intestinal lymphangiectasia secondary to neuroblastoma. *Can J Gastroenterol.* 1994;8(1):49-51. doi:10.1155/1994/621375

Zheng HL, Maruyama T, Matsuda S, et al. Neuroblastoma presenting with the nephrotic syndrome. *J Pediatr Surg.* 1979;14(4):414-419. doi:10.1016/s0022-3468(79)80003-2

64

Botulism to Abuse

Marie L. Batty

CHIEF COMPLAINT

Respiratory distress

HISTORY OF PRESENT ILLNESS

A 5-month-old girl presented to a local emergency room (ER) from her pediatrician's office for respiratory distress. She developed a cough 1 week ago, her abdomen appeared more distended, and she was stooling less frequently. A few days prior to presentation, she developed temperature lability with maximum temperature of 102.8 °F and minimum of 95.8 °F. On the day of presentation, she developed belly breathing and had decreased PO intake. In her pediatrician's office, she had increased work of breathing on examination and desaturated to 70% in the office. She was transported to the local ER for further evaluation. Also, she seemed to be moving her lower extremities less than normal over the prior 4 days, which mom attributed to her being sick.

In the ER, she had several bradycardic episodes to the 40 seconds with desaturations to the 60 seconds. A chest x-ray with right upper lobe (RUL) infiltrate suggested pneumonia, for which she received a dose of ceftriaxone. Respiratory viral panel was negative. She was admitted to her local hospital and started on high-flow nasal cannula of 6 L without improvement in her work of breathing. Given worsening respiratory status, she was transferred to the nearest tertiary hospital and admitted to the pediatric intensive care unit (PICU). En route, she continued to have episodes of bradycardia while asleep.

PAST MEDICAL HISTORY

Born at 39 weeks via vaginal delivery after uncomplicated pregnancy. Sustained collarbone fracture during delivery, which healed nonoperatively. No prior hospitalizations. Immunizations up-to-date. Formula fed, recently started taking table foods. At baseline, she has good head control and can roll in one direction.

Medications

Cough syrup for cough and congestion

Family/Social History

- She is the parents' first baby.
- No history of SIDS.
- Family lives in the city, and they drink city water.

EXAMINATION

- Vitals: T 37.2 °C, HR 110, RR 49, BP 113/57, O_2 saturation 100% on 21% FiO_2.
- General: Pale appearing, lethargic, and minimally reactive to interventions. Weak cry, difficult to hear at times. Crying with few tears.
- HEENT: Normocephalic, atraumatic, anterior fontanelle open, soft, and flat. Dry lips.

- Lungs: Clear to auscultation, diminished breath sounds in right upper lobe. Subcostal retractions with belly breathing. Weak cough, wet sounding, nonproductive.
- Heart: Heart rate 120 seconds when upset, 70 to 90 seconds when calm. Regular rhythm, no murmur.
- Abdomen: Distended abdomen. Soft, nontender, normoactive bowel sounds throughout.
- GU: Normal external female genitalia.
- Extremity: Warm and well perfused.
- Back: Spine straight, no sacral abnormality.
- Skin: Scab-like lesion on posterior scalp with surrounding seborrheic dermatitis. Café au lait macule on right inner thigh. No bruising.
- Neurologic: Alert but sleepy appearing. Face symmetric. Bilateral ptosis with incomplete lid closure while asleep. EOMI, PERRL. Weak cough and cry. Strong suck. Able to reach for things with upper extremities but minimal movement of lower extremities. Will withdraw lower extremities to pain. Decreased axial and appendicular tone with minimal head lag. Does not bear weight on lower extremities when held in standing position. Reflexes 1+ in right biceps, absent at left biceps, 1+ at right patella, absent at left patella, absent at bilateral ankles.

DIAGNOSTIC CONSIDERATIONS

- Sepsis
- CNS infection
- Infant botulism
- Guillain-Barre syndrome
- Transverse myelitis
- Congenital myasthenia gravis
- Intracranial hemorrhage
- Spinal muscular atrophy
- Inborn error of metabolism

Investigation and Results

- CBC: WBC 10 (81.5%N, 14.9%L), Hgb 10.3, Hct 31.3, **Plt 435**
- CMP: Na 137, K 4.6, Cl 107, **CO_2 19**, BUN 8, Cr 0.17, glucose 120, Ca 9.9, Alk phos 195, AST 28, ALT 28, Alb 3.9
- Capillary blood gas: pH 7.45, pCO_2 36, pO_2 64, BE 0.8
- TSH, free T4 normal
- Ammonia 30
- Cortisol 11.4
- Urine drug screen negative
- CSF studies:
  - Cell count: 8 nucleated cells, 113 RBCs
  - Protein 67
  - Glucose 74
  - CSF culture with no growth after 5 days
- *Clostridium* botulism culture and toxin assay sent

With progressive respiratory distress and examination findings of lethargy, bilateral ptosis, weak cry, hypotonia, and diminished reflexes, the leading diagnosis was **infantile botulism**, despite the parents' insistence that she had not had honey and had not been exposed to soil or construction. Neurology consultation confirmed this possibility, and efforts were made to obtain BabyBIG (botulism immune globulin) as treatment for presumed infantile botulism.

Meanwhile, a head ultrasound was obtained and was overall normal, with small asymmetry favored to represent artifact. Chest x-ray showed right upper lobe atelectasis, along with a cortical irregularity of the right humerus, possibly representing a fracture. A skeletal survey was then obtained based on this finding, and it showed many fractures of varying ages. Old fractures were noted of the right humerus and left clavicle. Multiple fractures were noted in the lower extremities, including distal left femur, distal right femur, distal left tibia and fibula, and distal right tibia, and they appeared to be of different ages. Brain MRI showed thin retroclival and bilateral tentorial extra-axial hemorrhage without mass effect. C-spine MRI showed ligamentous and cord injury at C7-T1, along with an epidural hematoma causing severe cord compression. A fracture of the T9 vertebral body was present. CT scan confirmed the T9 fracture and did not show intra-abdominal injury.

DIAGNOSIS

1. Child abuse, physical
2. Spinal shock

Treatment/Follow-up

Once the fractures and spinal cord injury were seen on imaging, a diagnosis of nonaccidental trauma (NAT) was made and infantile botulism was thought to be unlikely. BIG was canceled.

Neurosurgery and General Surgery were consulted. Her injuries were deemed nonoperative, and she was closely monitored. Over her month-long hospitalization, her examination improved to include movements of her lower extremities to light touch within the plane of the bed and wiggling of her toes. She moved her upper extremities spontaneously, could reach for items, and transfer items between her hands.

Imaging on admission showed right upper lobe consolidation and multifocal atelectasis. The location of the infiltrate was consistent with aspiration pneumonia, and she was treated with ampicillin-sulbactam with radiographic improvement. However, with continued respiratory distress, she was treated with bilevel positive airway pressure (BiPAP) but was ultimately intubated by the second day of hospitalization. She failed several trials of extubation and underwent tracheostomy for respiratory failure secondary to spinal cord injury.

During her PICU stay, she had bradycardia to the 50 seconds and received an epinephrine infusion for several days, thought to be due to spinal shock. She was gradually weaned off vasoactive medications. She was able to tolerate oral feeds by the time of discharge but was given supplemental nasogastric (NG) feeds overnight for increased calorie intake.

Child Protection Team, Social Work and Law Enforcement were involved with this patient and her family. Child Protective Services ultimately took custody of the patient. She was discharged after a month-long hospitalization to a rehabilitation facility for continued neurorehabilitation.

TEACHING POINTS

Child abuse, often called NAT, affects nine out of every 1000 children in the United States each year. NAT occurs in children of all ages, but children between the ages of 0 and 3 years are at the greatest risk and account for 77% of all NAT-related deaths. A review of the National Trauma Data Bank containing over 19,000 patients with nonaccidental injuries found traumatic brain injuries to be the most common presenting injury, occurring in over 50% of children with NAT. Soft-tissue injuries such as abrasions and contusions were seen in 38% of patients, and extremity fractures were present in 35% of cases. Traumatic brain injuries are the leading cause of death in children younger than 2 years. Additionally, there is significant morbidity associated with NAT, with the aforementioned study finding 11% of children hospitalized for NAT being discharged to intermediate- or long-term care facilities, as our patient was.

Children with symptoms due to NAT can often present nonspecifically at first. In patients with abusive head trauma, they often do not present with a clear history of head trauma. As in our case, a patient's symptoms may be nonspecific, with lethargy, irritability, poor feeding, hypotonia, and vomiting being the presenting signs.

One case report in *Pediatric Emergency Care* by Sagar, Shukla, and Bradley-Dodds described a 10-week-old infant with respiratory distress and a large pleural effusion from NAT. However, the patient was initially admitted with suspicion for infantile botulism, as he also had constipation and hypotonia on examination, in addition to his respiratory distress. In this case report, thoracic trauma was thought to be the mechanism by which this patient developed a large pleural effusion requiring chest tube drainage. In our patient, spinal cord injury was thought to be the cause of her respiratory failure requiring intubation and eventual tracheostomy.

Suggested Readings

Paul A, Adamo M. Non-accidental trauma in pediatric patients: a review of epidemiology, pathophysiology, diagnosis and treatment. *Transl Pediatr*. 2014;3(4):195-207. doi:10.3978/j.issn.2224-4336.2014.06.01

Rosenfeld EH, Johnson B, Wesson DE, et al. Understanding non-accidental trauma in the United States: a National Trauma Databank study. *J Pediatr Surg*. 2020;55(4):693-697. doi:10.1016/j.jpedsurg.2019.03.024

Sagar M, Shukla S, Bradley-Dodds K. Nonaccidental trauma presenting with respiratory distress and pleural effusion. *Pediatr Emerg Care*. 2012;28(1):61-63.

65

Prescreen
Sara Procknow

CHIEF COMPLAINT

Lethargy and poor feeding

HISTORY OF PRESENT ILLNESS

A 3-day-old full-term girl with an unremarkable pregnancy and birth arrived to the emergency department (ED) from home due to lethargy and poor feeding. She had been refusing to feed since yesterday and has not had a wet diaper in 24 hours. On arrival to the ED, she was somnolent and in respiratory distress.

PAST MEDICAL HISTORY

- Full-term
- No pregnancy or delivery complications

Family/Social History

She lives at home with her parents and four older siblings, all of whom are healthy. There is no family history of epilepsy, metabolic disorders, or consanguinity.

EXAMINATION

- Vitals: Temp 35.7, HR 88, Resp 4, BP 110/82, SpO_2 99%.
- General: Sleeping, but awakens with a strong cry. Barely breathing.
- Head: Normocephalic, atraumatic. Anterior fontanelle is flat.
- Eyes: No drainage. Pupils are equal, round, and reactive to light.
- Ears: Normally formed and positioned.
- Nose: No drainage.
- Mouth: Palate intact. Mucus membranes are moist.
- Pulmonary: Normal breath sounds; no wheezing, rhonchi, or rales. No increased work of breathing or tachypnea.
- Cardiovascular: Bradycardic with regular rhythm. No murmurs. Well perfused.
- Abdomen: Soft and flat. Bowel sounds present. No hepatosplenomegaly.
- Back: Spine straight, no sacral dimples or tufts.
- Extremities: Normally formed. No tenderness or deformity.
- Skin: Capillary refill < 2 seconds. Normal turgor. No rash or petechiae.
- Neurologic: Quiet with few spontaneous movements. Normal strength and tone. Symmetric Moro reflex.

DIAGNOSTIC CONSIDERATIONS

Lethargy and poor feeding in an infant are concerning for infection, asphyxiation, hypoxic-ischemic encephalopathy (HIE), or inborn error of metabolism. Trauma, including abuse, and ingestion also need to be considered.

Investigation

- Initial laboratory tests: CBC, blood culture, capillary blood gas, respiratory pathogen PCR, blood glucose, UA, CXR
- 10 mL/kg NS bolus and 2 L oxygen via nasal canula
- Ampicillin and gentamicin
- Laboratory tests: Lactate, pyruvate, ammonia, CK, metabolic laboratory tests (acylcarnitines, carnitine profile, serum amino acids, urine organic acids)

Results

- Blood culture: No growth
- CBG: 7.45/29/68/20/-3
- CBC: Normal
- Respiratory pathogen PCR: Negative
- Glucose: 65
- UA: Cloudy, 2+ protein, 2+ bacteria
- Lactate: 3.5 (normal 0.7-2.0), pyruvate: 0.13 (normal 0.03-0.1), ratio 13
- CK: 515 (normal < 300)
- **Ammonia: 1122** (normal for age < 100)
- Acylcarnitine profile: Accumulation of C4-OH carnitine and multiple long-chain esters consistent with ketogenesis
- Carnitine profile: Reduced total and free carnitine with mild accumulation of esterified carnitine likely reflecting ketogenesis
- Serum amino acids: Elevated citrulline without detectable argininosuccinic acid, elevated glutamine
- Urine organic acids: 2+ peak of orotic acid

DIAGNOSIS

Citrullinemia Type 1, due to arginosuccinate synthetase deficiency

Treatment/Follow-up

She was started immediately on continuous renal replacement therapy, sodium benzoate and sodium phenylacetate (Ammonul, an ammonia scavenger), and arginine. After the ammonia level improved and was stabilized, she was switched to oral ammonia scavengers, had a G-tube placed, and was discharged home. At home, however, she had several hyperammonemic crises with each viral infection, and she was eventually admitted to await liver transplantation.

TEACHING POINTS

While rare, inborn errors of metabolism should be considered on the differential for any newborn presenting with poor feeding, lethargy, or persistent tachypnea. Newborn screening has greatly improved the detection of inborn errors of metabolism in the neonatal period, but some diseases, particularly urea cycle disorders, **will manifest before the newborn screen is analyzed.** Laboratory investigations are required for diagnosis but will take time to complete. Treatment should be started as soon as an inborn error of metabolism is suspected. Prompt recognition and treatment can ameliorate the neurotoxicity associated with hyperammonemia. In addition to ammonia scavengers, preventing catabolism with high dextrose-containing fluids is key for any patient with a diagnosed or suspected inborn error of metabolism. Liver transplantation is curative for patients with urea cycle disorders, although they may continue to require dietary supplementation due to a small amount of urea cycle activity in peripheral tissues.

Suggested Readings

Ah Mew N, Simpson KL, Gropman AL, et al. Urea cycle disorders overview. In: Adam MP, Ardinger HH, Pagon RA, et al, eds. *GeneReviews®* [Internet]. University of Washington; 2017:1993-2020.

Del Re S, Empain A, Vicinanza A, et al. Irritability, poor feeding and respiratory alkalosis in newborns: think about metabolic emergencies. A brief summary of hyperammonemia management. *Pediatr Rep*. 2020;12:77-85.

Häberle J, Burlina A, Chakrapani A, et al. Suggested guidelines for the diagnosis and management of urea cycle disorders: first revision. *J Inherit Metab Dis*. 2019;42:1192-1230.

66

PET Positive

Rachel C. Orscheln

CHIEF COMPLAINT

Fever and weight loss in a heart transplant recipient

HISTORY OF PRESENT ILLNESS

A 11-year-old boy who underwent a heart transplant as an infant, on tacrolimus and mycophenolate mofetil, was referred to the pediatric infectious disease service for fevers for 2 weeks. He had a sore throat at the onset of the illness and a mild cough but no rhinorrhea. He had diarrhea for 1 day and occasional vomiting. He had a decreased appetite with a 3 lb weight loss. One week earlier, he had been seen at another hospital with an evaluation that included the following testing:

* Flu A/B antigen: Negative
* Throat culture: Negative for GABHS
* UA: Negative
* CBC: Normal except slightly low platelets of 129
* He had mild transaminase elevation of AST/ALT 75/82, respectively

He was treated with an empiric course of amoxicillin but had no improvement.

PAST MEDICAL HISTORY

* Dilated cardiomyopathy
* Orthotopic heart transplant
* CMV reactivation after transplant

Family/Social History

He lives with his family in a rural home with two dogs and two kittens, and he is scratched frequently. There are no other animal exposures. The family went spelunking months ago. Hepatitis (unknown type) in father. No other medical problems in the family, and no other family members are ill.

EXAMINATION

* General: Appears tired but smiles and answers questions appropriately.
* Head: Scabbing cat scratch on chin.
* Eye: Conjunctivae clear.
* Ears: Normal TMs.
* Nose: No rhinorrhea.
* Oropharynx: Mild posterior pharynx erythema, no tonsillar enlargement or exudate.
* Neck: Neck supple with shotty lymphadenopathy.
* Lungs: Clear to auscultation bilaterally, normal WOB, and good air movement.
* Heart: Regular rate and rhythm without murmurs, rubs, or gallops.
* Chest: Healed postsurgical scars.

- Abdomen: Soft, nondistended with no splenomegaly. Liver edge palpable 1 cm below costal margin.
- Extremity: Warm and well perfused, no edema, and no joint tenderness or swelling. No adenopathy. Healing cat scratches over forearms.
- Pulses: 2+ pulses and symmetric. Cap refill <2 seconds.
- Skin: No other rashes or lesions and no jaundice.
- Neurologic: Alert and interactive.

Diagnostic Considerations

- Viral infection such as EBV, CMV, or adenovirus
- Zoonotic infection such as *Toxoplasma* sp. or *Bartonella* sp. infection
- Endemic mycosis such as infection with *Histoplasma* sp. or *Blastomyces* sp.
- Posttransplant malignancy such as PTLD

Investigation and Results

At his initial visit, a limited evaluation was performed due to a high clinical suspicion for cat scratch disease. A CBC was normal with the exception of increased variant lymphs of 8%. EBV antibodies showed past infection, and EBV and CMV PCR testing were negative. A CXR was normal. *Bartonella* sp. antibodies were sent and were ultimately negative. He was started on an empiric course of azithromycin but returned to clinic 1 week later due to persistent fever. A more extensive infectious workup was performed including the following:

- NP swab for respiratory pathogens
- Adenovirus PCR
- HSV PCR
- Parvovirus PCR
- Viral hepatitis panel
- *Histoplasma* urine antigen and antibodies
- *Blastomyces* antibodies
- *Toxoplasma* antibodies
- Blood culture

Due to a heightened concern for PTLD, a PET scan was performed which demonstrated:

- Hypermetabolic splenomegaly with hypermetabolic cervical, mediastinal, and periportal lymph nodes highly suspicious for posttransplant lymphoproliferative disease.
- Right upper lobe pulmonary ground-glass opacity with FDG activity, could be infectious or inflammatory.

A *Histoplasma* urine antigen returned as positive at a level of 19.2 ng/mL.

Diagnosis

Histoplasmosis, disseminated

Treatment/Follow-up

He was admitted to the hospital and given a single dose of amphotericin with prompt resolution of his fever, but with a bump in his creatinine. He was switched to oral itraconazole with continued clinical improvement and improvement in renal function.

In follow-up after 2½ weeks of antifungal therapy, his urine *Histoplasma* antigen had decreased to 2.4 ng/mL.

Teaching Points

Histoplasmosis is the most common endemic mycosis diagnosed in the United States. Historically, the condition is felt to be most common in the region of the Ohio and Mississippi River Valleys due to soil and environmental conditions which favor the replication of the organism. However, the geographic distribution of infection may be wider than previously thought and may be expanding. Diagnosis of histoplasmosis can be challenging due to the overlap of symptoms with other clinical conditions, and the diagnosis of histoplasmosis is often delayed. Timely diagnosis is necessary in patients at risk for severe disease such as patients receiving oncological or biological treatment, patients with congenital or acquired immune deficiency, and patients who have received solid organ or stem cell transplant. In immunocompetent patients with mild symptoms, treatment with antifungals is not necessary. However, administration of antifungal treatment is necessary in patients with immunocompromising conditions or moderate to severe symptomatic disease.

Suggested Readings

Benedict K, Beer KD, Jackson BR. Histoplasmosis-related healthcare use, diagnosis, and treatment in a commercially insured population, United States. *Clin Infect Dis*. 2020;70(6):1003-1010. doi:10.1093/cid/ciz324

McKinsey DS, Pappas PG. Histoplasmosis: time to redraw the map and up our game. *Clin Infect Dis*. 2019;70(6):1011-1013. doi:10.1093/cid/ciz327

Ouellette CP, Stanek JR, Leber A, Ardura MI. Pediatric histoplasmosis in an area of endemicity: a contemporary analysis. *J Pediatric Infect Dis Soc*. 2019;8(5):400-407. doi:10.1093/jpids/piy073

Wheat LJ, Azar MM, Bahr NC, Spec A, Relich RF, Hage C. Histoplasmosis. *Infect Dis Clin North Am*. 2016;30(1):207-227. doi:10.1016/j.idc.2015.10.009

Wheat LJ, Freifeld AG, Kleiman MB, et al. Clinical practice guidelines for the management of patients with histoplasmosis: 2007 update by the Infectious Diseases Society of America. *Clin Infect Dis*. 2007;45(7):807-825. doi:10.1086/521259

67

Constipated Thinking

Julianne Ivy

CHIEF COMPLAINT

Needs a clean out

HISTORY OF PRESENT ILLNESS

A 10-year-old boy presented as a transfer from an outside hospital for 2 days of abdominal pain. The pain was primarily located in the right lower quadrant, was described as sharp and crampy in quality, and was worse with movement. It had become increasingly severe over the previous 2 days. The patient had a mildly decreased appetite but no nausea, vomiting, or diarrhea. He had no fevers. He did have constipation, and his last bowel movement was 5 days prior to presentation. His parents had been giving him Miralax twice daily for the previous 3 days, without any noticeable effect. At the outside hospital emergency department, a CT scan of the abdomen and pelvis was obtained, which was read as "a large stool burden...and a normal appendix." He was transferred for a bowel clean out.

PAST MEDICAL HISTORY

- Strabismus surgery at 2 years of age
- Chronic constipation

Medications

Miralax PRN

Family/Social History

Mother and paternal grandmother had hypothyroidism. Mother also had a deep vein thrombosis with pulmonary embolism after a long car ride. Maternal aunt had a deep vein thrombosis following immobilization after surgery.

EXAMINATION

- Vitals: T 36.3, HR 123, RR 24, BP 130/85, SpO$_2$ 96%, BMI 26 (98th percentile for age)
- General: Alert, well-appearing, no distress
- Abdomen: Soft, nondistended, markedly tender to palpation in the right upper and lower quadrants with voluntary guarding, no rebound tenderness, no palpable masses, bowel sounds present and normoactive

DIAGNOSTIC CONSIDERATIONS

- Constipation
- Appendicitis
- Mesenteric lymphadenitis

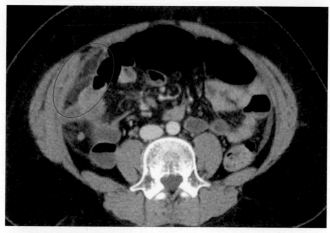

FIGURE 67.1 Axial abdominal CT scan.

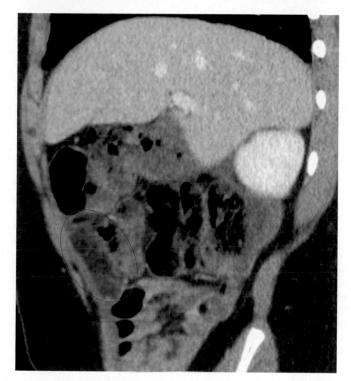

FIGURE 67.2 Coronal abdominal CT scan.

Investigation

- Laboratory workup: CBC, CMP, thyroid studies
- Consider repeat CT scan of abdomen and pelvis

Results

The laboratory workup was largely unremarkable, other than a slightly elevated white blood cell count of 13.8 k/mm³. However, the abdominal CT scan from the other institution was reviewed and showed an omental infarction (Figures 67.1 and 67.2).

DIAGNOSIS

Omental infarction

Treatment/Follow-up

The omental infarction was managed with acetaminophen and ketorolac. The patient's pain resolved by day 2 of hospitalization, and he was discharged home. A thrombophilia workup was performed given the presence of the omental infarction with a family history of deep vein thromboses, but it did not reveal an underlying predisposition to clotting. The patient and his family were counseled on making healthy choices regarding diet and exercise.

TEACHING POINTS

Omental infarction is a rare cause of acute abdominal pain in children, best known for being a sneaky mimicker of appendicitis. The precise pathogenesis of this condition is unknown, but in 90% of cases, the infarction involves the right epiploic vessels. The most well-established risk factor for omental infarction is obesity, specifically an increased amount of fat on the omentum. Infarction also tends to occur more frequently in males than females and more often in adults than children.

The typical presentation of omental infarction is 2 to 3 days of acute right lower quadrant abdominal pain. Additional gastrointestinal symptoms such as nausea, vomiting, anorexia, or diarrhea are present in anywhere from one-quarter to one-third of patients. Only a minority of patients present with peritoneal signs or fever.

Omental infarction can be diagnosed on imaging, but being such a rare diagnosis, it is frequently missed. Ultrasound shows an echogenic mass in the omental fat, and CT scan shows a triangular or oval-shaped heterogeneous mass, sometimes with surrounding inflammatory changes such as fat stranding. The diagnosis can also be made during surgery, with gross findings of infarction that are subsequently confirmed on histopathology.

In previous decades, surgical resection was performed on almost every case of known omental infarction. Additionally, many cases of omental infarction were not diagnosed until the patient was brought to the operating room for suspected appendicitis—only to find an infarcted omentum instead of an inflamed appendix. In those cases, patients typically underwent an appendectomy anyway, as well as surgical resection of the affected omentum. Currently, however, nonsurgical management is preferred. In a recent review of 10 patients with omental infarction, three patients went immediately to laparoscopy because there were signs of peritonitis, three patients were started on pain management alone but proceeded to surgery after persistent pain (lasting an average of 3 days), and four patients were successfully managed with nonsurgical measures, that is, analgesics plus antibiotics for abscess prophylaxis. All four of the latter patients had resolution of their symptoms and were discharged on day 4 of their hospital stay.

There is speculation that this rare diagnosis will become more common as obesity in children rises. Therefore, omental infarction should remain an important diagnostic consideration in pediatric patients presenting with acute abdominal pain. Constipation rarely, if ever, is a cause of severe abdominal pain, and the finding of a large stool burden is often a red herring.

Suggested Readings

Helmrath MA, Dorfman SR, Minifee PK, Bloss RS, Brandt ML, DeBakey ME. Right lower quadrant pain in children caused by omental infarction. *Am J Surg*. 2001;182(6):729-732.

Loh MH, Chan Chui H, Yap T-L, et al. Omental infarction—a mimicker of acute appendicitis in children. *J Pediatr Surg*. 2005;40(8):1224-1226.

Nubi A, McBride W, Stringel G. Primary omental infarct: conservative vs operative management in the era of ultrasound, computerized tomography, and laparoscopy. *J Pediatr Surg*. 2009;44(5):953-956.

Rimon A, Daneman A, Gerstle JT, et al. Omental infarction in children. *J Pediatr*. 2009;155(3):427-431.e1.

68

I Heard GERD

Julianne Ivy

CHIEF COMPLAINT

"Choking"

HISTORY OF PRESENT ILLNESS

A 5-month-old full-term infant presented to the emergency department with chronic choking episodes related to feeding, which have been occurring since birth. At 1 month of age, she was admitted to another hospital for bronchiolitis, and at that time, her mom was told that the choking was likely due to the infant's infection. However, the feeding intolerance continued to worsen steadily despite resolution of the viral infection. She now takes 3 to 4 oz every 2 hours while awake and has choking episodes with every few feeds. She sometimes chokes on her own saliva. One or two times a week, the choking episodes are severe enough that she turns purple.

Initially, she was exclusively breastfed, but around 3 months of age, her mom transitioned her to formula, thinking that the choking could be related to breastfeeding. Several different formulas have been tried without improvement. Most recently, she switched to an organic goat milk formula, which the baby seemed to tolerate slightly better. Mom has also tried a variety of bottles and nipples, with slightly more success with a preemie slow-flow nipple. Additionally, her mom experimented with different feeding positions, with only mild improvement noted in a semi–side-lying position.

PAST MEDICAL HISTORY

She was born full term following an uncomplicated pregnancy and delivery. She was briefly hospitalized at 1 month of age for bronchiolitis. She has been tracking along her growth curve. She has been meeting all of her developmental milestones appropriately.

Medications

Simethicone drops PRN

Family/Social History

Mother has celiac disease.

She lives with her father, who is in the military, and her mother, who is a stay-at-home mom. She does not attend daycare.

EXAMINATION

- Vitals: T 36.1, HR 140, RR 38, BP 92/74, SpO_2 100%
- Growth chart: Weight: 7.65 kg, 73rd percentile; length: 66 cm, 76th percentile; OFC: 43 cm, 69th percentile
- General: Well-appearing, well-nourished, nondysmorphic
- Head: Normocephalic, atraumatic, anterior fontanelle soft and flat
- Throat: Strong suck, no tongue-tie, bifid uvula, intact hard palate, 2+ nonobstructing tonsils

- Neck: Supple, no adenopathy, no palpable masses
- Respiratory: Breathing comfortably on room air, no stridor or wheezing
- Cardiovascular: Normal rate and regular rhythm, normal S1 and S2, no murmurs, peripheral pulses 2+ and equal bilaterally, no cyanosis
- Neuro: Appropriately interactive for age, good tone in upper and lower extremities

DIAGNOSTIC CONSIDERATIONS

- Infantile regurgitation, physiologic
- Gastroesophageal reflux disease (the term mom heard the most)
- Overfeeding
- Recurrent viral upper respiratory infection
- Laryngomalacia
- Laryngeal cleft
- Tracheoesophageal fistula
- Neuromuscular disorder

Investigation

- Respiratory viral multiplex swab
- Observation of patient's feeds
- Swallow study
- Laryngoscopy and bronchoscopy

Results

The patient's respiratory viral multiplex swab was negative. During admission, several different care providers witnessed the patient choking during feeds, sometimes with associated cyanosis. A barium swallow study was performed, which showed (1) a coordinated oral phase with organized suck and integrated oral motor reflexes and (2) aspiration and laryngeal penetration with thin and thick liquids. Subsequent laryngoscopy and bronchoscopy was notable for a deep interarytenoid groove at the level of the posterior commissure, that is, a type 1 laryngeal cleft.

DIAGNOSIS

Type 1 laryngeal cleft

Treatment/Follow-up

During the laryngoscopy, injection augmentation of the interarytenoid groove was performed. This involved injecting a filler material around the site of the cleft in order to close up the space connecting the larynx and esophagus. The patient was also placed on a thickened formula diet to help prevent aspiration until the full efficacy of the procedure could be assessed a few weeks later. She was discharged home with plans for a follow-up barium swallow study in a month.

TEACHING POINTS

A laryngeal cleft is an abnormal passageway between the larynx/trachea and the esophagus. This rare congenital malformation appears to occur when, in embryologic development, the septum that should form between the trachea and the esophagus does not fully close up, leaving an opening between these two tubes at their proximal ends. Most proximally, this also includes a failure of the cricoid lamina to fuse. The consequence is that food can pass from the upper esophagus into the airway.

These malformations are typically divided into four types. Type 1 refers to those clefts that are exclusively located above the vocal cords, while types 2 to 4 are characterized by progressive extension of the cleft into the esophagus and trachea. Severe type 4 clefts may extend as far as the carina.

The estimated incidence of laryngeal clefts is 1 in 10,000 to 20,000 live births. However, the true incidence is almost certainly higher because many mild cases go undiagnosed. In one study, the oldest patient with this congenital malformation was not diagnosed until 12 years of age.

Laryngeal clefts typically present with nonspecific feeding or respiratory symptoms, such as choking or cyanotic episodes during feeds, stridor, chronic cough, or recurrent pneumonia.

Initial management for type 1 laryngeal cleft patients mainly involves using thickened formulas, modified feeding positions, and high dose anti-reflux medication. In one retrospective study, 36% of patients were successfully treated with these measures alone; in another, it was 31%. For type 1 patients who fail these initial measures or any patient with a type 2 to 4 cleft, surgical repair is the next step.

Success rates after surgery are variable, and it often takes a few weeks to months for the full effect of surgery to be realized. In one study, at 12 months postoperation, 44% of type 1 patients no longer aspirated at all on swallow study, 33% had partial improvement in aspiration, and 22% continued to aspirate with all liquid consistencies. Interestingly, all of the latter patients underwent a repeat endoscopy that showed that their laryngeal cleft was successfully healed. These results underscore a major frustration in treating laryngeal clefts; up to half of patients have additional comorbidities that cause similar symptoms, such as laryngomalacia or tracheomalacia, tracheoesophageal fistulas, gastroesophageal reflux disorder, and neurodevelopmental disorders. Even when the cleft is treated, feeding intolerance may persist. For both families and caregivers, this can be a difficult prognosis to swallow.

Suggested Readings

Leboulanger N, Garabédian E-N. Laryngo-tracheo-oesophageal clefts. *Orphanet J Rare Dis.* 2011;6(1):81.

Ojha S, Ashland JE, Hersh C, et al. Type 1 laryngeal cleft: a multidimensional management algorithm. *JAMA Otolaryngol Head Neck Surg.* 2014;140(1):34-40.

Rahbar R, Rouillon I, Roger G, et al. The presentation and management of laryngeal cleft: a 10-year experience. *Arch Otolaryngol Head Neck Surg.* 2006;132(12):1335-1341.

Strychowsky JE, Dodrill P, Moritz E, Perez J, Rahbar R. Swallowing dysfunction among patients with laryngeal cleft: more than just aspiration? *Int J Pediatr Otorhinolaryngol.* 2016;82:38-42.

69

July 1st Disease

Patrick J. Reich

CHIEF COMPLAINT

"Bad summer cold"

HISTORY OF PRESENT ILLNESS

Five days prior to presentation, a 15-month-old boy had fever in the morning to 102 °F and was given ibuprofen every 6 hours. A bad runny nose and draining, red eyes were also present. The parents were unable to keep neither his eyes nor his nose clear from discharge. These symptoms worsened for the next 2 days, and he then developed a cough and started breathing fast.

Three days prior, he was taken to the emergency department (ED) where he was diagnosed with an upper respiratory tract infection and sent home. He saw his pediatrician the next day and was diagnosed with otitis media and started on antibiotics.

Two days prior, a small red rash was noticed on his cheek near his eye. The fevers, cough, and conjunctivitis continued. Over the next 24 hours, the rash spread.

On the day of admission, the rash now included most of his body and had progressed from the head to toe.

Review of systems:

- Positive: Fever, cough, tachypnea, red eyes, rash, decreased appetite, malaise, irritability, dry diapers, and cracked lips.
- Negative: Diarrhea, vomiting, seizures, puffy hands, and peeling skin.
- Labs: A nasopharyngeal swab for viruses was negative. WBC 6.2, hemoglobin 10.5, and platelets 218, with 7% bands, 69% neutrophils, and 19% lymphocytes.

PAST MEDICAL HISTORY

- Human metapneumovirus infection, 4 months ago.
- Otitis media × 3.
- Immunizations are up to date and include recent Varivax and MMR, given 10 days ago.

Medications

Amoxicillin

Family/Social History

The family returned 14 days ago from Turkey. All family members and recent travelers are symptom free.

EXAMINATION

He is febrile to nearly 40°, tachycardic to the 170s, tachypneic, and hypoxic to the mid 80s on room air. He is extremely fussy and irritable and difficult to console. He has exudative conjunctivitis. His nares demonstrate copious dried rhinorrhea. His oral mucosa is dry and his lips are cracked. Inspection inside of his mouth does not demonstrate any lesions or spots. The left tympanic membrane is bulging and distorted. There are no murmurs. His lungs are without wheezes and breath sounds are diffusely coarse, with fair air movement and with some mild accessory muscle use. His abdominal examination is benign. His genitourinary examination is normal. His musculoskeletal examination is normal. Skin has a diffuse, blanching, erythematous, papular rash with coalescing lesions on his scalp, face, and trunk. His neurologic examination, aside from his fussiness and irritability, is normal. He is moving all extremities well and has good tone.

DIAGNOSTIC CONSIDERATIONS

Based on symptoms (cough, coryza, conjunctivitis), descending rash, and recent travel, the intern considered measles a likely diagnosis.

Investigation

- Negative-pressure isolation room.
- Measles IgM and IgG, urine viral culture, measles FA, and repeat nasopharyngeal swab.
- Vitamin A, 200,000 IU daily for 2 days, to limit the risk of blindness and other neurological complications; a second dose should be given in 28 days.
- Ophthalmologic evaluation to assess for ocular complications from measles.
- Report case to the city health department and also to the infection prevention team (concerned with preventing infection spread to other patients) and occupational health team (concerned with preventing spread to workers and staff).
- Contacts from his prior ED visit, as well as the contacts in his pediatrician's office, need to be tracked down and assessed.

DIAGNOSIS

The **measles** testing returned positive.

TEACHING POINTS

Measles (aka rubeola, aka first disease) is the first of the childhood exanthems and has been recognized for centuries, but due to successful vaccination programs, it has been in dramatic decline. Prior to the release of the vaccine in 1963, there were approximately 500,000 cases each year in the United States, but this number decreased to only a handful of cases. Recently, however, there has been an increase in both the number of cases and the number of outbreaks, stemming from decreasing vaccination rates. During 2011, a total of 222 measles cases (incidence rate: 0.7 per one million population) and 17 measles outbreaks (defined as three or more cases linked in time or place) were reported to CDC, compared with a median of 60 (range: 37-140) cases and four (range: 2-10) outbreaks reported annually during 2001 to 2010. (Compare this to the number of cases of ehrlichiosis reported to the CDC in 2000, which was 200.)

Many cases of measles in the United States are "imported," picked up from exposure in endemic areas while traveling, but these index cases are then spread locally in outbreaks to other unimmunized individuals.

From the CDC website, http://www.cdc.gov/measles, "Even in previously healthy children, measles can be a serious illness requiring hospitalization. As many as 1 out of every 20 children with measles gets pneumonia, and about 1 child in every 1000 who get measles will develop encephalitis. (This is an inflammation of the brain that can lead to convulsions, and can leave the child deaf or with cognitive deficits.) For every 1000 children who get measles, 1 or 2 will die from it. Measles may cause a pregnant woman to have a miscarriage, give birth prematurely, or have a low-birth-weight baby. In developing countries, where malnutrition and vitamin A deficiency are common, measles has been known to kill as many as one out of four people. It is the leading cause of blindness among African children. Measles (*still*) kills almost 1 million children in the world each year."

Suggested Readings

Centers for Disease Control and Prevention. *Measles (Rubeola)*. 2020. http://www.cdc.gov/measles.
Moss WJ. Measles. *Lancet*. 2017;390(10111):2490-2502.
Paules CI, Marston HD, Fauci AS. Measles in 2019—Going backward. *N Engl J Med*. 2019;380(23):2185-2187.

70

The Eyes Have It

Andrew J. White

CHIEF COMPLAINT

Nausea and yellow eyes

HISTORY OF PRESENT ILLNESS

For the past 3 weeks, a 16-year-old girl has been nauseous, which gets better with eating. However, she has had less and less of an appetite and is becoming increasingly fatigued. Five days ago, she had nonbloody, nonbilious vomiting, which improved her nausea. The day prior to admission, she noticed her eyes turning yellow. Her urine was tea colored. The Monospot was negative. Hepatitis A, B, and C titers were negative. A friend of hers from school has been vomiting and has had some diarrhea.

Review of systems:

- Positive for yellow nail beds for about 2 weeks and dark urine.
- Denies fever, diarrhea, change in stool color, dysuria, SOB, or chest pain.

PAST MEDICAL HISTORY

- Mono in 2005
- No history of jaundice

Medications

- Mononessa (estradiol and norgestimate OCP)

Family/Social History

Family history:

- Mother with factor V Leiden and protein S deficiency
- Maternal grandmother underwent s/p cholecystectomy

Social history:

- Junior in high school
- No drugs, alcohol, cigarettes, or sexual activity

EXAMINATION

- Vitals: Weight 64 kg, height 170 cm, T 37.9, P 84, RR 20, BP 128/62, saturation 99% room air.
- General: Comfortable and in no acute distress.
- Eyes: Scleral icterus.
- Head: Normocephalic, atraumatic.
- Throat: No erythema, exudate, or lesions.
- Neck: Supple, no lymphadenopathy, thyroid not enlarged.
- Lungs: Clear to auscultation bilaterally, no wheezes or consolidations.
- Heart: RRR and no murmurs, rubs, or gallops.

- Abdomen: Soft, nontender, no hepatosplenomegaly.
- Extremities: No clubbing, cyanosis, or edema.
- Skin: Diffusely jaundiced. No spider angiomata.
- Neuro: Alert, answering questions appropriately. No abnormal movements or tone. 2+ reflexes, 5/5 strength.

DIAGNOSTIC CONSIDERATIONS

- Hemolytic disease with a viral or autoimmune hepatitis
- Gilbert syndrome
- OCP side effect
- Acetaminophen overdose
- Gallstones
- Wilson disease

Investigation and Results

- **Hb 9.2 g/dL**, WBCs 22.3, platelets 168. **AST 178 U/mL, ALT 34 U/mL**, alk phos 22 **IU/L** (low), **total bili 17.6 mg/dL, direct bili 9, PT 17.0** (slightly elevated), **INR 1.45**, albumin 3.3, acetaminophen level <5. Direct and indirect **Coombs negative**.

    The following day, laboratory tests were repeated:

- **Hb 5.6 g/dL**, direct bili **14 mg/dL**

    A repeat examination of the eyes was performed, acknowledging the apparent scleral icterus, but looking at the peripheral edges of the iris (Figure 70.1).

DIAGNOSIS

Hepatolenticular degeneration (Wilson disease)

Treatment/Follow-up

- Diagnostic labs: Urine copper 11,694 µg/L (normal 15-60), serum copper 1.66 µg/mL (normal 0.75-1.45), ceruloplasmin 10.5 (low).

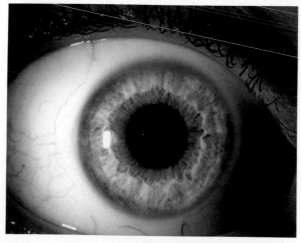

FIGURE 70.1 A repeat examination of the eyes revealed the presence of a Kayser-Fleischer ring, the brownish indistinct ring in the peripheral iris.

TEACHING POINTS

Wilson disease is an autosomal recessive disorder that affects copper metabolism. A defect in the ATP7B copper-transporting gene, located on the long arm of chromosome 13, leads to excessive copper deposition in the liver. One in 90 people in the United States carry one defective gene, and the incidence of Wilson disease is 1 in 30,000 to 40,000. Over 500 different mutations of the gene have been reported, and many individuals are compound heterozygotes. Therefore, presentation of Wilson disease can take many distinct forms.

In healthy individuals, ATPase 2 (encoded by ATP7B) serves two functions. First, in the hepatocyte's Golgi apparatus, it loads copper onto ceruloplasmin for transportation to other organs. Second, if the liver copper load is high, the ATPase 2 transports copper into vesicles for secretion in the bile. If copper accumulates in the liver and cannot be released into the bile, it eventually reaches cytotoxic levels and is released into the blood stream where it travels to other organs.

Most patients with Wilson disease present with hepatic, neurologic, and/or psychiatric symptoms. In the first 2 decades of life, children typically present with hepatic manifestations. These can range from incidentally found abnormal laboratory values to fulminant hepatic failure, as was the case in this patient. If the patient does present with liver failure, then Coombs negative hemolytic anemia is a well-described finding. The exact etiology of the anemia is unclear, but it is thought to be due to oxidative injury to erythrocytes from excess copper release from hepatocytes.

Kayser-Fleischer rings, low ceruloplasmin, and neurologic changes suggest a diagnosis of Wilson disease, but the gold standard is liver biopsy with quantitative copper level. Without intervention, Wilson disease is almost uniformly fatal. Treatment is chelation therapy. Penicillamine is the first-line choice for chelation therapy. It works by binding copper, gold, mercury, and arsenic and excreting them in the urine. Patients must also be started on zinc. Zinc binds to the same transporters as copper in the gastrointestinal tract and helps decrease the absorption of copper. Both medications are lifelong. Side effects of penicillamine include worsening neurologic symptoms, diarrhea, rash, thrombocytopenia, and leukopenia. Up to 30% of patients with Wilson disease are unable to tolerate the side effects and are switched to trientine, another copper-chelating agent.

Suggested Readings

Gilroy R. Wilson Disease. 2013. emedicine.medscape.com
Houchens N, Dhaliwal G, Askari F, Kim B, Saint S. Clinical problem-solving: the essential element. *N Engl J Med*. 2013;368:1345-1351.
Schilsky ML. Wilson disease: diagnosis, treatment, and follow-up. *Clin Liver Dis*. 2017;21(4):755-767.
Weiss K. Zinc monotherapy is not as effective as chelating agents in treatment of Wilson disease. *Gastroenterology*. 2011;140(4):1189.e1-1198.e1.

71

Out of Shape

Itay Marmor

CHIEF COMPLAINT

Cough and shortness of breath on exertion

HISTORY OF PRESENT ILLNESS

An 11-year-old African American boy with morbid obesity presented for evaluation of 6 months of shortness of breath with exertion. He said he knew that he was "out of shape." He also had a cough and some occasional night sweats, but no fevers, weight loss, joint pain, weakness, rash, ulcers, dry mouth or eyes, or any other symptom. He did not have any serious infections in childhood, and there is no family history of an immunodeficiency.

Prior outside workup included chest x-rays that showed bilateral patchy opacities and atelectasis. A chest CT scan showed multifocal bilateral airspace and ground-glass opacities with small nodules, as well as bilateral mediastinal and hilar lymphadenopathy. Bronchoscopy showed slight edema of his epiglottis, arytenoids, and vocal cord, and marked edema of the subglottis and trachea, increased vascularization, and severe inflammation and secretions, consistent with diffuse bronchitis. Infectious workup (including a BAL) was negative for viral, bacterial, fungal, and mycobacterial infections. Rheumatologic evaluation included an elevation of inflammatory markers (ESR, CRP, leukocytosis, thrombocytosis), a positive ANA at a dilution of 1:160, negative ENA, negative ANCA, normal ACE, elevated IgG (2234 IU/mL) and IgE (555), normal IgM and IgA, normal T-cell counts, and elevated B-cell count (CD19 1371).

He was treated with several courses of empiric antimicrobials, including an antifungal for 6 weeks (itraconazole), with no improvement. His symptoms were not responsive to a beta-agonist inhaler.

PAST MEDICAL HISTORY

- Morbid obesity (BMI 40)
- Eczema

Medications

None

Family/Social History

- Asthma—Brother, mother
- Obesity—Brother, mother

EXAMINATION

- Vitals: BP 110/64, HR 82, T 36 °C (96.8 °F), RR 18, Spo$_2$ 96% (on room air).
- General: No acute distress, no labored breathing while resting, but quickly becomes dyspneic after walking in the room.
- HEENT: Pupils equal, round, reactive to light, no synechiae, extraocular movements intact, oropharynx without erythema, mucous membranes moist.

- Lymph: No lymphadenopathy.
- Lungs: Decreased bilateral breath sounds.
- Cardiac: There are no murmurs, rubs, or gallops audible.
- Abdomen: Normal bowel sounds, soft, nondistended, no mass, no organomegaly.
- Skin: No rash or discoloration, normal turgor, no nailfold telangiectases, no nail pits or ridging, no digital ulcerations, normal capillary refill, and no sclerodactyly.
- Neuro: CN II to XII grossly intact, 5/5 UE and LE strength.
- Musculoskeletal: Full range of motion of all joints without tenderness, erythema, warmth, or effusion.

DIAGNOSTIC CONSIDERATIONS

Given the presentation of a chronic lung disease, chest CT findings of ground-glass opacities and bilateral hilar lymphadenopathy, a completely negative infectious workup (including a negative BAL), and no response to antimicrobials, several conditions were considered: sarcoidosis, inflammatory myositis–associated lung disease, small-vessel vasculitis, systemic lupus erythematosus, chronic granulomatous disease, common variable immunodeficiency, tuberculosis (TB), and histoplasmosis.

Investigation

- Lab workup
- Pulmonary function tests
- Chest CT
- Ultrasound-guided transbronchial biopsy of the lung (EBUS)

Results

- **Labs**: ESR 49, CRP 5.2 mg/L, WBC 9.8, platelets 611K, Hb 12.6. Normal CMP, CK, aldolase, LDH, C3, C4, CH50, IgG 1675, IgE 418, normal IgM, IgA, vitamin D-25-OH and 1,25-di-OH, ACE level, vaccine titers, DHR, UA, negative histoplasmosis, and TB.
- **PFTs**: Mixed restrictive and obstructive lung disease with air trapping.
- **Chest CT**: Extensive multifocal, predominantly lower lobe consolidations with ground-glass and peribronchovascular opacities and mediastinal and hilar lymphadenopathy.
- **Lung biopsy**: Noncaseating granulomas. Negative bacterial, fungal, and mycobacterial cultures.

DIAGNOSIS

Sarcoidosis

Treatment/Follow-up

- Oral steroids
- Anti-TNF: adalimumab
- Methotrexate

TEACHING POINTS

Pediatric-onset "adult-type" sarcoidosis is usually characterized by systemic manifestations (fever, malaise, weight loss) and pulmonary disease, associated with bilateral hilar adenopathy. Other manifestations may include liver involvement, splenomegaly, peripheral lymphadenopathy, skin lesions (eg, erythema nodosum), uveitis, and central nervous system involvement (neurosarcoid). Screening labs include ACE, vitamin D, and calcium, but these are neither sensitive nor specific. When suspected, the diagnosis is established with a transbronchial lymph node and lung tissue biopsy, showing evidence of noncaseating granulomas. Open lung biopsy is often necessary to identify the granulomata.

Early-onset sarcoidosis, often called Blau syndrome, presents usually before the age of ₅ years and typically with a granulomatous dermatitis. Other symptoms include arthritis and uveitis, but not pulmonary disease. Both early-onset and familial sarcoidosis are due to mutations in the NOD2 gene and were clinically described by James P. Keating in 1973, a decade earlier than Blau's description in 1985.

Suggested Readings

Blau EB. Familial granulomatous arthritis, iritis and rash. *J Pediatr*. 1985;107:689-693.

Chiu B, Chan J, Das S, Alshamma Z, Sergi C. Pediatric sarcoidosis: a review with emphasis on early onset and high-risk sarcoidosis and diagnostic challenges. *Diagnostics (Basel)*. 2019;9(4):160.

Keating JP, Weissbluth M, Ratzan SK, Barton LL. Familial sarcoidosis. *Am J Dis Child*. 1973;126(5): 644-647. PMID: 4745156.

Pattishall EN, Kendig EL Jr. Sarcoidosis in children. *Pediatr Pulmonol*. 1996;22(3):195-203.

Petty R, Laxer R, Lindsley C, Wedderburn L. *Textbook of Pediatric Rheumatology*. 7th ed. Elsevier Saunders; 2015.

72 Routine

Andrew J. White

CHIEF COMPLAINT

Her sats are low.

HISTORY OF PRESENT ILLNESS

A 10-year-old girl was sent to the emergency room from radiology, where she was scheduled for an elective magnetic resonance imaging (MRI) to evaluate a hemangioma on her neck. However, during the presedation evaluation, her O_2 sats were 85% and her lips appeared blue. She had no recent upper respiratory infection symptoms, nor fever, but does say that she has always had episodes of blue lips when she gets cold or agitated. She thinks she has less exercise tolerance compared to her classmates. She takes no medications.

PAST MEDICAL HISTORY

- She was a 33-week premature infant but was not given a diagnosis of chronic lung disease.
- Pneumonia, 2 years ago. Chest radiograph raised the possibility of tuberculosis or granulomatous disease, but the PPD was negative.
- Hemangioma, lateral neck. Originally thought to be a reactive lymph node, an ultrasound performed 1 month ago demonstrated a 2 × 2 cm hypervascular mass consistent with a hemangioma. The MRI scheduled for today was to further characterize this hemangioma.

Family/Social History

Family history: Sister with Wolff-Parkinson-White syndrome, and another sister with Chiari malformation. Father is deceased from melanoma.

Social history: There is an old furnace at home, but no carbon monoxide monitor.

EXAMINATION

- Vitals: HR 96, RR 22, T 36.6, BP 100/68, Spo$_2$ 84%.
- General appearance: Comfortable, but anxious and tearful.
- Skin: Skin warm and dry, no rash, and capillary refill <2 seconds.
- HEENT:
  - Head: Normocephalic, atraumatic.
  - Eyes: Conjunctiva clear, no drainage or injection. No scleral icterus.
  - Left ear: No preauricular pits, normal auricle, clear and intact TM, patent EAC.
  - Right ear: No preauricular pits, normal auricle, clear and intact TM, patent EAC.
  - Nasal examination:
    - The nasal bridge was straight without deformity.
    - The nasal cavity showed no drainage and no masses and was patent.
    - The septum was midline and intact.
  - Oral cavity/oropharynx:
    - The palate was intact, and the uvula was normal.
    - The tonsils were 2+ and nonobstructing.

- Neck examination: 2.5 cm mobile/soft mass anterior to the SCM (level II). Nontender to palpation without overlying skin changes. Auscultation revealed a bruit over the lesion.
- Pulmonary: Clear with no wheezing, rales, or rhonchi; no use of accessory muscles and no retractions.
- Cardiovascular: Regular rate and rhythm; no murmurs, rubs, or gallops; normal S1 and S2; 2+ distal pulses.
- Abdomen: Soft, nondistended, nontender, no hepatosplenomegaly, no masses palpated.
- Back: Spine straight with no deformities.
- Extremities: No clubbing, cyanosis, or edema.
- Neurologic: Mental status: Awake, alert, and answers questions appropriately for age.
- Cranial nerves: PERRL, EOMI, face symmetric, and tongue midline.
- Motor: Moves all four extremities.

DIAGNOSTIC CONSIDERATIONS

- Hypoxemia
- Mass in neck, presumed hemangioma
- Granulomatous disease, pulmonary, presumed histoplasmosis

Diagnostic considerations in the emergency department: "Given patient's hypoxemia of unclear etiology we considered diagnoses such as methemoglobinemia, CO poisoning, pulmonary fibrosis, intracardiac shunt, or pulmonary hypertension. Pulmonary sequestration, or an intrapulmonary inflammatory process such as healed granulomatous nodules, sarcoidosis, histoplasmosis, or tuberculosis."

Investigation

- 15 L O_2 NRB and then placed on 10 L high-flow nasal cannula.
- CBC and electrolytes were unremarkable. The methemoglobin level was normal.
- A respiratory viral multiplex swab was negative.
- Exclude TB: PPD, IGRA-TB, AFB.
- CXR.

Results

Chest x-ray (Figure 72.1): Diffuse miliary pulmonary nodules with questionable mediastinal lymph nodes are favored to represent a granulomatous process like sarcoidosis. A healed granulomatous infection is another consideration. Chest CT is recommended.

CT (Figure 72.2) read: There are innumerable tiny nodules scattered throughout the lungs with a miliary pattern. This appears to have progressed since the radiograph of 2015. There is no confluent airspace consolidation. There is no pleural effusion or pneumothorax. The heart size is normal. There is mild widening of the right paratracheal stripe and mild fullness of the left hilum, which may be a reflection of lymphadenopathy.

Impression: Diffuse miliary pulmonary nodules with questionable mediastinal lymph nodes are favored to represent a granulomatous process like sarcoidosis.

The unusual appearance of the lung parenchyma and lack of explanation, but consideration of sarcoidosis, led to the diagnostic procedure: an open lung biopsy.

Figure 72.3 is a photo of the surface of the lung showing numerous vascular appearing macules, which were biopsied.

Revised/Additional Diagnostic Considerations

- Sarcoidosis
- Hemorrhagic hereditary telangiectasia
- Vasculitis (eg, granulomatosis with polyangiitis)

DIAGNOSIS

Pathology from the lung biopsy provided the correct final diagnosis: **thyroid carcinoma, papillary.**

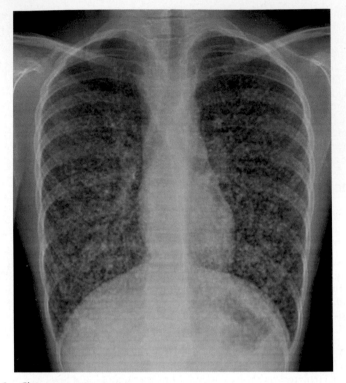

FIGURE 72.1   Chest x-ray.

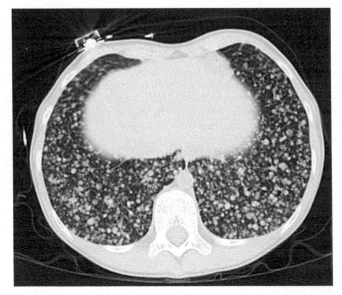

FIGURE 72.2   Chest CT scan.

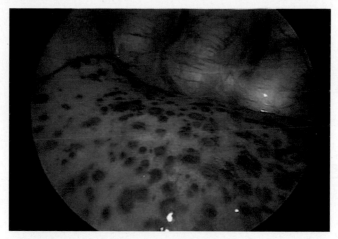

FIGURE 72.3 A photo of the surface of the lung showing numerous vascular appearing macules, which were biopsied.

Treatment/Follow-up

1. Resection of neck mass and thyroid gland, with neck dissection
2. I-131 (radioactive iodine)

TEACHING POINTS

Papillary thyroid carcinoma is the most common form of thyroid cancer, typically affecting middle-aged women. It is quick to spread to the neck lymph nodes and may metastasize to the lungs or bone. The cure rate is excellent with radioactive iodine, depending on how avidly the tumor cells take up iodine. It appears to be increasing in incidence in the United States, but the cause is unknown. The delay in diagnosis is not unusual.

Prognosis is generally favorable. The father's history of melanoma raises the possibility of a familial predisposition to malignancy.

Suggested Readings

Ho WL, Zacharin MR. Thyroid carcinoma in children, adolescents and adults, both spontaneous and after childhood radiation exposure. *Eur J Pediatr*. 2016;175(5):677-683.

Ozkan E, Soydal C, Araz M, Kucuk NO. Differentiated thyroid carcinomas in childhood: clinicopathologic results of 26 patients. *J Pediatr Endocrinol Metab*. 2011;24(9-10):739-742.

Spinelli C, Strambi S, Rossi L, et al. Surgical management of papillary thyroid carcinoma in childhood and adolescence: an Italian multicenter study on 250 patients. *J Endocrinol Invest*. 2016;39(9):1055-1059.

73

It's All in Your Head

Amanda Reis Dube, Jennifer Martens Dunn

CHIEF COMPLAINT

Vomiting and weight loss

HISTORY OF PRESENT ILLNESS

A 10-year-old girl presents to the emergency unit with 4 days of vomiting and 7 months of decreased appetite. She does not have abdominal pain but says that she feels full all the time. She has lost 15 lb in the last year. Speaking to the patient alone, she is tearful but denies thoughts of depression or wanting to hurt herself. She states that she eats three meals a day but has tried to become a vegetarian since losing her appetite. Parents do not think she is eating all three meals and that she has always been a picky eater, but recently, she has been refusing to eat foods that she used to love. They think that she worries a lot and sometimes has trouble falling asleep at night. She denies recent fevers, headaches, cough, rhinorrhea, or sore throat.

PAST MEDICAL HISTORY

- Intermittent constipation
- Up-to-date on vaccinations

Medications

None

Family/Social History

- Paternal grandfather with colon cancer and thyroid disease
- No family history of celiac disease or inflammatory bowel disease

EXAMINATION

- Vitals: T 98.3, HR 106, RR 20, BP 100/65, SpO$_2$ 99%, Wt 32.5 kg (71 lb; 46th percentile), Ht 146 cm (4′9″; 87th percentile), BMI 15.4 (22nd percentile)
- Gen: Thin girl in no acute distress, lying on bed, quiet but responsive to questions
- HEENT: Mucous membranes moist, no rhinorrhea
- Neck: Supple with no lymphadenopathy
- CV: RRR; no murmurs, gallops, or rubs
- Lungs: Clear with no retractions or tachypnea
- Abd: Normoactive bowel sounds, soft, nontender, nondistended, no masses or hepatosplenomegaly
- Ext: Warm, well-perfused, moves all extremities equally
- Neuro: PERRL, EOMI, alert and appropriately answers questions, face symmetric, balance normal

DIAGNOSTIC CONSIDERATIONS

Initially, the diagnostic considerations included constipation and anorexia nervosa.

Investigation

She was discharged from her initial emergency department visit with ondansetron of 4 mg TID PRN and Miralax 1 tsp per day. She followed up with her primary care physician (PCP) who documented continued episodes of vomiting, often in the mornings but sometimes in the afternoons. Thyroid studies, electrolytes, and urinalysis were normal. She continued to feel anxious with trouble falling asleep and had trouble ingesting enough Miralax to help with her constipation. Her physical examination remained unremarkable aside from low BMI. She was specifically noted to have clear sharp disks on fundoscopic examination, confirmed by two medical doctors at her PCP office. Head imaging was discussed but deferred. She was prescribed antacids and PediaSure and was referred to a counselor and gastroenterologist.

She was evaluated by GI and underwent an upper endoscopy with biopsy, upper GI with small bowel follow through, abdominal ultrasound, and celiac screen, all of which were normal. She also met with a counselor and followed up with a nurse practitioner at her PCP office, who referred her to an eating disorder treatment facility. After undergoing evaluation there, it was recommended that she enter the inpatient program. Her parents instead opted for outpatient treatment. She was started on mirtazapine, which initially increased her appetite, but the effect was not sustained. She completed the intensive outpatient program. However, she had lost another 10 lb. She went to see her PCP with a new complaint of 2 days bilateral throbbing headaches in addition to continued appetite loss and vomiting generally in the mornings. The PCP arranged for her to be directly admitted to the hospital. On admission, her BMI was 13.9, and her examination was notable for some truncal ataxia with positive Romberg sign.

That night, frequent neuro checks were ordered and performed. At 4 AM, her mental status was normal, but by 5:45, she was not responsive to commands with sluggish pupils and an R lateral gaze palsy. She was transferred to the pediatric intensive care unit (PICU) and a STAT head computed tomography (CT) was performed.

Results

Head CT showed a large posterior fossa mass with obstructive hydrocephalus, transependymal flow, and edema. Magnetic resonance imaging showed a 4.3 × 4.0 × 4.1 cm posterior fossa mass arising from the fourth ventricle with no spinal metastasis.

Diagnosis

Medulloblastoma, grade IV, standard risk

Treatment/Follow-up

In the PICU, she was given mannitol and was hyperventilated. A bedside external ventricular drain was placed, which resulted in improved mental status. Four days later, she went to the operating room for tumor removal. She recovered well from the surgery and had a rapid increase in appetite. She successfully completed chemotherapy.

She recovered well from her course of treatment although she has some residual high-frequency hearing loss and takes levothyroxine for management of mild radiation-induced hypothyroidism. She is getting excellent grades in honors and advanced courses at her middle school.

Teaching Points

Tumors of the central nervous system may present with weight loss and poor appetite. There can be a latency of many months to years between symptom onset and diagnosis due to the lack of neurologic examination findings such as cranial nerve palsies or headaches. Often, other diagnoses are pursued. In younger children, the differential may focus on more common causes of failure to thrive such as poor feeding or genetic/metabolic disorders. In older children and adolescents, GI causes as well as psychiatric causes such as anorexia nervosa are often suspected. There have been several case reports and case series reporting older children and adolescents presenting with weight loss that was initially suspected or diagnosed as an eating disorder until subsequent imaging revealed an intracranial mass. Medulloblastoma is the most common malignant pediatric brain tumor. Older children (older than 3-5 years) tend to have better prognoses than younger children. Optimal treatment combines surgical resection, radiation therapy, and adjuvant chemotherapy. Eating disorders are a relatively common pathology in adolescent females and should be considered in the differential of an adolescent with weight loss. However, for patients without body dysmorphia, other differential diagnoses should also be entertained. It is possible for brain tumors to grow to a substantial size while only producing nonspecific symptoms. Thus, it is important to exclude intracranial pathology in not only infants but also older children who present with decreased appetite, weight loss, and/or failure to thrive.

Suggested Readings

Chipkevitch E. Brain tumors and anorexia nervosa syndrome. *Brain Dev*. 1994;16(3):175-179.

Chipkevitch E, Fernandes ACL. Hypothalamic tumor associated with atypical forms of anorexia nervosa and diencephalic syndrome. *Arq Neuropsiquiatr*. 1993;51(2):270-274.

Distelmaier F, Janssen G, Mayatepek E, Schaper J, Göbel U, Rosenbaum T. Disseminated pilocytic astrocytoma involving brain stem and diencephalon: a history of atypical eating disorder and diagnostic delay. *J Neurooncol*. 2006;79(2):197.

Fleischman A, Brue C, Poussaint TY, et al. Diencephalic syndrome: a cause of failure to thrive and a model of partial growth hormone resistance. *Pediatrics*. 2005;115(6):e742-e748.

Krugman SD, Dubowitz H. Failure to thrive. *Am Fam Physician*. 2003;68(5):879-884.

Poussaint TY, Barnes PD, Nichols K, et al. Diencephalic syndrome: clinical features and imaging findings. *AJNR Am J Neuroradiol*. 1997;18(8):1499-1505.

Rohrer TR, Fahlbusch R, Buchfelder M, Dörr HG. Craniopharyngioma in a female adolescent presenting with symptoms of anorexia nervosa. *Klin Pädiatr*. 2006;218(02):67-71.

Roussel MF, Hatten ME. Cerebellum: development and medulloblastoma. *Curr Top Dev Biol*. 2011;94:235-282.

Taylor RE, Bailey CC, Robinson K, et al. Results of a randomized study of preradiation chemotherapy versus radiotherapy alone for nonmetastatic medulloblastoma: the International Society of Paediatric Oncology/United Kingdom Children's Cancer Study Group PNET-3 study. *J Clin Oncol*. 2003;21(8):1581-1591.

Zeltzer PM, Boyett JM, Finlay JL, et al. Metastasis stage, adjuvant treatment, and residual tumor are prognostic factors for medulloblastoma in children: conclusions from the Children's Cancer Group 921 randomized phase III study. *J Clin Oncol*. 1999;17(3):832-845.

74

Too Much of a Good Thing

Anne Marie Anderson

CHIEF COMPLAINT

Vomiting and weight loss

HISTORY OF PRESENT ILLNESS

A 4-month-old infant presented to the emergency room with vomiting and failure to gain weight. She was born at an estimated gestational age of 40 weeks and 2 days, weighing 3.317 kg, at the 38th percentile. The nursery course was uncomplicated, and she went home on a diet of breastfeeding and expressed breast milk. For the first 3 months of life, she was feeding well and growing appropriately. Mom fed every 2.5 to 3 hours, either spending 20 minutes at the breast or receiving 3 to 4 oz of expressed breast milk via bottle.

At 3 months of age, mom returned to work, and the infant was placed in daycare. The infant's average intake dropped to 1 to 2 oz per feed. One week prior to presentation, she began having one to two episodes of large-volume, nonbloody, nonbilious emesis per day. At her 4-month well-child check, she weighed 4.763 kg, at the 1st percentile. This was her heaviest recorded weight. The pediatrician was worried about her growth velocity and recommended that the infant receive at minimum 24 oz of expressed breast milk per day. Mom began offering bottles of expressed breast milk every 1 to 2 hours, but the infant would turn her head and cough with each attempt at feeding. Her emesis persisted. One week later she was again seen where her weight was down to 4.706 kg, and she was started on ranitidine. Mom discontinued attempts at breastfeeding, offering only expressed breast milk. She produced at least 16 oz/d but had a stored supply adequate enough to meet the 24 oz/d goal. In the 2 days prior to presentation, the infant took on average 13.5 oz of breast milk per day. In those 2 days, the baby was sleepy and had decreased urine output with about five diapers per day, down from an average of seven per day.

She had normal, regular stools and had no sweating or increased work of breathing with feeds. There were no upper respiratory infection symptoms nor fevers.

PAST MEDICAL HISTORY

She was born at 40 weeks, 2 days. There were no pregnancy complications. Mom was group B strep (GBS) negative. The infant went home from the hospital on day of life 2. She had a bowel movement in the first 24 hours of life. Her newborn screen was normal. She was up-to-date on her 4-month vaccinations. At 4 months, the infant was rolling, tolerating tummy time, moving objects from hand to hand, smiling, tracking, and babbling.

Medications

Vitamin D

Family/Social History

Family history: Dad with a history of type 1 diabetes.
Social history: She is an only child and lives with mom and dad. She attends daycare.

EXAMINATION

- Vitals: Weight: 4.536 kg (0.55%), HR 130, BP 110/83, RR 40, SpO$_2$ 96%, temp: 36.6 °C (97.9 °F).
- Constitutional: Alert, smiling, interactive. *Cachectic-appearing.*
- Head: *Anterior fontanelle sunken.* No cranial deformity. Ears: tympanic membranes without fluid or erythema.
- Nose: Nose normal. No nasal discharge
- Oropharynx: *Dry mucous membranes.*
- Eyes: No conjunctival infection. Red reflex is present bilaterally. PEERL, EOMI.
- Neck: Normal range of motion, neck supple, no lymphadenopathy
- Cardiovascular: Normal rate, regular rhythm, S1 normal and S2 normal. No murmur. Femoral pulses 2+.
- Pulmonary/chest: Lungs clear to auscultation bilaterally. No increased work of breathing.
- Abdominal: Scaphoid and soft. Normal bowel sounds, no tenderness, no hepatosplenomegaly. Genitourinary: Tanner 1 female.
- Musculoskeletal: Negative Ortolani and Barlow maneuvers.
- Neurological: Alert. Suck normal. Appropriate tone but *slight head lag present.*
- Skin: Mottled. *Capillary refill 2 to 3 seconds.* No rash or jaundice.

DIAGNOSTIC CONSIDERATIONS

At presentation, the differential diagnosis for the infant was broad in including inadequate intake, metabolic abnormality, pyloric stenosis, neonatal diabetes, oropharyngeal dysfunction, cystic fibrosis, milk protein intolerance, reflux, and neurologic abnormality.

Investigation

Initial laboratory evaluation included complete blood count (CBC), comprehensive metabolic panel (CMP), urinalysis (UA), thyroid-stimulating hormone (TSH) and free T4, ammonia, lactate, pyruvate, C-reactive protein (CRP), chest x-ray, and pyloric ultrasound. An IV was placed, and she was given a normal saline bolus.

Her initial laboratory tests demonstrated a normal glucose, hyponatremia, hypochloremia, and a slight leukocytosis. She had a mildly elevated TSH with a normal free T4 and normal lactate, pyruvate, and ammonia. Her chest x-ray and pyloric ultrasound were normal.

Prior to admission from the ER to the general pediatrics floor, the laboratory called reporting a critical calcium value on the CMP of greater than 15 mg/dL which was thought to be spurious. An ionized calcium was obtained and also resulted as critically high at >8 mg/ dL. Endocrine was consulted and recommended obtaining parathyroid hormone (PTH), 1,25(OH)$_2$ vitamin D, 25(OH) vitamin D, magnesium, phosphorus, random urine calcium, and creatinine.

Results

Pertinent results, normal values in parentheses:

- *Na:* 131 mmol/L (135-135 mmol/L)
- *Cl:* 96 mmol/L (100-114 mmol/L)
- *WBC:* 19.5 K/mm^3 (100-114 mmol/L)
- *TSH:* 6.03 µL U/mL (0.3-4.2 µL U/mL)
- *Free T4:* 1.61 ng/dL (0.9-1.7 ng/dL)
- *Calcium:* >15 mg/dL, upon further testing by lab 18.6 mg/dL (8.6-11.0 mg/dL)
- *Ionized calcium:* >8 mg/dL (3.8-5.2 mg/dL)
- *PTH:* <5 pg/mL (14-72 pg/mL)
- *1,25(OH)$_2$ Vitamin D:* 76 ng/dL, (24-86 ng/dL)
- *25(OH) Vitamin D:* >96 ng/dL, upon further laboratory testing **430 ng/dL** (20-100 ng/dL)
- *Urinary calcium/creatinine ratio:* 3.44 (<0.14)

DIAGNOSIS

Hypervitaminosis D

The infant was given IV furosemide in the ED and was admitted to the pediatric intensive care unit (PICU) for telemetry monitoring, receiving fluid resuscitation combined with diuresis to treat the hypercalcemia, thought to be secondary to vitamin D toxicity. Upon further discussion with parents, for 3 months the infant had been receiving vitamin D Hi-Po Emulsi-D3 drops purchased on Amazon which have 2000 international units of vitamin D per drop. Parents had been giving about 0.25 to 0.50 mL/d or about 7 to 15 drops, equivalent to about 14,000 to 30,000 IU/d. Mom was also taking vitamin D supplementation while breastfeeding. Further laboratory testing determined the infant's calcium was 18.6 mg/dL and baseline 25-OH vitamin D was elevated at 430 ng/dL. Renal ultrasound demonstrated bilateral medullary nephrocalcinosis.

Treatment/Follow-up

She was started on Calcilo formula, a low-calcium feed. Prednisolone was also started as an adjuvant therapy to prevent intestinal calcium reabsorption. Consideration was given to administering calcitonin or bisphosphonates, but these therapies were not needed. Furosemide and steroids were continued for 3 days until her calcium was less than 11.5 mg/dL. As her calcium levels dropped, her oral intake and emesis improved. During a 1-week hospitalization, she demonstrated weight gain and stabilization of her calcium and was ultimately discharged on Calcilo. Ionized calcium at the time of discharge was 5.58 mg/dL. Over the next 2 months, the calcium normalized and she was able to transition off Calcilo to regular formula.

TEACHING POINTS

Vitamin D supplementation for infants has become an important consideration in the last few decades with pediatricians increasingly advocating for exclusive breastfeeding. In response to a resurgence in vitamin D deficiency and rickets, particularly in exclusively breastfed infants with darker skin, the American Academy of Pediatrics increased its recommendation for vitamin D supplementation from 200 to 400 IU/d in 2008.

Vitamin D supplementation is widely available in over-the-counter preparations with the most common being D-Vi-Sol, a formulation of cholecalciferol, D3, which contains 400 IU per 1 mL. However, many case reports of hypervitaminosis D in infants have brought awareness to the variable concentrations of these products. Even when 400 IU is the intended dosing, many preparations contain 400 IU per drop, instead of per milliliter. A parent may confuse these concentrations and instead give 1 mL, equivalent to about 30 drops, and infants could instead receive 12,000 IU daily. The maximum recommended dose for infants less than 6 months is 1000 IU. Furthermore, recent studies have suggested that in adult preparations of vitamin D supplementation, only one-third of the compounded pills met the US Pharmacopeial Convention standards containing 90% to 110% of the active ingredient, whereas the rest had either higher or lower concentrations than expected.

The signs and symptoms of vitamin D toxicity can be nonspecific in neonates and may include poor feeding, feeding intolerance, constipation, polyuria, dehydration, lethargy, irritability, failure to thrive, emesis, and diarrhea, all resulting from hypercalcemia. The degree of symptoms usually correlates with increasing levels of hypercalcemia. The excess calcium load filtered through the kidneys leads to hypercalciuria. Prolonged hypercalciuria leads to polyuria due to decreased concentrating ability. Nephrolithiasis can also result, as did in this patient.

The pharmacokinetics of vitamin D contribute to its toxicity. Because D3 is fat soluble, it can be stored in adipose tissues for up to 2 months at a time. D3 is then hydroxylated in the liver to form 25-hydroxyvitamin D_3 or 25(OH)D which is also fat soluble and can be stored for months at a time. 25(OH)D then binds to vitamin D binding protein (DBP) which slows excretion by the kidney. The kidney ultimately hydroxylates 25(OH)D to its active form, $1,25(OH)_2D$, known as calcitriol. Calcitriol mediates increased intestinal absorption of calcium, leading to hypercalcemia. Patients with hypervitaminosis D typically have elevated 25(OH) D levels, reflecting elevated vitamin D stores. $1,25(OH)_2D$ levels, however, may be increased or normal due to feedback and regulation from PTH and calcium. In this patient, 25(OH) D was markedly elevated at 430 ng/dL, but levels of $1,25(OH)_2D$ were within normal range, reflecting her undetectable PTH level. Therefore, with excessive 25(OH)D stores existing in adipose tissues for months, simply discontinuing vitamin D supplementation is insufficient.

This case highlights the importance of parental, and physician, education regarding over-the-counter products on the market. While a simple medication reconciliation often assumes that infants on vitamin D supplements are taking the recommended 400 IU, the extra step of asking parents about specific formulations and dosing methods can be critical to making the diagnosis. Pediatricians often consider vitamin D to be a harmless and essential supplement for breastfeeding infants to prevent vitamin D deficiency and rickets. However, as with most good things in life, moderation is key.

Suggested Readings

Bilbao NA. Vitamin D toxicity in young breastfed infants: report of 2 cases. *Glob Pediatr Health*. 2017;4:1-5.
LeBlanc ES, Perrin N, Johnson JD. Over-the-counter and compounded vitamin D: is potency what we expect? *JAMA Intern Med*. 2013;173(7):585-586.
Rajakumar K, Reis EC, Holick MF. Dosing errors with the over-the-counter vitamin D supplementation: a risk for vitamin D toxicity in infants. *Clin Pediatr (Phila)*. 2013;52(1):82-85.
Smollin C, Srisansanee W. Vitamin D toxicity in an infant: case files of the University of California, San Francisco medical Toxicology Fellowship. *J Med Toxicol*. 2014;10(2):190-193.
Vogiatzi MG, Jaconson-Dickman E, DeBoer MD. Vitamin D supplementation and risk of toxicity in pediatrics: a review of current literature. *J Clin Endocrinol Metab*. 2014;99(1):1132-1141.

75

Insufficient

Mary E. Fournier

CHIEF COMPLAINT

"She hasn't had a period in over a year."

HISTORY OF PRESENT ILLNESS

A 12-year-old girl reached menarche at the age of 10 years and has a current gynecologic age of 2 years. Periods were initially irregular, occurring every 1 to 3 months, lasting 5 days, with moderate flow requiring three to four pads per day. She denied any history of associated cramping or any other menstrual symptoms. She had three to four periods over the first 8 months following menarche and has had no menstrual bleeding or spotting since. Last menstrual period (LMP) was 16 months ago. She was seen by her primary care provider (PCP) after 8 months of no bleeding and was assured that irregular periods are typical in young adolescents. No further evaluation was done at that time and watchful waiting was recommended.

PAST MEDICAL HISTORY

Occasional headaches

Medications

None

Family/Social History

She is in the sixth grade and is described as a quiet child by her mother. She lives with her mother and maternal aunt; father is not involved. Family history is significant only for obesity in mother and stroke in maternal great-grandmother. No family history of menstrual irregularities or infertility.

EXAMINATION

- General: Well appearing, obese, no acute distress.
- Skin: Dark, thickened, velvety skin noted along the posterior neck consistent with acanthosis nigricans. No evidence of abnormal hair growth or acne.
- HEENT: Eyes are PERRLA and EOMI, ears are normal, TMs clear, nares clear, oral pharynx normal, moist mucus membranes.
- Neck: Supple, no masses, no thyromegaly or lymphadenopathy.
- Resp: Clear to auscultation bilaterally, no wheezes or crackles.
- C/V: Regular rate and rhythm, no murmurs, rubs, or gallops.
- GI: Abdomen soft, nontender, no masses or hepatosplenomegaly, normal bowel sounds.
- Breasts: Normal female, SMR IV.
- Genitalia: Normal external female, no lesions or discharge, pubic hair SMR V, pelvic examination deferred.
- Extremities: No clubbing, cyanosis, or edema.
- Neuro: CNs 2 to 10 intact, strength 5/5, reflexes equal bilaterally.

DIAGNOSTIC CONSIDERATIONS

This patient's menstrual pattern is consistent with secondary amenorrhea, described as absence of menses for more than 3 months in girls who previously had regular menstrual cycles or 6 months in girls who had irregular menses. While girls often have irregular periods during the first 2 years following menarche, lack of menses for more than 3 to 6 months warrants investigation. Diagnostic considerations include delayed maturation of the hypothalamic-pituitary-gonadal axis, hormonal abnormality such as thyroid disease, hyperprolactinemia, polycystic ovarian syndrome, ovarian insufficiency, hypogonadotropic hypogonadism, and late-onset congenital adrenal hyperplasia.

Investigation

- Urine HCG negative
- Thyroid disease excluded with normal TSH and free T4
- Prolactin, DHEA-sulfate, and early morning 17-hydroxyprogesterone
- Gonadotropin and ovarian hormones
- Progesterone challenge
- Pelvic ultrasound

Results

Gonadotropin levels were obtained and were significantly elevated with luteinizing hormone (LH) 51.2 U/L and follicle-stimulating hormone (FSH) >100 U/L. Ovarian hormones including estradiol and free and total testosterone were lower than expected for current SMR stage.

Transabdominal pelvic ultrasound shows a small uterus, measuring 5.8 × 2.9 × 1.9 cm. The endometrial stripe is minimal and measures 3 mm in thickness. The ovaries are normal in appearance; the left ovary measures 2.2 × 1.2 × 2.0 cm for a volume of 3 mL; the right ovary measures 1.4 × 1.7 × 1.5 cm for a volume of 2 mL. No follicles are seen in either ovary. IMPRESSION: The ovaries and uterus appear understimulated. They are small, no follicles are seen in the ovaries, and the endometrial stripe is 3 mm thick.

Patient was given oral medroxyprogesterone 10 mg daily for 10 days. Withdrawal bleed was expected within 1 week of cessation of the hormones but did not occur.

DIAGNOSIS

Primary ovarian insufficiency

Treatment/Follow-up

1. Thoughtful and careful disclosure of diagnosis to adolescent and parent with direct, developmentally appropriate language and resources, allowing sufficient time for questions and support
2. Chromosomal analysis to evaluate for Turner syndrome
3. DEXA scan to evaluate bone health associated with estrogen deficiency
4. Evaluation for adrenal autoantibodies
5. Hormone replacement therapy for preservation of cardiovascular and bone health as well as sexual function

TEACHING POINTS

Primary ovarian insufficiency (POI), previously described as premature menopause or premature ovarian failure, is the development of hypergonadotropic hypogonadism prior to the age of 40 years. Studies have shown the incidence of spontaneous POI in adolescents and young women to be approximately 1 in 10,000. Patients typically present with concerns for irregular or absent menstrual cycles, including primary amenorrhea. Other symptoms are generally associated with estrogen deficiency and include hot flashes, vaginal dryness, sexual dysfunction, and concern for bone loss, including increased fracture rate. POI is associated with significant vascular endothelial dysfunction which increases the patient's risk of cardio-vascular disease and mortality. Young women with POI also often have significant emotional sequelae following diagnosis including depression and anxiety.

Diagnosis is made by gonadotropins, particularly FSH, measured in the menopausal range. Patients with POI might have intermittent ovarian function, so repeated measurements and corresponding estradiol levels are helpful in the diagnosis. Other causes of oligo- and amenorrhea should be ruled out. Once a diagnosis is made, further evaluation is needed to assess for underlying etiology as well as commonly associated disorders. In particular, patients should be evaluated for chromosomal and autoimmune disorders.

Management of POI primarily involves hormone replacement therapy with estrogen and progestin. For young adolescents with primary amenorrhea who have not fully developed secondary sex characteristics, lower estrogen doses with gradual increases are necessary to mimic gradual pubertal maturation. For patients with secondary amenorrhea, higher replacement doses of estradiol with cyclic progestin are required. Alternatively, combined oral contraceptive pills might be used. Hormone replacement therapy should be continued until the age of typical menopause, around 50 to 51 years.

Suggested Readings

Committee Opinion No. 605: primary ovarian insufficiency in adolescents and young women. *Obstet Gynecol.* 2014;124:193-197.

Committee Opinion No. 698: hormone therapy in primary ovarian insufficiency. *Obstet Gynecol.* 2017;129(5):e134-e141 [Reaffirmed 2020].

Coulam CB, Adamson SC, Annegers JF. Incidence of premature ovarian failure. *Obstet Gynecol.* 1986;67:604-606.

Covington SN, Hillard PJ, Sterling EW, Nelson LM; Primary Ovarian Insufficiency Recovery Group. A family systems approach to primary ovarian insufficiency. *J Pediatr Adolesc Gynecol.* 2011;24:137-141.

de Almeida DM, Benetti-Pinto CL, Makuch MY. Sexual function of women with premature ovarian failure. *Menopause.* 2011;18:262-266.

De Vos M, Devroey P, Fause BC. Primary ovarian insufficiency. *Lancet.* 2010;376:911-921.

Kalantaridou SN, Naka KK, Papanikolaou E, et al. Impaired endothelial function in young women with premature ovarian failure: normalization with hormone therapy. *J Clin Endocrinol Metab.* 2004;89:3907-3913.

Nelson LM. Primary ovarian insufficiency. *N Engl J Med.* 2009;360:606-614.

Popat VB, Calis KA, Kalantaridou SN, et al. Bone mineral density in young women with primary ovarian insufficiency: results of a three-year randomized controlled trial of physiological transdermal estradiol and testosterone replacement. *J Clin Endocrinol Metab.* 2014;99:3418-3426.

Popat VB, Calis KA, Vanderhoof VH, et al. Bone mineral density in estrogen-deficient young women. *J Clin Endocrinol Metab.* 2009;94(7):2277-2283.

76 ICP

Farid Farkouh

CHIEF COMPLAINT

"She was totally out of it."

HISTORY OF PRESENT ILLNESS

A 17-year-old girl was brought to the emergency department (ED) after experiencing an episode of loss of consciousness. She woke up that morning with a headache, which was typical for her the last several months, and she went to school after eating breakfast. After school, however, she had some blurry vision and dizziness for about 20 minutes and then she lost consciousness. She was unarousable for about 10 minutes, as estimated by her friends, who said "She was totally out of it." Upon regaining consciousness, she felt nauseous and had return of a headache, but her mental status was back to her normal baseline. She had no recent head trauma, no abnormal limb movements, and no abnormal eye movements or tongue biting during the episode, and she was breathing regularly throughout. She had no fevers, no rashes, and no diarrhea.

PAST MEDICAL HISTORY

- Obesity
- Chronic nausea for months
- Chronic headaches for months
- Anxiety

Medications

- Escitalopram 20 mg once daily
- Oral contraceptive

Family/Social History

She denies anxiety, depression, or suicidal ideations. She does not use alcohol, tobacco, or other drugs.

EXAMINATION

- Vitals: T 36.1 °C, HR 88, BP 103/71, RR 22, Spo$_2$ 99%. Weight 99.6 kg, BMI 37.5 kg/m^2.
- General: Obese, but chatty and unhappy about the episode.
- HEENT: Normocephalic, atraumatic, no conjunctival injection, mucous membrane moist.
- Resp: Comfortable work of breathing with clear symmetric breath sounds, no crackles.
- CV: Regular rate and rhythm, no murmur.
- Abd: Nondistended, nontender.
- Extremities: Warm and well-perfused.
- Skin: No rash.
- Neurological examination: Alert and oriented. CN II-XII intact with normal visual acuity, normal fundoscopic examination with sharp margins of optic discs and full visual fields

bilaterally. No nystagmus. Normal muscle bulk and strength throughout. Sensation intact to light touch. Reflexes 2+ at knees and ankles and forearms; toes are down-going with plantar stimulation. No dysmetria with finger-nose-finger testing. Normal gait.

DIAGNOSTIC CONSIDERATIONS

- Syncope, vasovagal
- Intracranial mass (tumor)
- Obstruction of CNS venous outflow (eg, venous sinus thrombosis, jugular vein compression)
- Migraine
- Meningitis, doubt
- Idiopathic intracranial hypertension

Investigation and Results

- Glucose was 68 in the ED.
- Orthostatic vital signs repeated on several occasions: Normal.
- Head MRI: Normal MRI of the brain with normal ventricles and no evidence of hydrocephalus or cranial masses.

After excluding the most likely causes, a lumbar puncture was performed, with a recorded opening pressure of 27 cm H_2O. The CSF was crystal and colorless and had zero nucleated cells and no RBCs.

DIAGNOSIS

Idiopathic intracranial hypertension without papilledema (IIHWOP)

Treatment/Follow-up

She was started on acetazolamide, a carbonic anhydrase inhibitor that reduces the rate of CSF production and has been associated with improved outcomes in patients with idiopathic intracranial hypertension (IIH). She was also strongly encouraged to start a weight loss program. The episode of loss of consciousness was probably due to a transient, spike, or higher elevation of intracranial pressure (ICP), as the episode has not recurred after initiating treatment with acetazolamide.

TEACHING POINTS[1-6]

IIH, also known as pseudotumor cerebri, is a condition of unknown etiology that manifests with chronically elevated ICP with normal brain parenchyma but without ventriculomegaly, mass lesion, or underlying infection or malignancy. A variant of IIH called idiopathic intracranial hypertension without papilledema (IIHWOP) has been described as a rare cause of chronic headache of unknown origin. Permanent vision loss is the major morbidity associated with IIH. A study that followed 57 patients for 5 to 41 years found that 24% developed blindness or severe visual impairment.

IIH predominantly affects obese young women and is also associated with certain drugs (vitamin A, tetracycline, growth hormones). There is some evidence that oral hormonal contraceptives increase the risk of IIH, but a recent study found no significant association between incidence of IIH and use of hormonal contraceptives.

Symptoms include diffuse headaches, visual symptoms such as transient vision loss, photopsia, diplopia, retrobulbar pain, and pulsatile tinnitus.

The pathophysiology is due to mismatch between production and resorption of CSF, which leads to increased ICP, causing damage to structures of the CNS and especially to the optical nerve fibers. A proposed mechanism of the pathophysiology: venous sinus stenosis → venous outflow obstruction → venous hypertension → decreased CSF absorption → increased ICP → venous sinus compression, which leads to a vicious cycle of worsening the venous sinus stenosis further. Some studies have utilized electroencephalogram (EEG) to continuously monitor

ICP and found that there are transient spikes in the ICP of patients with IIH. These spikes could lead to a decrease in cerebral blood flow (CBF), which could be the cause of syncope.

Required for diagnosis of IIH:

- Papilledema (not necessary for diagnosis of IIHWOP)
- Normal neurologic examination, except for cranial nerve abnormalities
- Neuroimaging: Normal brain parenchyma without evidence of hydrocephalus, mass, or structural lesions and no abnormal meningeal enhancement on MRI
- Normal CSF composition
- Elevated lumbar puncture opening pressure (≥25 in adults and ≥28 cm in children)

Treatment has two goals: The alleviation of symptoms (headache) and the preservation of vision.

- Discontinue any potential causative medications, if possible.
- Implement weight loss strategies.
- First-line therapy is acetazolamide, with the addition of furosemide if needed.
- Consider surgery if medical measures fail:
  - Optic nerve sheath fenestration, which is the removal of small patches of dura surrounding the optic nerve to allow CSF to drain into the periorbital fat.
  - CSF shunt, typically ventriculoperitoneal.
- Serial lumbar punctures are not recommended as the CSF typically reaccumulates within 6 hours, making this treatment of short-term duration only.

Suggested Readings

Corbett JJ, Savino PJ, Thompson HS, et al. Visual loss in pseudotumor cerebri. Follow-up of 57 patients from five to 41 years and a profile of 14 patients with permanent severe visual loss. *Arch Neurol.* 1982;39(8):461-474.

Kilgore KP, Lee MS, Leavitt JA, Frank RD, Mcclelland CM, Chen JJ. A population-based, case-control evaluation of the association between hormonal contraceptives and idiopathic intracranial hypertension. *Am J Ophthalmol.* 2019;197:74-79.

Larimer P, Mcdermott M, Scott B, Shih T, Poisson S. Recurrent syncope due to refractory cerebral venous sinus thrombosis and transient elevations of intracranial pressure. *Neurohospitalist.* 2013;4(1):18-21.

Matheos K, Dai S. Idiopathic intracranial hypertension without papilledema in children: a case series. *Adv Pediatr Res.* 2015;2:14.

Simone RD, Ranieri A. Commentary: idiopathic intracranial hypertension without papilledema (IIHWOP) in chronic refractory headache. *Front Neurol.* 2019;10:39.

Simone RD, Romigi A, Albanese M, et al. Revised diagnostic criteria for the pseudotumor cerebri syndrome in adults and children. *Neurology.* 2014;82(19):1752-1753.

77

Hard Stop

Shelley C. Choudhury, Shruti Sakhuja

CHIEF COMPLAINT

"Not having stools regularly"

HISTORY OF PRESENT ILLNESS

A 16-month-old boy presented to the emergency department after 3 weeks without producing any stool. Interventions prior to this visit included daily juice intake, one suppository with a resulting small bowel movement weeks ago, and one-time laxative use. He has had occasional streaks of nonbloody stool in the past, but never constipation for this long. The day prior to presentation, he spiked a fever to 101° F, started vomiting, and developed abdominal distention. He has had decreased appetite and increased sleepiness. An abdominal x-ray was obtained and suggested bowel obstruction.

PAST MEDICAL HISTORY

- Iron deficiency anemia diagnosed at age 14 months
- Born at 35 weeks, twin delivery, admitted to neonatal intensive care unit for 1.5 weeks, and passed meconium within first 24 hours

Medications

Ferrous sulfate

Family/Social History

- Constipation in mother
- Lives with parents
- Up-to-date on immunizations

EXAMINATION

- Vitals: HR 115, RR 30, O$_2$ 100%, T 38.1, BP 113/85
- General: In no discomfort, not acutely distressed
- Skin: Warm and dry, no rash
- HEENT: Normocephalic, MMM, no congestion/rhinorrhea, no scleral icterus, TMs clear
- Neck: No cervical adenopathy, thyroid nonenlarged
- CV: Tachycardic, regular rhythm, no murmur, intact distal pulses
- Respiratory: Clear bilaterally, no increased work of breathing, no wheezes
- Abdomen: Moderately distended and firm but not hard, diffusely tender to palpation
- MSK: Normal ROM
- Neuro: Alert, appropriate for age

TABLE 77.1 Initial Laboratory Workup

Laboratory Workup
UA—1 + LE, negative nitrites
Urine culture—no growth
WBC 12.2 cells/mm³
Hemoglobin 9.9 g/dL
Creatinine 1.1 mg/dL
CO_2 15 mEq/L
Uric acid 10.6 mg/dL
LDH 407 U/L
AFP 4.0 ng/mL
Beta hCG <5 mIU/mL

AFP, alpha fetoprotein; hCG, human chorionic gonadotropin; LDH, lactate dehydrogenase; UA, urinalysis; WBC, white blood cell.

DIAGNOSTIC CONSIDERATIONS

Differential diagnosis for a patient with difficulty stooling includes chronic idiopathic constipation, bowel obstruction, congenital anomalies such as Hirschsprung disease, underlying endocrinopathies such as hypothyroidism, celiac disease, or neoplasia.

Investigation

- CBC
- CMP
- UA
- LDH
- Uric acid
- AFP
- Serum beta hCG
- Biopsy
- Abdominal plain film
- Abdominal ultrasound
- CT of abdomen/pelvis
- MRI of abdomen/pelvis
- PET scan

Results (Tables 77.1 and 77.2; Figures 77.1-77.3)

Imaging reveals a large mass consistent with a malignancy. The child was taken to the operation room for biopsy/resection and pathology revealed a high-grade embryonal rhabdomyosarcoma—with extensive anaplasia, mitotic figures, and necrosis. It was positive for vimentin, desmin, and WT-1. Fluorescent in situ hybridization is negative for FOXO1.

DIAGNOSIS

1. **High-grade embryonal rhabdomyosarcoma**, group III, stage 2, intermediate risk
2. **Bilateral hydronephrosis** secondary to bladder outlet obstruction
3. **Acute kidney injury** secondary to bladder outlet obstruction
4. **Normocytic anemia**

Treatment/Follow-up

He was evaluated by urology, oncology, and pediatric surgery and underwent cystoscopy with ureteral stent placement and laparoscopic incisional biopsy. The right ureter was inadvertently

TABLE 77.2 Initial Imaging Studies

Imaging Studies	
Abdominal plain film	Distended loops of air-filled bowel with a paucity of air in the midabdomen obstruction vs ileus. Masslike radiodensity in the lower abdomen.
Abdominal ultrasound	Echogenic mass with internal vascularity posterior to the bladder. Markedly distended bladder and bilateral hydronephrosis.
CT of abdomen/pelvis	1. Large presacral heterogeneously enhancing mass with internal cystic areas resulting in mass effect on the rectum, colon, and bladder. Likely arising from bladder base or prostate. Diagnostic considerations include neuroblastoma, sarcoma, and sacrococcygeal teratoma. 2. Bilateral moderate hydronephrosis with bladder outlet obstruction and thickening of bladder wall. 3. Right-sided thoracic aorta.
MRI of abdomen/pelvis	1. Large heterogeneous pelvic mass (4.9 × 4.6 × 4.8 cm), arising from bladder neck, urethra, or prostate suggestive of pelvic rhabdomyosarcoma. 2. Thickened bladder wall, likely superimposed cystitis. 3. No lymphadenopathy.
PET	Relative increase in tumor size, no metastatic disease.

CT, computed tomography; MRI, magnetic resonance imaging; PET, positron emission tomography.

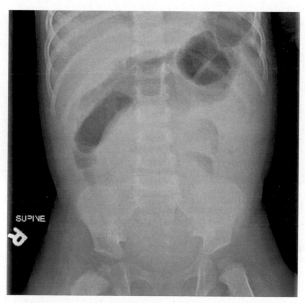

FIGURE 77.1 Plain film showing paucity of gas in lower abdomen.

transected during the procedure, and the procedure was converted to open with suprapubic catheter placement in addition to port-a-cath placement. A diverting colostomy was placed after development of worsening abdominal distention and bilious emesis secondary to obstruction. The cancer was treated with a combination of vincristine, irinotecan, dactinomycin, cytoxan, and radiation. His course was complicated by persistent urinary candidiasis and neuropathy secondary to both nerve compression and chemotherapy.

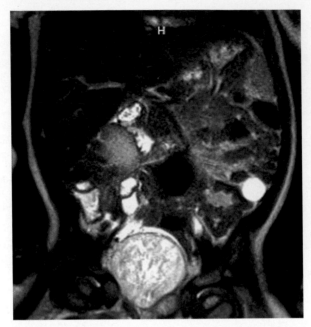

FIGURE 77.2 Magnetic resonance imaging findings of abdomen/pelvis, coronal view, showing enhancing tumor.

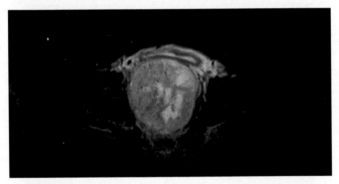

FIGURE 77.3 Magnetic resonance imaging findings of abdomen/pelvis, axial view, showing compression of rectum.

TEACHING POINTS

The differential diagnosis of constipation in pediatric patients is broad, but extrinsic causes (think compression) should also be considered along with intrinsic causes, particularly if there is no history of chronic constipation. Rhabdomyosarcomas (RMS) are the most common soft-tissue sarcomas in childhood, but they have a variable presentation based on their location and mass effect. The majority of genitourinary tract RMS are of the embryonal type (embryonal rhabdomyosarcomas, ERMS), differentiated from alveolar RMS by immunohisto-chemistry staining; ERMS can be associated with neurofibromatosis 1, Beckwith-Wiedemann, Li-Fraumeni, DICER1, and Costello syndrome but is usually sporadic. Diagnosis is made by biopsy. For staging evaluation, patients should undergo CT or MRI of the mass and surrounding structures. Anatomic boundaries of the tumor (which determine stage, risk stratification, and treatment) should be documented prior to starting therapy. Complexities of pelvic anatomy will automatically increase risk stratification of bladder/prostate origin tumors and can lead to urinary, gastrointestinal, reproductive, and neurological complications from mass effect, local tumor invasion, and subsequent surgical interventions. Management has shifted from radical excision to primarily chemotherapy and radiation. Long-term complications include bowel and bladder dysfunction, cardiac dysfunction secondary to chemotherapy effects, and secondary tumors.

Suggested Readings

Alexander N, Lane S, Hitchcock R. What is the evidence for radical surgery in the management of localized embryonal bladder/prostate rhabdomyosarcoma? *Pediatr Blood Cancer*. 2012;58(6):833-835.

Parham DM, Barr FG. Classification of rhabdomyosarcoma and its molecular basis. *Adv Anat Pathol*. 2013;20(6):387-397.

Perez EA, Kassira N, Cheung MC, Koniaris LG, Neville HL, Sola JE. Rhabdomyosarcoma in children: a SEER population based study. *J Surg Res*. 2011;17(2):e243-e251.

78 The Usual Suspects

Andrew J. White

CHIEF COMPLAINT

Painful rash and a fever

HISTORY OF PRESENT ILLNESS

An 8-year-old boy presented with 9 days of fever and a painful rash.

Nine days ago, his first symptoms were chest pain with deep breaths and a headache. At an outside hospital emergency department (ED), he was tested for flu and strep, which were both normal. He was diagnosed with a upper respiratory infection (URI)/bronchitis and sent home with 5 days of azithromycin. After his first dose of azithromycin, he vomited and he has continued to have painful episodes of emesis daily, preceded by intense chills, rigors, and fevers as high as 103.

Six days ago, grandmother noticed a **rash** on his abdomen and face. He went to his pediatrician and the azithromycin was discontinued. A complete blood count (CBC) and a comprehensive metabolic panel (CMP) were obtained and were both normal. The chest pain and headache had resolved.

Five days ago, the rash spread across his entire trunk, all four extremities, and his back and became very painful, tender to touch, and itchy.

On the day of admission, he returned to the outside hospital ED because of fever, chills, emesis, and the rash that had spread. CMP, CBC, and urinalysis (UA) were unremarkable.

PAST MEDICAL HISTORY

Healthy

Medications

Recent azithromycin, none in last 6 days

Family/Social History

He has exposure to the following potential sources of infection:

- Chickens, pigeons, goats, dogs, horses, cows.
- Stray cat with kittens in the barn attic; he has been scratched.
- Hunts deer, rabbit, turkey, but not in a few months.
- Eats turkey, rabbit, and squirrel, but not in the last few months.
- Prefers his deer meat rare to medium rare.
- No unpasteurized dairy.
- Helped clear rubble on a burned down property, sweeping up ashes and using a Bobcat.
- Mosquitos, of course.
- Ticks but no recent bites.
- Swims in the Black River.

EXAMINATION

Comfortable and in no acute distress.

- Vitals: T 37.5, HR 100, RR 32, blood pressure 104/69, pulse oximetry 96%.
- Skin
  - A tender to touch diffuse, blanching, macular rash is present over trunk, arms, legs, cheeks, and buttocks, sparing palms and soles.
  - No mucosal membrane involvement or desquamation.
- HEENT
  - Head: Normocephalic, atraumatic.
  - Eyes: Conjunctivae clear. No drainage or injection. No scleral icterus.
  - Nose: No drainage. No masses visualized.
  - Mouth: Posterior pharynx clear. Mucous membranes moist. No oral lesions.
  - Throat: No tonsillar hypertrophy.
  - Neck: Supple. No lymphadenopathy.
- Pulmonary: Clear to auscultation bilaterally. No wheezes, rales, or rhonchi.
- Cardiovascular: Regular rate and rhythm. No rubs or gallops, 2/6 systolic murmur. Normal S1 and S2, 2+ distal pulses.
- Abdomen: Soft, nondistended, nontender, no hepatosplenomegaly, no masses palpated, normoactive bowel sounds.

DIAGNOSTIC CONSIDERATIONS

The admitting team's diagnostic thoughts (ie, *the usual suspects*)

- Serum sickness/drug rash/DRESS
- Rocky Mountain spotted fever
- *Bartonella*
- Ehrlichiosis
- Histoplasmosis
- Glandular tularemia
- Q fever (added by infectious disease team)
- Arboviral illness
- EBV, CMV, enterovirus, Coxsackie virus, adenovirus
- *Mycoplasma*
- Endocarditis
- Kawasaki disease, or other vasculitis
- Brucellosis (home-prepared meat)

Investigation

Tests were sent for the usual suspects. The initial laboratory results returned:

- Monospot negative.
- Urinalysis normal.
- ESR 12, CRP 30.9, CMP normal.

Results

Most tests returned negative; however,

- *Coxiella burnetii* (Q fever) ab, IgG, phase **I 1:256** (Normal is <1:16 titer)
- *Coxiella burnetii* (Q fever) ab, IgM, phase I < 1:16 (Normal is <1:16 titer)
- *Coxiella burnetii* (Q fever) ab, IgG, phase II **1:128** (Normal is <1:16 titer)
- *Coxiella burnetii* (Q fever) ab, IgM, phase II < 1:16 (Normal is <1:16 titer)

DIAGNOSIS

Q fever

Treatment/Follow-up

Doxycycline 100 mg po 2 times a day

TEACHING POINTS

Q fever was first recognized as a human disease in 1935 after an outback of a febrile illness among slaughterhouse workers in Queensland, Australia.

The name "Q" came from "query" as the cause was unknown. It is now known to be caused by the intracellular bacterium, *Coxiella burnetii*. (Coxiella, after Harold Rea Cox, a bacteriologist from the Johns Hopkins School of Public Health, and burnetii, after Frank Macfarlane Burnet, an Australian virologist who won the Nobel prize for his work in immunology, specifically regarding tolerance.)

It is commonly transmitted to humans from cattle, sheep and goats, especially when they are giving birth.

Infection usually occurs from aerosols, or occasionally the gastrointestinal (GI) tract, or percutaneous exposure. The incubation period is approximately 20 days (range 14-39).

The illness manifests as fever with signs of pneumonia (cough, dyspnea, sputum), increased transaminases, and thrombocytopenia.

More severe presentations include meningitis, meningoencephalitis, pericarditis, myocarditis, cholecystitis, and adenitis.

Chronic Q fever is diagnosed in patients whose symptoms last for more than 6 months (1%-5% of pts).

C. burnetii does not grow in routine blood cultures.

The most common method used to make the diagnosis is using immunofluorescence assay (IFA) against the *C. burnetii* antigens.

C. burnetii has two distinct antigens called phase I and phase II.

Antibodies directed toward phase II develop after antibodies directed to phase I.

A fourfold rise in anti-phase II IgG from the acute and convalescent time points taken 3 to 6 weeks apart is diagnostic.

Treatment: Doxycycline. If there is Q fever endocarditis—doxycycline and hydroxychloroquine for a minimum of 18 months.

If the patient has Q fever meningoencephalitis, use fluoroquinolones because they have better cerebrospinal fluid (CSF) penetration. If the patient is pregnant, use cotrimoxazole.

While some of the presenting features of this patients' illness are atypical for Q fever, the rather broad exposure history, fever with chills and rigors, and tantalizing initial serology make this diagnosis most likely. Repeat serologic testing will be of utmost importance to confirm the diagnosis.

"Sometimes when you round up the usual suspects, you find Keyser Söze."

Suggested Readings

Anderson A, Bijlmer H, Fournier PE, et al. Diagnosis and management of Q fever—United States, 2013: recommendations from CDC and the Q fever working group. *MMWR Recomm Rep.* 2013;62:1-30.

Centers for Disease Control and Prevention. *National Center for Emerging and Zoonotic Infectious Diseases (NCEZID) Division of Vector-Borne Diseases (DVBD).* 2013.

Dahlgren F, McQuiston J, Massung R, et al. Q fever in the United States: summary of case reports from two national surveillance systems, 2000-2012. *Am J Trop Med Hyg.* 2015;92(2):247-255.

Million M, Raoult D. *Recent Advances in the Study of Q Fever Epidemiology, Diagnosis and Management.* Elsevier; 2015.

79

Too Low to Blow

Robert D. Williams, Ana S. Solís Zavala

CHIEF COMPLAINT

Low oxygen

HISTORY OF PRESENT ILLNESS

An 8-day-old boy was admitted for respiratory distress syndrome (RDS).

He was born at 36 weeks 4 days via C-section to a G2P2 mother, complicated by intra-uterine growth restriction (IUGR) and maternal exposure to COVID-19. At birth, Apgar scores were 8 and 8, but he had retractions and nasal flaring, developed desaturations, and was placed on 1 L of O_2 via nasal cannula. Ampicillin and gentamicin were started. A COVID swab was negative.

From day of life (DOL) 3 to 7, the supplemental oxygen was successfully decreased, but he fed poorly. He was treated with phototherapy for unconjugated hyperbilirubinemia, which resolved in 2 days.

The comprehensive metabolic panel was flagged for a low **alkaline phosphatase** of 12 U/L.

A chest radiograph showed normal-appearing heart and lungs but generalized decreased mineralization.

INITIAL LABORATORY RESULTS

- Electrolytes were within normal limits
- Calcium 10.5 mg/dL (normal)
- Phosphorous 7.2 mg/dL (normal limits)
- Repeat **alkaline phosphatase: 17 U/L (low)**

Family/Social History

- Mother with delayed dentition and learning disability
- Sister with delayed dentition and short stature
- Other family members with delayed dentition, cavities, and short stature

EXAMINATION

- Vitals: Temp 36.9 °C, pulse 160, Resp 36, BP 54/35, SpO_2 100%.
- Length was 1%, weight 10%, and OFC 4%.
- General: Consistent with estimated gestational age but small and hypotonic.
- Skin: Pink, no rash.
- Head: Large anterior fontanelle soft, open, flat, no molding, bogginess over the skull, soft skull.
- Eyes: Normally spaced, open spontaneously.
- Ears/nose/throat/palate: No ear pits or tags, nares appear patent, palate intact.
- Respiratory: Clear to auscultation bilaterally, no retractions, good air exchange.
- Cardiovascular: Regular rate and rhythm, no murmurs, adequate lower extremity pulses equal bilaterally, normal capillary refill.
- Abdomen: Round, soft, nontender, nondistended, no organomegaly.

- Genitalia: Male—normal phallus, bilateral descended testes, normal genitalia for gestational age.
- Anus: Patent.
- Spine: Straight and intact, no sacral dimple or tuft.
- Extremities: No clavicular crepitus, hips stable with no clicks or clunks; widening of wrists and bowing of the right tibia.
- Neurologic: Awake; tone, reactivity, suck, and grasp appropriate for gestational age; complete Moro.

DIAGNOSTIC CONSIDERATIONS

- Osteogenesis imperfecta: A group of genetic disorders leading to imperfect bone formation at increased risk of fractures
- Achondrogenesis: Disorders affecting cartilage and bone development, leading to short limbs and other skeletal abnormalities
- Hypophosphatasia: Genetic disorder characterized by abnormal development of bones and teeth due to defective mineralization

Investigation and Results

- Radiographs (Figures 79.1 and 79.2).
- **Diagnostic Test: DNA sequencing.** The results showed that he is compound heterozygous for two changes in ALPL (c.881A > C transversion in exon 9 and c.892G > A transition in exon 9), confirming the diagnosis of perinatal hypophosphatasia.

DIAGNOSIS

Hypophosphatasia, perinatal

Treatment/Follow-up

- Asfotase alfa is the enzyme replacement of tissue nonspecific alkaline phosphatase.
- Laboratory tests checked 48 hours after initiation of therapy showed (appropriately) elevated alkaline phosphatase level of 3099 U/L, ionized calcium 5.48 mg/dL, phosphorous of 7.4 mg/dL, and low vitamin B6 at <2 µg/L.

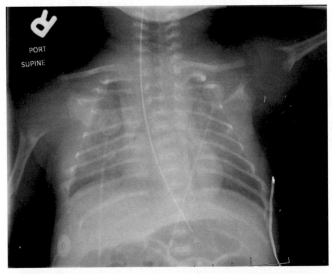

FIGURE 79.1 Chest x-ray shows generalized demineralization and abnormal, eroded metaphyses.

- Breast milk fortification with human milk fortifier to provide supplemental vitamin B6 (392 µg) was initiated for vitamin B6 profile with undetectable levels of pyridoxal-5-phosphate and pyridoxic acid at <2 µg/L.
- Repeat laboratory tests 2 weeks later showed improved level of pyridoxal-5 phosphate of 54 µg/L and pyridoxic acid level of 35 µg/L.
- Repeat imaging approximately 1 month after initiation of therapy showed significant improvement with increased mineralization of ribs, wrists, and knees.

TEACHING POINTS

Hypophosphatasia is a genetic disorder characterized by abnormal development of bones and teeth. The disease is caused by mutations in the ALPL gene that is responsible for encoding tissue-nonspecific alkaline phosphatase (TNSALP) enzymes. Mutations in the gene lead to insufficient levels of TNSALP enzymes which leads to defective mineralization in which bones and teeth are unable to properly uptake minerals such as calcium and phosphorous. Hypophosphatasia has a range in severity of presentation and there have been six major clinical forms identified. The varying clinical forms are mostly based on the age of onset of symptoms and diagnosis and are as follows: perinatal, infantile, childhood, adult, and odon-tohypophosphatasia. Severity of the disease in general is correlated to the residual alkaline phosphatase activity in the body.

Perinatal hypophosphatasia is characterized by improper skeleton formation in utero and often results in stillbirth. Other time, newborns may survive for several days and pass away due to respiratory failure in the setting of chest deformities and underdeveloped lungs. Infantile hypophosphatasia often does not have any noticeable abnormalities at birth, but symptoms such as failure to thrive and craniosynostosis develop by 6 months of age. Infants affected by the infantile form have softened, weakened bones leading to the skeletal malformations of rickets such as bowing deformities or chest, wrist, and ankle joint deformities. It is important to note that due to the presence of chest deformities, infants are at increased risk of acquiring pneumonia and have varying degrees of pulmonary insufficiency that can lead to respiratory failure.

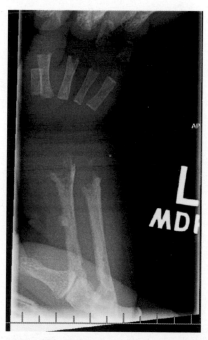

FIGURE 79.2 Wrist radiograph with demineralization and bone resorption.

Hypercalcemia is another complication that can be seen with hypophosphatasia. It can lead to symptoms including vomiting, constipation, weakness, poor feeding, and nephrocalcinosis due to the increased excretion of calcium by the kidneys.

Treatment of perinatal and infantile hypophosphatasia is with asfotase alfa enzyme replacement therapy that is injected subcutaneously. It is important to ensure that you rotate injection sites to avoid lipohypertrophy.

Suggested Reading

Whyte MP. Enzyme-replacement therapy in life-threatening hypophosphatasia. *N Engl J Med.* 2012;366:904-913.

80

I'm From the Future

Shruti Sakhuja, Rachel Zolno

CHIEF COMPLAINT

Altered mental status

HISTORY OF PRESENT ILLNESS

A 13-year-old girl presents with 3 months of depressive symptoms. Initially, she only expressed anxiety regarding school performance, but she progressively developed poor sleep, irritability, anhedonia, decreased appetite, and suicidality. She was taken to an outside hospital where her workup, including head computed tomography (CT), was normal and was admitted to an inpatient psychiatric facility, where she began to develop auditory and visual hallucinations and difficulty speaking. She was diagnosed with major depressive disorder with psychotic features and eventually discharged home on Lexapro and Seroquel. Two days after discharge, she again experienced auditory and visual hallucinations, hyperactivity, and hypersexuality. She displayed episodes of aggressive behaviors at home including cursing, biting herself and others, thrashing, emptying drawers, and knocking over a stereo. She attempted to elope from home, saying "I'm from the future" and "I don't belong here," prompting her family to again bring her to the emergency room (ER).

She has not had fevers, rhinorrhea, congestion, headaches, chest pain, nausea, vomiting, diarrhea, joint pain, rashes, change in appetite, or change in weight.

PAST MEDICAL HISTORY

Healthy

Medications

- Lexapro 10 mg daily
- Seroquel 25 mg/25 mg/100 mg

Family/Social History

She does not use alcohol or tobacco or take drugs. She lives at home with mom, maternal grandparents, and two younger siblings. She is in seventh grade.

There is a strong family history of psychiatric disorders including depression, anxiety, and bipolar disorder, on both maternal and paternal sides of the family. Mom has systemic lupus erythematosus and lupus nephritis.

EXAMINATION

- Vital signs: T 36.4 C, HR 136, BP 122/96, R 20, O_2 sat 100% on room air.
- General: Wandering around the room, occasionally mumbles and makes small vocalizations, speech dysarthric
- Head: Normocephalic, atraumatic.

- Eyes: Conjunctivae clear bilaterally, extraocular movements intact, pupils dilated 5 mm equally round and reactive.
- Neck: Neck supple, no lymphadenopathy.
- Heart: Regular rate and rhythm, no murmurs, normal S1 and S2.
- Lungs: Clear to auscultation bilaterally, good air movement.
- Abdomen: Soft, nondistended, nontender, no hepatosplenomegaly.
- Extremity: Extremities warm and well perfused, no edema, no joint tenderness, or swelling.
- Skin: No rashes or lesions, no jaundice, no cuts/bruises.
- Neurologic: Awake, pacing around the room, mumbling about "returning from time traveling," repeatedly saying "no it's not my birthday, I'm older than everyone in the world." Cranial nerves intact. Making persistent chewing movements. Poor eye contact. Minimal interaction with the examiner. Follows simple commands intermittently and with repeated prompting. 5/5 strength in all extremities. Sensation grossly intact throughout. Unsteady gait. No dysmetria or intention tremor. Mild dystonia of left hand. Reflexes 2+ throughout.

DIAGNOSTIC CONSIDERATIONS

An acute onset of altered mental status with psychosis suggests diagnoses that include intoxication or ingestion, a primary psychiatric condition such as early-onset schizophrenia, or mood disorder with psychotic features, CNS lupus, autoimmune encephalitis, or a metabolic encephalopathy.

Investigation

Psychiatry and Toxicology were consulted and recommended discontinuing all psychiatric medications for the possibility of a drug-induced delirium. Neurology was also consulted to exclude organic causes.

Initial laboratory investigations included

- CBC
- CMP
- Folic acid level
- Vitamin B12 level
- Urine drug screen
- Urinalysis
- Urine beta hCG
- Ethanol level
- Salicylate level
- Acetaminophen level
- ESR, CRP
- HIV, RPR
- TSH, free T4
- Ceruloplasmin, copper level
- Serum autoimmune encephalitis panel
- ANA, ENA

A brain magnetic resonance image (MRI) with and without contrast was performed, along with chest CT to search for a tumor that might cause a paraneoplastic syndrome. Routine electroencephalogram (EEG) was performed.

Over the next 2 days, her physical examination included waxing and waning alertness and mental status, the development of mutism, trouble swallowing, insomnia, twitching of her arms, a shuffling gait with freezing, upper extremity rigidity, hyperreflexia, and right gaze preference. She also exhibited blood pressure lability. There was increasing suspicion for encephalopathy given the deterioration in her neurological examination, so a repeat routine EEG was performed.

A lumbar puncture (LP) was performed, and cerebrospinal fluid (CSF) studies including cell count and differential, protein, glucose, culture, autoimmune encephalopathy panel, IgG index, oligoclonal bands, and neopterin were sent.

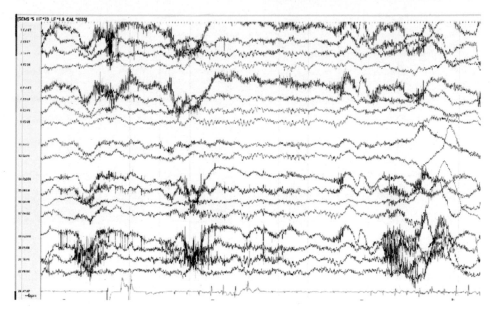

FIGURE 80.1 Routine electroencephalogram (EEG)—normal.

Results

- Brain MRI: Normal venous and arterial flow. Normal corpus callosum. Posterior fossa is unremarkable. Pituitary and sella are normal. Brainstem is normal. Ventricles are normal in size and position without evidence of hydrocephalus. Impression: No intracranial abnormality.
- Chest, abdomen, pelvic CT: Lungs clear, central airways patent. No pleural effusion or pneumothorax. Heart is normal in size without pericardial effusion. No lymphadenopathy in chest. Liver, gallbladder, spleen, pancreas, adrenal glands, and kidneys are normal. There is no lymphadenopathy in the abdomen. No bowel obstruction. No pelvic mass. Impression: No evidence of malignancy within chest, abdomen, or pelvis.
- Routine EEG (Figure 80.1): EEG in awake-only state is normal for age. No background or epileptiform abnormalities were identified.
- Repeat routine EEG (Figure 80.2): Background activity contained excessive generalized delta activity with a frontal predominant, lacked normal waking patterns, and lacked reactivity to finger pinch. These findings indicate moderate generalized cerebral dysfunction of any etiology. Periodic oral automatisms present in the EEG.
- CSF analysis: 2 nucleated cells, 0 RBCs, 90% lymphocytes, protein 15, glucose 68, gram stain and culture negative, 6 oligoclonal bands, normal IgG index, positive NMDA receptor antibodies

DIAGNOSIS

Anti-NMDA receptor encephalitis

Treatment/Follow-up

She was started on risperidone for psychotic symptoms, but this was discontinued due to excessive sedation. She was then started on clonidine for agitation. The autoimmune encephalitis was treated with a total of 5 g IV methylprednisolone, five cycles of plasmapheresis, and rituximab. She was discharged home after a 1-month inpatient stay, during which time she participated in rehabilitation services, with the plan to continue outpatient therapy and outpatient counseling. She was discharged home on clonidine, zolpidem (to help with sleep), and a prolonged steroid taper.

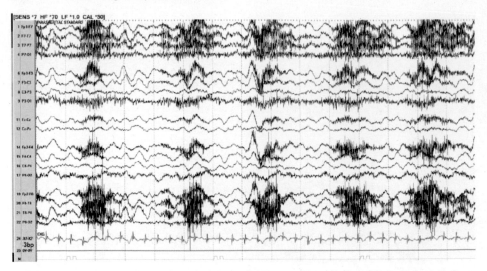

FIGURE 80.2 Routine electroencephalogram (EEG)—moderate generalized cerebral dysfunction with periodic oral automatisms.

An MRI chest/abdomen/pelvis with and without contrast was performed 2 days after discharge and showed no evidence of teratoma or other malignancy. She was seen in Neurology clinic 2 months later, at which time her examination had returned to baseline.

Teaching Points

Anti-NMDA receptor encephalitis is a form of autoimmune encephalitis, resulting in psychiatric symptoms, memory and cognitive deficits, dyskinesias, seizures, language dysfunction, and autonomic dysfunction. Diagnosis is confirmed by detection of IgG antibodies to GluN1 subunit of the NMDA receptor in CSF or serum. CSF IgG antibody testing is highly sensitive and specific to the disease. About 50% of women older than 18 years have associated ovarian teratoma, while less than 9% of girls younger than 14 years have a teratoma. African-American women, in particular, have a stronger association between anti-NMDA receptor encephalitis and teratoma.

Treatment involves immunosuppression (IV methylprednisolone, plasmapheresis, or IVIG) and tumor resection if present. Immunotherapy may be started prior to antibody results if anti-NMDA encephalitis is suspected. Probable criteria include rapid onset of abnormal behavior, speech dysfunction, seizures, movement disorders, decreased consciousness, and autonomic dysfunction; abnormal EEG or CSF pleocytosis/oligoclonal bands; and exclusion of other disorders. Second-line therapies include rituximab and/or cyclophosphamide. Long-term follow-up involves physical rehabilitation and psychiatric management of protracted behavioral symptoms. Most patients will have complete resolution of symptoms by 24 months. Relapse can occur in 15% to 24% of patients.

Suggested Readings

Dalmau J, Tüzün E, Wu HY, et al. Paraneoplastic anti-NMDA receptor encephalitis associated with ovarian teratoma. *Ann Neurol*. 2007;6(1):25.

Gable M, Glaser C. Anti-NMDA receptor encephalitis appearing as a new-onset psychosis: disease course in children and adolescents within the California Encephalitis Project. *Pediatr Neurol*. 2017;72:25-30.

Graus F, Titulaer M, Balu R, et al. A clinical approach to diagnosis of autoimmune encephalitis. *Lancet Neurol*. 2016;15(4):391-404.

Nichols T. Anti-NMDA receptor encephalitis: an emerging differential diagnosis in the psychiatric community. *Ment Health Clin*. 2016;6(6):297-303.

Pruetarat N, Netbaramee W, Pattharathitikul S, Veeravigrom M. Clinical manifestations, treatment, and prognostic factors of pediatric anti-NMDA receptor encephalitis in tertiary care hospitals: a multicenter retrospective/cohort study. *Brain Dev*. 2019;41(5):436-442.

81

Social History—Contributory

Andrew J. White

CHIEF COMPLAINT

"No weight gain for a year"

HISTORY OF PRESENT ILLNESS

For 6 months or longer, this 26-month-old has gained no weight despite having an "excessive" appetite. He has been in the care of mom and stepdad for 13 months. They are concerned that he eats excessive amounts of food "more than an adult" at a sitting and will continue to eat, taking food from others' plates if allowed to do so. He has episodes of abdominal bloating (abdomen swells up with air and perhaps food) that last for several days and resolve without intervention.

He drinks a lot of water. He will drink all the water in the toilet bowl, flush, and drink it dry again. He drinks his bathwater and creek, puddle, and river water. They keep the bathroom door locked to control this behavior. He is allowed to have large amounts of juice, soda, and vitamin water.

His stools are described as extremely foul smelling and greasy and occur four to five times a day. No vomiting, melena, or bloody stools.

PAST MEDICAL HISTORY

- Birth: 32-week twin A on supplemental O_2 for 2 days after delivery. He was discharged home from the neonatal intensive care unit at 1 month of age, no complications. Twin B is growing well.
- Pneumonia: Once at 13 months of age; no recurrent pneumonia or sinusitis.

Family/Social History

The twin is doing well and does not have these problems.

The father (and namesake of this boy) committed suicide shortly after the time of his conception. He shot himself in the head with a gun in front of mom's other children. She found him, and them, together afterward covered in blood and called an ambulance, but he was pronounced dead on arrival. He was the third-generation male (father, his father, and his grandfather) to commit suicide, and when asked, she agreed that he (and likely they) was alcoholic.

Mother became aware of her pregnancy 1 day after the father's funeral, and she reports extreme emotional difficulty ("I lost it") during the time of pregnancy and immediately after delivery of the twins. She received psychotherapy or counseling during her pregnancy and after for about a year. She denies hospitalization or electroconvulsive therapy (ECT).

He, his twin, and siblings were removed from mother's care when he was 3 months of age. The rest of the children were returned to her care when he was 14 months old. Mom and stepdad describe him as being withdrawn and "like his father."

EXAMINATION

He is a watchful, marasmic boy with a classic wasted, malnourished appearance due to reduced mass of muscles and absence or severe reduction of the fat layer. Weight = 9.8 kg (less than 5%; 50th percentile 12-month-old), length = 87.5 cm (25th percentile), and OFC = 49.8 cm (50th percentile). His face is thin and triangular with temporal wasting and thin hair. No murmurs or crackles; no clubbing, pallor, jaundice, or cyanosis. Abdomen was mildly protuberant; no hepatosplenomegaly and no masses. He had no inguinal or axillary adenopathy.

He was limp when lifted. When not moved by the examiners, he lay motionless except for ventilatory muscles and eye movements ("vigilant"). When moved or rolled by examiner, he accepted whatever position in which he was placed without complaint or effort to reposition himself. He did not have waxy immobility. The hypotonia which was apparent when he was handled included his truncal and appendicular musculature. When placed in a standing position in the middle of the floor he had a slow, unsteady, wide-based gait. CN II-XII were intact. Glossal mass was normal without fasciculations. Lanugo-like hair was present along the dorsal aspects of his arms and trunk. Optic fundi normal. DTRs l+.

DIAGNOSTIC CONSIDERATIONS

- Psychosocial dwarfism
- Other consideration (unlikely but will be assessed):
  - Cystic fibrosis
  - Diabetes insipidus, central or nephrogenic
  - Gluten-sensitive enteropathy, celiac disease unlikely
  - Diencephalic syndrome (brain tumor)

Investigation

1. CBC with diff, electrolytes.
2. Albumin, alkaline phosphatase, transaminases.
3. Calcium, phosphorus, amylase, and lipase.
4. Vitamin A, PT/PTT, cholesterol.
5. T4, TSH, free T4.
6. Sweat test.
7. Urinalysis.
8. X-ray for bone age.
9. X-ray of lumbar spine, PA, and lateral.
10. UGI/SBFT.
11. Skeletal survey/CT head/TTG antibody to exclude celiac.
12. Physical examination of siblings.
13. Obtain information concerning mother's earlier assessment from State Services.
14. Consultation with social work and child protection.
15. Report this as probable abuse/neglect to the Department of Child Protection, if above mentioned studies are consistent with diagnosis of psychosocial dwarfism.

Treatment/Follow-up

We explained to mother and stepfather the most likely cause of his cessation of growth and some less likely alternatives that we will test for. Mother said little; stepfather maintained the conversation, making the point that they have had many visits from DFS and homemakers and the latter person said they had a good home. He protested that she/they had worked hard to have a healthy home. He said, in a determined but not intimidating fashion, that he was angry. We explained that our primary responsibility is to the child and we could not fail in that responsibility even if it meant that we had to say things that are likely to be unacceptable to mother and stepfather.

TEACHING POINTS

Severe growth impairment commencing upon return to the care of his mother, bizarre eating and drinking behavior, hypotonia, developmental delay, malabsorption-type stools, and absent evidence of specific organ dysfunction or dysmorphic/genetic syndrome are classic findings of a child with psychosocial dwarfism, a profound and life-threatening failure of the development of the normal love bond of a child-mother pair. Children with this rare form of child abuse are at great risk to permanent nutritional and development disability or death if not permanently placed with a nurturing family. In a healthy home, or even in a nurturing institution, without other specific therapy all of the findings will revert to normal, and the child will be revealed to be mostly or entirely normal. The fact that other children (even the identical twin) are growing normally in the same home is not only **not inconsistent** with this diagnosis but occurs commonly. There often seems to be a special problem between the caretaker and the specific victim. In other instances, as in this case, the victimized child bears the name of the biological father, who has in some way victimized the mother.

Even in a busy children's hospital, such children are uncommonly seen, usually one every 1 to 2 years. There is often insufficient recognition of the nature of such children's true diagnosis and needed treatment. Furthermore, physicians and social workers, except for true experts in child abuse or growth assessment, fail to take the necessary information and arguments to the family, juvenile authorities, protective agency personnel, and, most importantly, the judge who must decide to abrogate parental rights and take custody of the child in the name of the state until an appropriate home is found for the child. If a second opinion is sought, it should be from a truly senior pediatrician who is on the staff of a center of excellence, where many children with growth problems are evaluated yearly.

Suggested Readings

Accardo P, Caul J, Whitman B. Excessive water drinking: a marker of caretaker interaction disturbance. *Clin. Pediatr (Phila)*. 1939;28:416-418.

Blizzard RM, Bulatovic A. Psychosocial short stature: a syndrome with many variables. *Bailliere Clin Endocrinol Metabol*. 1992;6:687-712.

Buda FB, Rothney WB, Rabe EF. Hypotonia and the maternal-child relationship. *Arn.J.Dis.Child.*. 1972;124:906-907.

Demb JM. Reported hyperphagia in foster children. *Child Abuse Negl*. 1991;15:77-88.

Green WH, Campbell M, David R. Psychosocial dwarfism: a critical review of the evidence. *J Am Acad Child Psychiatry*. 1984;23:39-48.

Hopwood NJ, Becker DJ. Psychosocial dwarfism: detection, evaluation and management. *Child Abuse Neglect*. 1979;3:439-448

Hopwood NJ, Powell GF. Emotional deprivation. Report of a case with features of leprechaunism. *Am J Dis Child*. 1974;127:892-894.

Money J. The syndrome of abuse dwarfism (psychosocial dwarfism or reversible hyposomatotropism). *Am J Dis Child*. 1977;131:508-513.

Money J. *The Kaspar Hauser Syndrome of "Psychosocial Dwarfism"; Deficient Statural, Intellectual, and Social Growth Induced by Child Abuse*. Prometheus Books; 1994:1-290.

Munoz-Hoyos A, Molina-Carballo A, Augustin_Morales M, et al. Psychosocial dwarfism: psychopathological aspects and putative neuroendocrine markers. *Psychiatry Res*. 2011;188(1):96-101.

Powell GF, Brasel JA, Raiti S, Blizzard RM. Emotional deprivation and growth retardation simulating idiopathic hypopituitarism. II. Endocrinologic evaluation of the syndrome. *N Engl J Med*. 1967;276:1279-1283.

Whitten CF, Pettit MG, Fischhoff J. Evidence that growth failure from maternal deprivation is secondary to undereating. *J Am Med Assoc*. 1969;209:1675-1682.

82

Better Get a Bucket

Andrew J. White

CHIEF COMPLAINT

A 14-year-old boy with a severe headache

HISTORY OF PRESENT ILLNESS

The family ate chicken sandwiches while the father was cleaning some rocks from his fish tank at the kitchen sink. He had taken these rocks out of the family aquarium (120 gallon, saltwater with fish and soft corals) outside to clean with the intention of ridding the tank of the zoanthid corals which were getting overgrown (Figure 82.1). Outside he used a small propane torch (*think crème brulee, not industrial welding*) on them, and then he placed them in a bucket in the kitchen sink in hot water. The patient, sister, and mother were sitting about 6 feet away, and father joined them for lunch, also eating a sandwich, which he thought tasted unusual. Thirty minutes later, the boy felt he needed to step outside as he was developing a severe headache and thought he might throw up. He was no better, and he went back inside to lie down on the couch and watch TV. He felt progressively more symptomatic with headache, shaking chills, cough, and general malaise. The father, mother, and sister also became symptomatic and headed to the local emergency department (ED). On the way, they did some *googling* and deduced they were poisoned from the coral in the bucket rather than the sandwiches.

In the ED, the boy was febrile 39.1, hypotensive (80/39 and was started on epinephrine), and persistently tachycardic with HR 127 to 153. He was saturating well on RA, but upon admission, his SpO_2 was low at 89%, which improved on 2 L NC of supplemental oxygen. He had a worsening cough but no shortness of breath (SOB).

Mother and father were both intubated for respiratory failure. The sister was admitted.

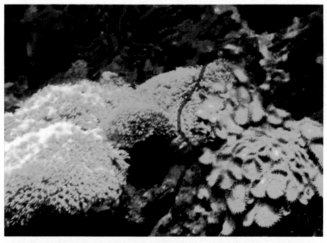

FIGURE 82.1 The family aquarium with zoanthid corals outlined in red.

PAST MEDICAL HISTORY

ADHD

Medications

Dexmethylphenidate

EXAMINATION

- Well-appearing; well-nourished; well-developed, but with frequent coughing
- Head: Normocephalic, atraumatic
- Eye: Conjunctivae clear, PERRL, EOMI
- Nose: No drainage
- Oropharynx: MMM
- Lungs: Clear to auscultation bilaterally, normal WOB, good air movement, and on 10 L nonrebreather
- Heart: Regular tachycardic, with normal S1 and S2 and no murmur, rubs, or gallops
- Abdomen: Soft, nontender, nondistended, bowel sounds present, no masses, and no organomegaly
- Extremity: Bilateral arms and legs with active movement, sensation to light touch, warm with flash capillary refill
- Pulses:2+ pulses and symmetric, pulses bounding
- Skin: No rashes or lesions and no jaundice
- Neurologic: Alert, face symmetric, PERRL, EOMI, moves all extremities and normal tone

Investigation and Results

- VBG: 7.42/48/37/31.
- Na 137, K 3.8, Cl 100, CO_2 26, BUN 13, Cr 0.8, CK, 137, WBC 13.3 K, Hgb 12.4, Plt 304.
- CXR: Interstitial opacities, bilateral.

DIAGNOSIS

1. Palytoxin poisoning, from zoanthid coral
2. Lung injury, due to #1
3. Respiratory failure due to #1, #2
4. Hypotension, due to #1

Treatment/Follow-up

The boy was admitted to the pediatric intensive care unit (PICU) where the hypotension was treated with vasopressors and his hypoxemia with supplemental oxygen.

He was not intubated. Over the course of a few days, his BP improved and his hypoxemia resolved. After a week in the hospital, all family members improved and were discharged home, but they complained of residual headaches for weeks.

TEACHING POINTS

Palytoxin is a potent vasoconstrictor found in some zoanthid corals, which are a family of colony-forming small anemones sometimes called button polyps, and often kept in marine aquaria. The toxin is potent and is considered to be one of the most poisonous nonprotein chemicals known. It has 64 chiral centers and was a challenge for synthetic organic chemists until Kishi succeeded in the synthesis in 1989, after previously synthesizing tetrodotoxin (27 chiral centers), another marine toxin, infamously present in puffer fish.

Palytoxin is not inactivated by heat, unlike some other common marine hazards, such as lionfish venom, and the attempt at destroying the coral with flame and hot water did not remove the toxin but did allow it to be aerosolized. It can be inhaled and is also readily absorbed through the skin. There is no known antidote, although vasodilators have a theoretical benefit. It may be inactivated with bleach and can be removed from the aquarium with activated charcoal. Exposures are more common than you might guess. A total of 171 cases were reported to the National Poison Data System most of which were minor, but 10 of whom were admitted to intensive care units. Severe symptoms generally include respiratory failure, rhabdomyolysis, and cardiac ischemia. It may be fatal in some cases.

They are popular corals for the home aquarium because they are attractive, readily available, and easy to keep alive. Whether most people know about the risks, however, is unclear. The owner of a local pet shop was well aware of the issue when contacted and thinks he himself had some mild poisoning in the past when getting new specimens into the shop. He no longer carries them anymore, intentionally.

An unresolved question is: How does a vasoconstrictor cause hypotension? The short and overly simple answer may be that palytoxin has other mechanisms of action.

Suggested Readings

Armstrong RW, Beau JM, Cheon SH, et al. Total synthesis of palytoxin carboxylic acid and palytoxin amid. *J Am Chem Soc.* 1989;111:7530-7533.

Murphy LT, Charlton NP. Prevalence and characteristics of inhalational and dermal palytoxin exposures reported to the National Poison Data System in the US. *Environ Toxicol Pharmacol.* 2017;55:107-109.

Schulz M, Łoś A, Szabelak A, Strachecka A. Inhalation poisoning with palytoxin from aquarium coral: case description and safety advice. *Arh Hig Rada Toksikol.* 2019;70(1):14-17.

Tartaglione L, Pelin M, Morpurgo M, et al. An aquarium hobbyist poisoning: identification of new palytoxins in Palythoa cf. toxica and complete detoxification of the aquarium water by activated carbon. *Toxicon.* 2019;161:44-49.

Thakur LK, Jha KK. Palytoxin induced acute respiratory failure. *Respir Med Case Rep.* 2016;20:4-6.

Violand N. *Palytoxin and You: How and Why to Avoid a Deadly Zoanthid Toxin.* Tropical Fish Hobbyist; 2008.

83

Don't Hold Your Breath

Andrew J. White

CHIEF COMPLAINT

A 23-month-old boy was found unresponsive by his sister.

HISTORY OF PRESENT ILLNESS

Dad came home from work and was in the backyard having a beer with his brother. The child's 9-year-old sister was asked to bring them some bug spray, and she did, and then went back to the front yard to play with her brother. A few minutes later, dad heard someone crying, so he walked into the house and saw the sister trying to awaken the patient, who was unresponsive on the couch. The sister said she was decorating a tree in the front yard and the brother was with her. Sister thinks he might have eaten a rock or maybe one of the tree decorations. Dad spent several minutes trying to awaken the child but did not check a pulse. He did not know how to perform cardiopulmonary resuscitation (CPR) and called emergency medical services (EMS). The child did not have any rhythmic jerking, color change, urinary/bowel incontinence, or tongue biting.

EMS arrived about 10 minutes later and provided bag-mask ventilation. The child was crying soon after EMS arrived, and they recorded that his lungs were clear on examination. After regaining consciousness, the child appeared to take a deep breath every few breaths. There was no emesis, cough, or congestion.

He was taken to the nearest hospital, where a head computed tomography (CT), chest x-ray (CXR), complete blood count (CBC), comprehensive metabolic panel (CMP), erythrocyte sedimentation rate (ESR) of 22, lactate of 4.1, urinalysis (UA), and urine drug screen were obtained and were essentially normal or nondiagnostic.

An electrocardiogram (ECG) demonstrated sinus rhythm.

The child was described as "wailing" in the ED for a long amount of time.

There were no medications in the house other than acetaminophen and ibuprofen. Dad does have fertilizer for his garden, but these are kept in a closed area in the backyard. The bug spray was at the father's side.

PAST MEDICAL HISTORY

He has no allergies.

He is up-to-date on immunizations.

Family/Social History

No one in the family has seizures. An older brother had a heart murmur.

EXAMINATION

- Vitals: BP 99/55, pulse 98, Temp 37 °C, Resp 22, Wt 13.6 kg, SpO$_2$ 100%
- General: Alert, well appearing, and no acute distress
- Head: Normocephalic, atraumatic
- Eyes: Conjunctivae clear, PERRL, EOMI
- Nose: No drainage

- Oropharynx: MMM, posterior pharynx clear and no cavities
- Neck: Neck supple and no lymphadenopathy
- Back: Spine straight and no CVA tenderness
- Lungs: Clear to auscultation bilaterally, normal WOB, and good air movement
- Heart: II/VI systolic murmur, regular rate and rhythm, normal S1 and S2
- Abdomen: Soft, nontender, nondistended
- Extremity: Extremities warm and well perfused, no edema and no joint tenderness or swelling
- Pulses: 2+ pulses and symmetric
- Skin: No rashes or lesions and no jaundice

Diagnostic Considerations

This several-minute episode of unresponsiveness was initially thought to be due to either:

- Breath-holding spell
- Choking on foreign body
- Toxic ingestion
- Nonaccidental trauma
- Seizures
- Arrhythmia

The sudden onset of altered mental status in combination with sister's thought that he might have ingested a small decorative object makes choking a likely culprit. It is also possible that this was a breath-holding spell, although there was no apparent loss of temper, screaming, or crying, until after he was in the ER. He does have a new murmur—or at least one that dad has not been told about before. The ECG at the outside hospital (OSH) is reassuring in regard to cardiac arrhythmia that could lead to sudden arrest. The fact that he is growing well and runs around and plays with his cousin and sister is reassuring from a cardiac perspective.

Investigation

An echocardiogram was ordered for the next morning based on the possibly new murmur.

Results

Echocardiogram:

- Normal segmental anatomy
- **Severe valvar and supravalvar aortic stenosis**, peak gradient 90 mm Hg, mean gradient 52 mm Hg.
- Thickened, dysplastic, trileaflet aortic valve
- Mildly hypoplastic sinotubular junction
- Trivial aortic insufficiency
- Mild increased flow velocity across aortic arch, 2.4 m/s (normal <2 m/s), without diastolic continuation pattern
- Normal LV size and systolic function

Diagnosis

Aortic stenosis

Treatment/Follow-up

Cardiology was consulted and made the following observations and comments:

"Normally active precordium. Normal S1, S2. No S3/S4/click/rub. Pulses 2+ in radial and femoral arteries. There is a harsh III/VI systolic ejection murmur at the right upper sternal border heard throughout the precordium. PMI is normal.

A 23-month-old boy with no known medical history who presents with a syncopal episode. An echocardiogram demonstrates aortic stenosis and supra valvar aortic stenosis. There is a peak gradient of 90 mm Hg and mean of 52 mm Hg. Typically we recommend intervention with aortic valvuloplasty in the cath lab for patient with a mean echo gradient of >50 mm Hg.

It is unusual that the patient has never been diagnosed prior to this admission as he has a prominent heart murmur. The patient has likely had an abnormal valve since birth, but the gradient across the valve was not significant enough to cause symptoms. He has no left ventricular hypertrophy or dilation which would suggest that the severity of the valve stenosis has worsened over a shorter time frame. He has no dysmorphic features on examination to suggest genetic etiology such as Williams syndrome. First-degree relatives should be screened as there is some increased incidence in family members."

Treatment: Aortic valvuloplasty (balloon) in the cath lab tomorrow.

TEACHING POINTS

Aortic stenosis is a rare condition that accounts for 3% to 6% of congenital heart defects.

It is more common in boys than girls (4:1), and it may occur with other conditions include patent ductus arteriosus (PDA), coarctation, and ventricular septal defect (VSD). Infants with aortic stenosis may present in heart failure or may be relatively asymptomatic, depending on the degree of stenosis. There are several morphological variants of aortic stenosis, often involving different valve anomalies (hence the term "valvular aortic stenosis"), and the most common (representing 90% of cases) is called type I. These cases involve bicuspid valve leaflets, which may be underformed, fused, anomalous, and which may degenerate over time. The classic finding for newborns is absent femoral pulses, but if the degree of stenosis is not severe, this physical finding may not be present.

If symptomatic, the clinical presentations may include a pale, mottled, hypotensive, or dyspneic infant. Systolic ejection murmurs are present. The lack of a documented murmur in this patient suggests either poor documentation, poor auscultation skills, or a progressive lesion.

In older children, dyspnea, angina, or syncope, particularly with exercise, may occur. The risk of sudden death has been between 1% and 10% between the ages of 5 and 15 years. The cause of syncope is not known, although decreased neurologic or cardiac perfusion is likely.

Balloon valvuloplasty remains the primary intervention, although repeated procedures are common, and surgical valvuloplasty or replacement is often performed.

Suggested Readings

Hoffman JIE, Christianson R. Congenital heart disease in a cohort of 19,502 births with long-term follow-up. *Am J Cardiol*. 1978;42:641-647.
Singh GK. Congenital aortic valve stenosis. *Children (Basel)*. 2019;6(5):69.

84

Basketball Player Down

Rachel Zolno

CHIEF COMPLAINT

Weak legs

HISTORY OF PRESENT ILLNESS

A 17-year-old girl presented with 1 month of bilateral lower extremity weakness and tingling after a flu-like illness. Initially, she described 3 days of constant lower extremity weakness and numbness and also had fevers, muscle aches, and vomiting. During this illness, she was unable to walk unassisted. She had one episode of urinary incontinence because she could not get to the bathroom quickly enough but has not had any bowel or bladder incontinence. These symptoms completely resolved after 3 days, and she resumed her normal activities.

One week later, she began to have paroxysmal bilateral lower extremity weakness and paresthesias again. These episodes occurred around four times a day with activity and lasted for several seconds at a time. Her knees would buckle, and she had difficulty walking due to a sensation of numbness and tingling from her knees down to her ankles. After falling down on the court during a school basketball game during one of these episodes, she was taken to the emergency room.

PAST MEDICAL HISTORY

Chronic neck and low-back pain, for which she has received physical therapy.

Medications

None

Family/Social History

She is in the 11th grade and lives with her parents and brother. She is a competitive basketball player and volleyball player. She does not use alcohol, tobacco, or drugs.

EXAMINATION

- Vitals: T 36.3 °C, HR 72, BP 122/78, R 16, O_2 sat 99% on room air
- General: In no acute distress, well-nourished, cooperative
- Head: Normocephalic, atraumatic
- Eyes: Conjunctivae clear bilaterally
- Neck: Neck supple, no lymphadenopathy
- Heart: Regular rate and rhythm, no murmurs, normal S1 and S2
- Lungs: Clear to auscultation bilaterally, normal respiratory effort, normal breath sounds
- Abdomen: Soft, nondistended, nontender, normal bowel sounds, no organomegaly
- Extremity: Extremities warm and well perfused, no edema, no joint tenderness or swelling
- Back: Tenderness to palpation over the bilateral lateral lumbar spine, spine straight
- Skin: No rashes or lesions

- Neurologic:
  - Mental status: Alert and oriented, follows commands, speech is fluent and articulate
  - Cranial nerves: Extraocular movements intact, pupils equally round and reactive, no afferent pupillary defect, facial sensation intact to light touch, face symmetric, unable to elicit ptosis with prolonged upward gaze, hearing intact, palate elevated symmetrically, tongue protrudes midline
  - Sensory: Sensation intact to light touch and temperature in all extremities, impaired proprioception in lower extremities, impaired vibratory sensation at the great toes, ankles, and patella bilaterally, Romberg with sway at ankles and knees
  - Motor: Normal muscle bulk and tone, 5/5 neck flexion and extension, 5/5 strength in upper and lower extremities with exception of 4+/5 strength hip flexion bilaterally, no abnormal movements
  - Reflexes: Trace patellar and Achilles reflexes bilaterally, brisk 2+ biceps and brachioradialis reflexes, no clonus at ankles, toes are upgoing bilaterally with plantar stimulation
  - Coordination: No dysmetria with finger-nose-finger
  - Gait: Normal-based gait, able to toe walk, difficulty with heel walk and tandem gait

DIAGNOSTIC CONSIDERATIONS

Postinfectious demyelinating processes such as Guillain-Barré syndrome, acute disseminated encephalomyelitis (ADEM), and transverse myelitis should be considered given the onset of her symptoms following a viral infection. The upper motor neuron findings on examination suggest a central nervous system process. Findings of decreased vibratory sense and proprioception with intact sensation to light touch and temperature suggest a dorsal column pathology. Diagnoses affecting the dorsal column include vitamin B12 deficiency, syphilis, or a spinal vascular insult. Other considerations for paroxysmal weakness include myasthenia gravis, central nervous system mass, an autoimmune process such as multiple sclerosis, heavy metal intoxication, or a functional syndrome.

Investigation

Laboratory investigation:

- CBC
- CMP
- Magnesium level
- Phosphorus level
- Ionized calcium
- Creatine kinase
- CRP, ESR
- Urine beta hCG
- Urinalysis
- Urine drug screen
- TSH, free T4
- Vitamin B12
- RPR, HIV
- Methylmalonic acid
- Homocysteine
- Folate acid level
- Vitamin E level
- Copper level
- Heavy metal screen
- Hemoglobin A1C

An MRI total spine with and without contrast was performed due to high suspicion for spinal cord pathology. On the spinal MRI, there was a possible pontine lesion. Therefore, an MRI of the brain with and without contrast was obtained the next day along with a lumbar puncture.

Results

- Initial laboratory evaluation was all within normal limits.
- MRI total spine (Figure 84.1): There is patchy diffuse cord signal abnormality throughout the entire spine, most prominent in the lower cervical region, midthoracic region, and near the conus. There is a possible pontine lesion, incompletely characterized.

    Impression: Diffuse patchy central and dorsolateral spinal cord signal abnormalities in the cervical, thoracic, and lumbar spine without enhancement. Differential includes demyelinating disease versus parainfectious/peri-inflammatory etiology.
- MRI brain (Figure 84.2): At least 30 foci of hyperintensity on FLAIR and T2-weighted images within the periventricular, juxtacortical, callosal, cerebellum, thalamus, and brainstem white matter. Increased FLAIR signal within the orbital segment of the right optic nerve suspicious for plaques. Impression: Multiple intracranial white matter lesions compatible with multiple sclerosis.
- CSF analysis: 28 nucleated cells, 7 RBCs, 97% lymphocytes, protein 18, glucose 50, Gram stain and culture negative, oligoclonal bands 21, positive IgG index 2.17, NMO IgG negative, and JC virus negative
- Serum NMO IgG negative
- Serum MOG IgG positive, 1:100

Diagnosis

Relapsing-remitting multiple sclerosis. Although serum MOG was slightly positive, presentation and MRI findings were consistent with multiple sclerosis.

Treatment/Follow-up

She was treated with a 5-day course of high-dose IV steroids while inpatient and was discharged home on a 2-week oral prednisone taper. At her follow-up appointment 2 weeks post discharge, her weakness and paresthesias had resolved and she denied any new symptoms. She

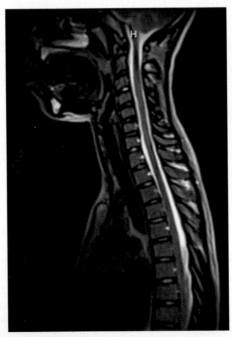

FIGURE 84.1   T2 upper spine magnetic resonance image (MRI), sagittal.

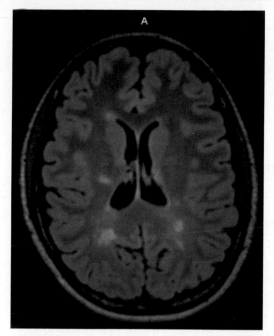

FIGURE 84.2 Fluid attenuated inversion recovery (FLAIR) brain magnetic resonance image (MRI), axial.

had a normal eye examination with ophthalmology. For long-term treatment, she was started on oral fingolimod, a sphingosine 1-phosphate receptor modulator.

TEACHING POINTS

Of all new-onset multiple sclerosis cases, only 2.0% to 4.0% occur in patients younger than 18 years old. The vast majority of pediatric multiple sclerosis diagnoses are relapsing-remitting (>90%), where patients have periods of acute symptoms followed by asymptomatic periods. In pediatric patients, relapse is more frequent and more likely to occur earlier on in the disease course. Initial clinical presentation is variable but can include optic neuritis, vertigo, ataxia, limb sensory loss, urinary incontinence, weakness, fatigue, or depression. Optic neuritis is most common.

The pathophysiology of multiple sclerosis involves a cell-mediated autoimmune response against oligodendrocytes. On MRI, this demyelination presents as ovoid foci. Diagnosis of multiple sclerosis can be made by imaging alone. Criteria for diagnosis involve lesions that are disseminated in both time and space. Typical multiple sclerosis lesions are located in the periventricular, juxtacortical, infratentorial regions and spinal cord. Initial management includes IV high-dose corticosteroids. Intravenous immunoglobulin (IVIG) and plasmapheresis can also be used. Long-term treatment involves immunomodulatory therapy. First-line therapy is either interferon beta or glatiramer acetate. Second-line therapies include natalizumab, fingolimod, mitoxantrone, cyclophosphamide, rituximab, and daclizumab.

Suggested Readings

Banwell B. Pediatric multiple sclerosis. *Handb Clin Neurol.* 2013;112(3):1263-1274.

Belman AL, Krupp L, Olsen CS, et al. Characteristics of children and adolescents with multiple sclerosis. *Pediatrics.* 2016;138(1):e20160120.

Brenton J, Banwell B. Therapeutic approach to the management of pediatric demyelinating disease: multiple sclerosis and acute disseminated encephalomyelitis. *Neurotherapeutics.* 2016;13:84-95.

Padilha I, Fonseca A, Pettengill ALM, et al. Pediatric multiple sclerosis: from clinical basis to imaging spectrum and differential diagnosis. *Pediatr Radiol.* 2020;50:776-792.

Waldman A, Ness J, Pohl D, et al. Pediatric multiple sclerosis: clinical features and outcome. *Neurology.* 2016;87(9 suppl 2):S74-S81.

85

1 mL/mile
David B. Wilson

CHIEF COMPLAINT

"Fatigue"

HISTORY OF PRESENT ILLNESS

The patient is a 16-year-old cross-country runner (logs about 40 miles/wk) who noticed a gradual decrease in her endurance. Her coach raised the possibility of iron deficiency anemia, prompting an evaluation by her pediatrician and a subsequent referral to hematology. She has had no alopecia, abdominal pain, hematochezia, melena, hematuria, menorrhagia, fear of gaining weight, or distorted perception of body habitus. She eats a diverse diet, including iron-rich foods.

PAST MEDICAL HISTORY

Keloid excision, earlobe

Medications

Combined (estrogen-progestin) oral contraceptive pill for irregular periods
No vitamin supplementation

Family/Social History

No anemia, no systemic lupus, no sickle cell disease

EXAMINATION

Vital signs were normal.
  She has a runner's physique—thin but fit. BMI = 17.3 kg/m².
  The remainder of her examination was unremarkable.

DIAGNOSTIC CONSIDERATIONS

- Iron deficiency anemia
- Celiac disease
- Hypothyroidism
- Systemic lupus erythematosus

Investigation and Results

Labs: WBC = 3.2 to 4.2, **Hb = 10.4 g/dL**, Plt = 219, **retic = 1%, MCV = 99, ferritin = 3**.
  Urinalysis, ANA, dsDNA, CMP, LDH, vitamin B_{12}, and folate levels were normal.
  Screening labs for hypothyroidism and celiac disease were negative.

DIAGNOSIS

Runner's anemia (a form of hemolytic anemia)

TEACHING POINTS

Runner's anemia is a result of mechanical hemolysis from the repetitive pounding of feet on pavement. This condition is akin to *march hemoglobinuria*—hemolysis caused by repeated mechanical injury to red blood cells during long-distance marches. Occult gastrointestinal blood loss (from a whole lotta shakin'...?) may also contribute to runner's anemia.

One study of 113 runners (men and women) documented systemic iron deficiency in 56%, although the degree of anemia was generally mild. Serum haptoglobin, Fe, and transferrin concentrations were low. A small subset of the study participants had plasma-free Hb levels measured immediately after a long run—the levels were markedly elevated.

Diagnostic pearl: The unusual combination of *macrocytosis* (presumably stress erythropoiesis), low retic count, and low serum ferritin may be seen in this condition.

A trial of oral Fe supplementation did not alleviate her symptoms (nor normalize her serum ferritin), but parenteral Fe supplementation did.

Based on her parenteral Fe infusion requirements over the past year, she loses ~40 mL of blood per week, equivalent to 1 mL/mile of running.

Suggested Readings

Dang CV. Runner's anemia. *J Am Med Assoc.* 2001;286:714-716.
Hunding A, Jordal R, Paulev PE. Runner's anemia and iron deficiency. *Acta Med Scand.* 1981;209:315-318.

86

Baby Blues
Elizabeth A. Daniels

CHIEF COMPLAINT

"My baby is blue."

HISTORY OF PRESENT ILLNESS

A 7-month-old former term baby boy with a history of colic presents with cyanosis. One month ago, he began to have increased fussiness, which was attributed to teething. However, over the last week, he has developed a progressive blue tinge to his skin, most prominent around his mouth and his nail beds. Additional symptoms include a recent decrease in energy. He has not had any recent fevers or respiratory symptoms. He has been gaining weight well and does not have any sweating or worsening cyanosis with feeds. He was seen by his pediatrician who measured his saturation by pulse oximetry at 85%, which did not improve with application of oxygen by nasal cannula. He was immediately sent to the nearest emergency department by ambulance. A blood gas was ordered, and the nursing staff noticed dark-colored blood while obtaining the lab tests.

PAST MEDICAL HISTORY

A murmur was heard in the newborn nursery; an echocardiogram was performed at 2 days of life and was normal.

Medications

None

Family/Social History

No one in the family has had congenital heart disease, methemoglobinemia, or episodes of hemolysis. He lives with his parents in an urban area. The house is not supplied by well water, and there are no known chemicals, including antifreeze, present in the home.

EXAMINATION

- General: Well-developed, well-nourished infant with obvious cyanosis, seems tired but is easily arousable.
- HEENT: Conjunctivae clear, anterior fontanelle soft and flat, nonsyndromic features.
- Lungs: Clear to auscultation bilaterally, normal work of breathing.
- Heart: Regular rate and rhythm, normal S1 and S2, and no murmur appreciated.
- Abdomen: Soft, nontender, no organomegaly.
- Extremity: Extremities warm with good capillary refill.
- Pulses: Symmetric, 2+ femoral pulses.
- Skin: Pale, blue-tinged skin more prominent around the lips and nail beds.
- Neurologic: Alert, face symmetric, intact grasp, Moro, and suck.

DIAGNOSTIC CONSIDERATIONS

The dark-colored blood and recent use of a teething agent led the physicians to immediately consider methemoglobinemia. When asked again about medications, the mother again said "none," but on more targeted and specific questioning, mother had indeed been applying a topical oral gel for the teething pain. She carried it in her purse, and when examined by the physician, it was confirmed to contain benzocaine.

Investigation and Results

Labs:

- Arterial blood gas with methemoglobin level of 17%
- CBC with normal hemoglobin
- G6PD negative

DIAGNOSIS

Methemoglobinemia, acquired, secondary to benzocaine.

Treatment/Follow-up

Discontinue benzocaine, and consider treatment with methylene blue.

TEACHING POINTS

Methemoglobin is an oxidized form of hemoglobin that cannot deliver oxygen to tissues. It has many causes, both congenital and acquired. Routine pulse oximetry cannot detect methemoglobin; blood with a large concentration of methemoglobin will always register an oxygen saturation of 85% due to the wavelength of light that it absorbs.

Most patients with congenital methemoglobinemia appear cyanotic but are often otherwise asymptomatic. This is because those with chronically increased methemoglobin levels can develop a compensatory erythrocytosis, enabling them to deliver sufficient oxygen to their tissues. Causes of congenital methemoglobinemia include cytochrome b5 reductase deficiency (Cyb5R is the enzyme that reduces ferric heme to ferrous heme in red blood cells), hemoglobin M disease (a disease in which patients have a fixed percentage of ferric hemoglobin due to an abnormal hemoglobin structure), and deficiency in cytochrome b5 (the electron receptor in the reaction mediated by Cyb5R).

In contrast, acquired methemoglobinemia can be serious and even fatal. Causes of acquired methemoglobinemia include exposure to medications such as topical anesthetics (especially benzocaine), dapsone, antimalarials such as chloroquine or primaquine, inhaled nitric oxide, substances containing high levels of nitrates and nitrites (including well water), aniline dyes and other chemicals, and even carrot juice. Because of the risk of acute toxic methemoglobinemia, the FDA issued a warning against benzocaine teething products in 2018.

Once the diagnosis is made, management includes discontinuation of triggering drug or medication and supportive care as needed. Depending on the severity of the case, one might also be treated with methylene blue. This is the treatment of choice for symptomatic acute toxic methemoglobinemia, but it cannot be used for individuals with G6PD deficiency. Ascorbic acid, exchange transfusion, hyperbaric oxygen, and blood transfusions are also therapeutic options.

Suggested Readings

Da-Silva SS, Sajan IS, Underwood JP III. Congenital methemoglobinemia: a rare cause of cyanosis in the newborn—a case report. *Pediatrics*. 2003;112(2):e158-e161.

Keating JP, Lell ME, Strauss AW, Zarkowsky H, Smith GE. Infantile methemoglobinemia caused by carrot juice. *N Engl J Med*. 1973;288(16):824-826.

87

MOG

Kimberly Wiltrout

CHIEF COMPLAINT

Eye pain and vision loss

HISTORY OF PRESENT ILLNESS

A 15-year-old boy presented with 3 weeks of progressively worsening pain and vision loss in his right eye. His course started with pain in the right eye and several days later the onset of eye pain. He also had blurring of vision in the right eye and color desaturation. His eye pain was worsened by moving the right eye in all directions. He also had a constant, sharp right frontal headache that did not improve with ibuprofen. He had no other associated neurologic or systemic symptoms.

PAST MEDICAL HISTORY

He has had no vision problems or other neurologic or autoimmune disease.

Family/Social History

He has not had any recent vaccinations or travel. There was no history of contact with a cat or fever to suspect cat scratch disease caused by *Bartonella henselae*. He had no family history of vision loss or neurologic disease.

EXAMINATION

His initial neurologic and ophthalmologic examination was significant for right eye visual acuity of 20/400+, with 20/20 visual acuity in the left eye. He had a right relative afferent pupillary defect (APD). He endorsed red desaturation in the right eye. He had optic disc edema with flame hemorrhages noted on funduscopic examination. His visual fields were intact, as were extraocular movements despite the pain with movement. The remainder of his neurologic examination was normal, including strength, sensation, deep tendon reflexes, and coordination.

DIAGNOSTIC CONSIDERATIONS

The history and physical examination localized his deficit to the right optic nerve and are consistent with optic neuritis. There are multiple etiologies for optic neuritis to consider: demyelinating diseases such as multiple sclerosis (MS) or neuromyelitis optica (NMO), autoimmune diseases such as systemic lupus erythematosus or sarcoidosis, infectious/parainfectious conditions such as *B. henselae*, or a postvaccination response. Also of consideration was a hereditary optic neuropathy, such as Leber hereditary optic neuropathy (LHON), although this typically presents as a subacute painless vision loss. Toxins and nutritional deficiencies such as B$_{12}$ deficiency can also lead to optic neuropathy.

This patient's history of painful eye movements and acute vision loss and examination with optic disc edema were consistent with optic neuritis rather than LHON or a nutritional deficiency. His history and examination were also negative for other systemic features suggestive of infectious or inflammatory/autoimmune etiologies, such as history of exposures,

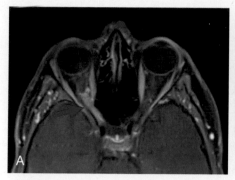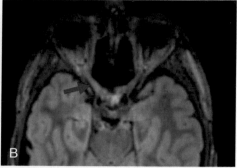

FIGURE 87.1 Patient's brain magnetic resonance image. A, Axial T1 postcontrast image with a red arrow pointing to contrast enhancement in right optic nerve. B, Axial T2 fluid-attenuated inversion recovery image with a red arrow pointing to the hyperintensity of the right optic nerve.

fevers, lymphadenopathy, and rash. To help confirm the presence of optic neuritis and to differentiate the various etiologies, a brain and cervical spine magnetic resonance imaging (MRI), serum serological tests, and lumbar puncture for cerebrospinal fluid (CSF) cell count, protein, glucose, and oligoclonal bands were performed next.

Investigation and Results

His evaluation included a brain and cervical spine MRI with and without contrast that was notable for T2 hyperintensity and contrast enhancement of the right optic nerve with the most distal aspect of the nerve spared (Figure 87.1). The right fovea appeared edematous, consistent with his clinical findings of optic disc edema.

The CSF studies included 5 nucleated cells with 1 red blood cell and protein of 33 and glucose of 55. He had no oligoclonal bands and an unremarkable IgG index. His serum NMO-IgG antibody was negative. The serum myelin oligodendrocyte glycoprotein (MOG) antibody was positive with 1:1000 titer. His vitamin D level was 35. He also had a normal C-reactive protein and negative HIV and rapid plasma reagin testing.

DIAGNOSIS

Optic neuritis, due to MOG antibody

Treatment/Follow-up

He was treated with 5 g intravenous methylprednisolone and a 2-week oral steroid taper after discharge from the hospital with significant improvement. His discharge examination from the hospital showed an improved visual acuity in the right eye of 20/25 with improved red desaturation. He continued to have a right APD. He had no pain with extraocular movements.

Repeat MOG antibody 6 months later continued to be positive with 1:100 titer. However, at his follow-up visits, his vision had returned to 20/20 in each eye with no further symptoms and normal neurologic examination with exception of mild right optic nerve pallor and subtle right APD.

TEACHING POINTS

As in his presentation, optic neuritis in children and adolescents typically presents with subacute onset of visual acuity deficits in one or both eyes, dyschromatopsia or red desaturation, pain with eye movements, and APD with optic disc edema noted on examination. Compared to adult presentations of optic neuritis, children are more likely to present with optic disc edema and can have peripapillary flame hemorrhages as this patient did. However, it is important to perform a complete neurologic examination in these patients as this may provide clues to alternative diagnoses, such as abnormal mental status raising concern for acute disseminated encephalomyelitis (ADEM) with optic neuritis or other neurologic deficits pointing to past or present additional demyelinating lesions suggesting diagnoses of MS or NMO, for example.

Etiologies of optic neuritis include demyelinating, systemic inflammatory, infectious, and parainfectious. Isolated optic neuritis is defined as a single and isolated episode of optic neuritis with evidence of inflammation of the optic nerve on MRI, but the brain and spinal cord imaging are typically normal with unremarkable laboratory evaluation. Optic neuritis may also be the initial presentation of demyelinating disease in children. Among the demyelinating etiologies are neuromyelitis optica–optic neuritis (NMO-ON), MS-associated optic neuritis, and MOG antibody–positive optic neuritis. There have been multiple studies evaluating risk of developing MS after a first presentation of pediatric optic neuritis. In these studies, the risk of developing MS varies between 13% and 36% between 2- and 10-year follow-up. The risk increases for older children, those with brain MRI abnormalities at presentation, and those with bilateral sequential or recurrent optic neuritis.

MOG is a protein located in the outermost surface of the myelin sheaths in the central nervous system and is therefore a biologically accessible antigenic target for circulating autoantibodies. In an analysis of serial evaluations of MOG antibodies starting at clinical onset and extending up to 13 years, MOG antibodies were positive at onset in 30% to 50% of pediatric acute demyelinating disease, especially in younger children and those presenting with optic neuritis and ADEM. MOG is helpful in prognostication as absence of anti–MOG antibody in a patient with isolated optic neuritis was associated with higher likelihood of a monophasic outcome. However, the presence of MOG antibody did not necessarily indicate a relapsing course, as 72% of the children who were MOG antibody positive at presentation had a monophasic course, supporting need for serial testing without initiation of a maintenance therapy at onset of disease. Children who did have relapse of disease tended to do so in a clinical pattern similar to NMO spectrum disorders.

An accepted treatment algorithm for MOG-positive optic neuritis is to treat with intravenous methylprednisolone at onset of disease with a prednisone taper. If there are signs of severe demyelinating disease, plasma exchange or intravenous immunoglobulin (IVIG) is recommended acutely. After recovery from the acute presentation, patients are monitored clinically, and MOG antibody is tested every 6 months. If there is relapse of disease, the acute treatment is repeated and maintenance therapy with IVIG is started for 12 to 24 months. Alternative treatments include rituximab, mycophenolate mofetil, and azathioprine, based on a study of more than 100 children with significant decreased annual relapse rate with use of these immunosuppressants.

In summary, pediatric optic neuritis typically presents with acute to subacute onset of visual acuity deficits in one or both eyes, red desaturation, pain with eye movements with APD, and optic disc edema noted on examination. Etiologies of optic neuritis include demyelinating, systemic inflammatory, infectious, and parainfectious and may be a single, isolated event. Demyelinating etiologies include NMO-ON, MS-associated optic neuritis, and MOG-positive optic neuritis. Serum MOG antibody testing can be helpful for prognostication of relapse of demyelinating diseases such as optic neuritis. It is currently acceptable to wait for relapse, prior to initiation of maintenance therapy for MOG antibody–positive optic neuritis, as most children will not have relapse.

Suggested Readings

Bonhomme GR, Waldman AT, Balcer LJ, et al. Pediatric optic neuritis: brain MRI abnormalities and risk of multiple sclerosis. *Neurology*. 2009;72(10):881-885.

Borchert M, Liu G, Pineles S, Waldman A. Pediatric optic neuritis: what is new. *J Neuroophthalmol*. 2017;37(suppl 1):S14-S22.

Hacohen Y, Wong YY, Lechner C, et al. Disease course and treatment responses in children with relapsing myelin oligodendrocyte glycoprotein antibody-associated disease. *JAMA Neurol*. 2018;75(4):478-487.

Hemmer B, Archelos J, Hartung H. New concepts in the immunopathogenesis of multiple sclerosis. *Nat Rev Neurosci*. 2002;3:291-301.

Lucchinetti CF, Kiers L, O'Duffy A, et al. Risk factors for developing multiple sclerosis after childhood optic neuritis. *Neurology*. 1997;49(5):1413-1418.

Petzold A, Wattjes MP, Costello F, et al. The investigation of acute optic neuritis: a review and proposed protocol. *Nat Rev Neurol*. 2014;10(8):447-458.

Waldman AT, Stull LB, Galetta SL, Balcer LJ, Liu GT. Pediatric optic neuritis and risk of multiple sclerosis: meta-analysis of observational studies. *J AAPOS*. 2011;15(5):441-446.

Waters P, Fadda G, Woodhall M, et al. Serial anti–myelin oligodendrocyte glycoprotein antibody analyses and outcomes in children with demyelinating syndromes. *JAMA Neurol*. 2020;77(1):82-93.

Wilejto M, Shroff M, Buncic JR, Kennedy J, Goia C, Banwell B. The clinical features, MRI findings, and outcome of optic neuritis in children. *Neurology*. 2006;67(2):258-262.

Zamvil SS, Slavin AJ. Does MOG Ig-positive AQP4-seronegative opticospinal inflammatory disease justify a diagnosis of NMO spectrum disorder? *Neurol Neuroimmunol Neuroinflamm*. 2015;2(1):e62.

Try Again

Miriam Ben Abdallah

CHIEF COMPLAINT

Bloody stool

HISTORY OF PRESENT ILLNESS

A 22-month-old boy presented with 2 days of painless hematochezia. Two days ago, he began having loose, watery stools with bright red blood without mucus, several times a day. The blood was mixed in with the diarrhea. He had a diverse diet of fruits and vegetables without recent changes or increase in red foods or juice. He did not have a history of constipation. He had no complaints of, or evidence of, abdominal pain before or after the bouts of diarrhea. He did not have any change in appetite, fatigue, vomiting, fevers, rash, change in urine output, hematuria, myalgias, or arthralgias. He had no recent travel, new food exposure, or sick contacts. He was not enrolled in daycare, nor had the family gone on any recent camping trips. He did not have any recent history of antibiotic use.

The persistence of the bloody diarrhea led the parents to take him to the emergency department where he was afebrile, mildly tachycardic with a heart rate of 130 beats per minute, and had a normal blood pressure of 82/56 mm Hg. He was breathing comfortably on room air with a normal respiratory rate and oxygen saturation. He was well appearing and well hydrated with normal capillary refill. The most recent diaper showed watery stool mixed with bright red blood.

PAST MEDICAL HISTORY

Healthy

Medications

None

Family/Social History

No inflammatory bowel disease in the immediate family

EXAMINATION

The abdominal examination included mild midline periumbilical tenderness with no rebound or guarding.

DIAGNOSTIC CONSIDERATIONS

A Meckel diverticulum (MD) was considered most likely, although infectious colitis was also high on the differential.

Investigation

Initial workup included a positive fecal occult blood test and negative gastrointestinal (GI) pathogen panel (which tests for multiple common bacterial and viral pathogens using polymerase chain reaction methodology), and a stool ova and parasite was sent and returned on hospital day 2 as negative.

A complete blood count showed a normal white blood cell count, mild normocytic anemia (hemoglobin 10.8 g/dL), and normal platelet count.

Initial chemistries were unremarkable with AST/ALT 28 U/L and 32 U/L, creatinine 0.3 mg/dL, and potassium of 3.7 mmol/L. LDH was 72 U/L.

An abdominal plain radiograph and ultrasound were negative for evidence of volvulus, intussusception, or appendicitis.

Pediatric gastroenterology was consulted and recommended initiation of cimetidine and a proton pump inhibitor (PPI) and a Meckel scan (technetium-99m pertechnetate scintigraphy) in the morning. The Meckel scan was performed on hospital day 2 and was negative.

Results

The negative Meckel scan and other nondiagnostic tests, as well as ongoing bloody diarrhea with decreasing hemoglobin levels, led the team to consult pediatric surgery. On hospital day 3, he was taken for a diagnostic laparoscopy during which a diverticulum of 4.8 cm was identified, located 50 cm from the ileocecal valve. The diverticulum was excised laparoscopically, and pathology demonstrated the presence of pancreatic heterotopic mucosa.

DIAGNOSIS

MD, with pancreatic tissue

TEACHING POINTS

MD is the most common congenital malformation of the GI tract and is frequently discussed as a common cause of painless GI bleeding in toddlers. It is a remnant of the omphalomesenteric duct, which connects the gut to the yolk sac in early embryology. The classical description of an MD is known as the "rule of twos":

- 2% of the population
- Presents around age 2 year
- 2:1 male:female ratio
- Often around 2-in long
- Found within 2 feet of ileocecal valve
- Two types of mucosa: heterotopic (atypical or misplaced histologically) and native intestinal mucosa

Gastric mucosa is the most common type of heterotopic tissue, but pancreatic and colonic mucosae are also possible. Both gastric and pancreatic mucosa can lead to GI bleeding due to ulceration caused from secretions produced by these tissues.

Suspicion for an MD should be high in any child with painless gastric bleeding younger than 10 years, but particularly in toddlers. For any child with intussusception, MD should be considered as a possible lead point. If a child presents with signs of appendicitis, but workup for appendicitis is negative, MD with inflammation or infection (known as Meckel diverticulitis) or ruptured MD should be considered as a possibility.

Diagnosis of an MD is typically performed through a Meckel scan, mesenteric arteriography, or exploratory laparoscopy. A Meckel scan is a nuclear medicine test in which technetium-99m pertechnetate, a radiopharmaceutical that has special affinity for gastric mucosa, is intravenously administered and localizes in areas of the body with gastric mucosa. It is thought to be up to 97% sensitive for MD and 95% specific in pediatric cases. However, in the instances where the MD does not contain gastric mucosa, this results in a falsely negative Meckel scan. Cimetidine, a histamine H2 receptor antagonist, can be used to increase retention of technetium-99m in gastric mucosa to increase sensitivity for an initial or repeat Meckel scan for stable patients with high suspicion.

Initial management of MD depends on the presenting symptoms. In the case of acute blood loss anemia, intravenous lines should be placed with blood, fluid, and electrolyte repletion as needed. GI bleeding should be started on a PPI for GI protection. Obstruction as a presenting sign may warrant nasogastric decompression. All patients with symptomatic MD will need definitive surgical management and should be made NPO for the procedure. In the case of an incidentally found MD on imaging, elective resection is not recommended in children. However, intraoperative incidentally found MD should be resected.

Suggested Readings

Francis A, Kantarovich D, Khoshnam N, Alazraki AL, Patel B, Shehata BM. Pediatric Meckel's diverticulum: report of 208 cases and review of the literature. *Fetal Pediatr Pathol.* 2016;35:199.

Park JJ, Wolff BG, Tollefson MK, Walsh EE, Larson DR. Meckel diverticulum: the Mayo Clinic experience with 1476 patients (1950-2002). *Ann Surg.* 2005;241:529.

Sagar J, Kumar V, Shah DK. Meckel's diverticulum: a systematic review. *J R Soc Med.* 2006;99:501-505.

St-Vil D, Brandt ML, Panic S, Bensoussan AL, Blanchard H. Meckel's diverticulum in children: a 20-year review. *J Pediatr Surg.* 1991;26:1289-1292.

Sinha CK, Pallewatte A, Easty M, et al. Meckel's scan in children: a review of 183 cases referred to two paediatric surgery specialist centres over 18 years. *Pediatr Surg Int.* 2013;29:511.

Turgeon DK, Barnett JL. Meckel's diverticulum. *Am J Gastroenterol.* 1990;85(7):777-781.

Zani A, Eaton S, Rees C, Pierro A. Incidentally detected Meckel diverticulum: to resect or not to resect? *Ann Surg.* 2008;247(2):276-281. doi:10.1097/SLA.0b013e31815aaaf8

Index

Note: Page numbers followed by "f" indicate figures and "t" indicate tables.